Tending Lives

NURSES ON THE MEDICAL FRONT

BY ECHO HERON

Published by The Ballantine Publishing Group

INTENSIVE CARE: THE STORY OF A NURSE

CONDITION CRITICAL: THE STORY OF A NURSE CONTINUES

MERCY

TENDING LIVES: NURSES ON THE MEDICAL FRONT

PULSE

A Fawcett Columbine Book
Published by The Ballantine Publishing Group

Copyright © 1998 by Echo Heron

http://www.randomhouse.com

LIBRARY OF CONGRESS CATALOGING-IN-PUBLICATION DATA
Heron, Echo.
    Tending lives : nurses on the medical front / Echo Heron.
    p. cm.
    ISBN 0-449-91076-8 (alk. paper)
    1. Nursing—Anecdotes. I. Title.
RT61.H46 1998
610.73—dc21   97-46103
                                                         CIP

Book design by Holly Johnson

Manufactured in the United States of America

First Edition: June 1998

10 9 8 7 6 5 4 3 2 1

Tending Lives

NURSES ON THE MEDICAL FRONT

Echo Heron

FAWCETT COLUMBINE
THE BALLANTINE PUBLISHING GROUP
NEW YORK

Author's Note

I have written this book to describe for the reader the experiences, thoughts, and feelings of many different nurses and other healthcare providers in many different situations. I have borrowed from true incidents and have based many of the scenes contained in this book on the real life events that I have seen or the contributors have described to me.

With the exception of the individuals named in the chapter about the Oklahoma City bombing, and me, I have used fictitious names and characteristics for all the patients, family members, doctors and other health-care providers, hospitals, schools, and institutions portrayed here. In some cases I have also combined characteristics of individuals and have altered the chronology and place of events. Thus, this book is not intended to record events as historical fact, nor is it meant to focus criticism on any particular group, individual, or institution. Any resemblances the reader may imagine they discern are unintended and entirely coincidental.

For the millions of nurses world wide
who dedicate themselves to the art of healing.

Contents

Acknowledgements

For their support, their technical advice, and for making their resources available to me, many thanks to Laura Gasparis Vonfrolio, Tom Meadoff, Ken Holmes, Nicole Leclair, Suzanne Gordon, Mary Dale and Jim Scheller, Linda Stone, Harold Stearley, Jane and Glen Justice, California Nurses Association, Peter Ramme, Catherine Murray Barnes, Linda Stone, Patrizia DiLucchio, Debra L. Nicholls, Connie Dahlin, Meghan Denzel, Martha Carnes, Rosette Silva, Valerie Jean Gonzales, Kellie Moore, and Scott Jones.

Contributors

These are the nurses who openly shared themselves and their world to make this book possible. They are the true authors.

I am deeply grateful to each of them.

From my heart—thank you.

Jacqueline C. Baldwin
Sue Blaisdell
Sarah Broecker
Katharine Cranwell
Steve Dee
LaNai Dohr
Dee Flanagan
Chris A. Floden
Kathleen C. Heron
L. Hinds
Bonnie G. Jacks
Mark Kobe
Kaye Manly-Hayes
Betsy Mazzoleni
Rita McClain
Bruce E. McLaughlin
Kathy Morelli
Laurel Nickerson
Courtney E. Nield
Terry Patrick
Lauren Rachow
Peter Ramme
Barbara Resnick

Zack Rinderer
Christine Lindstrom Schaeffer
Dana Scholl
Deena Scintilla
Kathy Sinnett
Jill Sproul
Sharon Squires
Harold Stearley
Jane Ramenofsky Stewart
Linda Stone
Elizabeth Vito
Georgia R. White
Janet R. Williams
And all those who wish to remain anonymous

Introduction

I believe that when a person becomes a nurse, they sign on for life. It doesn't seem to matter for how long, or in what branch of nursing one works; there is a certain quality—a spirit, a depth of soul—which is unique to the nurse.

At the risk of causing the elite of nursing's professional societies and academia to clench and grind their teeth, I also believe nursing is a calling, in that nurses possess an abundance of compassion—the wisdom born of the heart. Indeed, one of the basic rewards of nursing is the fulfillment which comes from the knowledge that one has made a positive, often profound, difference in another's life.

Nursing is most certainly a world unto itself. Nurses are the nitty-gritty of "hands-on" people. Those who choose this profession are not the type who shrink from adversity; they are as frontline as frontline gets. Let's face it—a person doesn't go through all those years of education and specialized training if they faint at the sight of blood, shrink from death, suffering, disease, overbearing doctors, and go squeamish at the thought of being smeared with various bodily fluids and solids.

What nurses witness and get involved with on a daily basis—death, birth, extreme despair, suffering, life-altering trauma, extreme joy, rage, disease—are phenomena most "normal" people experience only a few times during an entire lifetime. In the course of their typical workday, nurses deal with most—sometimes all—of those events.

The idea for this book came to me early one morning as I sat listening to a group of nurses swap "nurse stories." These were the kind of true medical tales which enthralled nonmedical personnel ("normal" people) and kept them riveted to their seats. I had written two books about my own experiences in nursing—why not broaden the brush and add more colors to the palette? I would invite nurses from every branch of nursing to share themselves and their stories—allow normal people in behind the closed doors and let them walk around in the nurses' shoes for a chapter or two.

Thinking in terms of *This is gonna be a piece of cake!* I took out ads in national nursing journals, newspaper classifieds, and the Web. So absolutely sure was I that I would receive an overwhelming response, I envisioned my local post office calling me to say that I needed a four-wheel-drive truck to pick up the hundreds of sacks of letters. I'd already decided to organize them by state and then by branch of nursing. Too, I calculated, it would probably require a full week just to download all the E-mail, let alone read and print it out.

Excuse me while I clear my throat and choke.

After three months, I had received a total of sixteen responses, not including those from my nurse friends whom I'd harangued on a daily basis. Eleven of the sixteen replies were from nurses claiming to be writing the same book. Of the remaining five, one upbraided me for "exploiting" the profession, one was from a physician wanting to know if he could get in on the act, two were legitimate, and one was from someone clearly not from anywhere on this planet or even California.

Time for new tactics. I sent copies of my ad to various nurse acquaintances asking them to post them in the nurses' lounges of every unit, ward, and medical floor of every hospital, clinic, and nursing registry in their area. Soon it was reported to me that within twenty minutes to twenty-four hours of posting, the ad would be taken down by management, and the warning issued that any nurse who replied to "that ad" would be suspended.

Because I had a difficult time believing this, I personally took "that ad" around to my local hospitals. Surely something so benign as wanting to interview nurses about their experiences couldn't be seen as a threat to management.

Again, give me a moment while I cough up a hair ball of naïveté.

The routine went something like this: I'd present myself to the director of nurses or one of the nurse managers, and as soon as they understood who I was and what I was trying to do, they would, one, start shaking their heads while they showed me the way out of the building; two (my favorite), tell me they did not want "their" nurses involved in any project which involved nurses discussing nursing, because it was "unethical" and in conflict with the interests of the administration and nursing in general; or three, laugh in my face and tell me to get real, get moving, and get lost before they called security. God forbid the spotlight of recognition should fall on nursing.

After a brief lapse into hopelessness, I pressed on only slightly daunted; I was a nurse on a mission, after all. I decided on the direct approach—armed with a phone and 103 phone numbers of "mover and shaker" nurses from Maine to Hawaii, Alaska to Key West, I began making calls. Once I had a nurse on the line (yes, it *was* rather like fishing), I would introduce myself, explain what I was trying to accomplish, and beg for interviews.

All were initially wary, a few hung up on me right off the bat, most listened politely until I was done, then employed the "Just Say No" method of refusal. After the first twenty-five calls and subsequent refusals, I got up the courage to start asking, "Why not?"

The most frequently given answer was: "I'm afraid." Or: "I can't afford to lose my job, and if the administration ever found out I spoke to you, I'd be fired immediately."

I walked on my hands and did somersaults at that point to assure each nurse of complete confidentiality. I promised I wasn't part of the CIA or a Neo-Nazi Nurse group trying to trap them into giving away secrets. Hell, they didn't have to breathe a word about their views on nursing politics and healthcare—I wanted to know why they became nurses in the first place and have them talk from the heart about their daily world.

But still, the threat of being fired or having some stigma placed on them by management was strong enough to keep most nurses silent. In this volume there are stories from several who made me promise that I would not use their names anywhere in the book. To inject a note of amusement here: One nurse even insisted on having her interview in an out-of-the-way parking lot, then arrived by taxi disguised in a wig and sunglasses. So terrified was she of being seen by someone from hospital management that I had to interview her in the back of the cab as we drove from one end of Chicago to the other.

By the time all was said and done, I had spoken directly to or corresponded with approximately four hundred nurses from every state in the union about being interviewed for this book. Of that number, I was granted approximately one hundred interviews. And of those one hundred interviews, less than half were willing to follow through and allow their stories to be published.

At first I was shocked and dismayed by the fear I heard and saw, even though I understood where it came from. Other times, I was so frustrated by it that I wanted to divorce the whole profession. But every time I conducted an interview or transcribed a tape, I came away with the same feelings about nurses that I have held for them from the beginning—respect, awe, and love for this family of extraordinary human beings.

Nurses are incredible people working in an incredible profession. Theirs is the face of human compassion. They have all saved lives and eased the fears and suffering of their fellow women and men. There is not one who can ever be correctly referred to as "just a nurse." Nurses are a far cry from the stereotypical images the media have been pushing on the American public since the profession began—the intellectually challenged, subservient inferior of the physician, or the oversexed slut in whites looking for a doctor to marry, or the pill-pushing, bedpan-wielding grunt, or the masculine, overweight, muscle-bound army nurse who wields her syringe like an M-14.

In this book alone, one of the contributors teaches ballet on the side, another is an attorney, another leads vision quests and teaches rock climbing, several have multiple master's degrees and doctorates, several are paramedics, one is a professional comedienne, another a professional seamstress. There's a weekend racecar driver, a weekend blues singer, a substitute violinist for a professional orchestra, a professional pilot, a publisher, an award-winning artist, a cartoonist, an inventor of medical equipment, a carpenter, a farmer, a diving instructor—and on and on.

Today nurses everywhere are angry, frustrated, and horrified by what the insurance companies and the hospital corporations are doing in the name of greed to their profession and to their patients. I could fill the pages with statistics and facts that would chill the average reader (and potential patient) to the bone and fill the average nurse with even more rage and helplessness than she or he feels already. But I did not want this book to be about politics. Rather, I want it to be used as admission into the nurse's world, to allow the reader to experience firsthand the soul of nurses as they go on about their business of caring.

In the following chapters you will hear the true voices of American healthcare. Compassionate healers and proven heroes—these are the nurses. Come, take a walk in their shoes.

—Echo Heron
San Francisco, May 1997

Laura T.

"It took me almost ten years of working with 'tragedy' patients before I learned how not to take them home," said Laura T., a critical care nurse for a Seattle-based nursing registry. "But every once in a while I'll care for a patient—like Matthew—who I not only take home, but make a permanent part of my life."

The forty-eight-year-old divorcée divides her time between nursing, photography, and working as a counselor in a battered women's shelter. She lives in a quiet suburb outside of Seattle, ten miles from her twenty-five-year-old son, Joshua.

She says she and Joshua are still riding the same bus.

I knew by the way the nurse avoided my eyes when she gave report that I had been assigned a tragedy. Nurses who worked through registries got used to caring for tragedies—those patients who would never get better, or wake up from their coma, or be weaned off the ventilator, or go home, no matter what we, the medical warriors, did for them.

Matthew was the ICU Tragedy of the Month. One by one, each staff nurse had had a chance to take care of him, and one by one, each nurse had come to the conclusion his case was hopeless.

Report on my other patients had been quick and painless: My twenty-eight-year-old unstable septic shock case was vented and receiving a variety of intravenous drugs which supported her blood pressure and cardiac rhythm. Mr. Mazzoni was considered semistable, though his eighty-four-year-old heart was giving us a hell of a run for our money by flipping in and out of ventricular fibrillation at will.

Julie, the nurse reporting off, searched through the card file until she came to the information card on my third patient. She cleared her throat. After that came the series of familiar nuances—the slight pause, the slow shake of the head, and the inability to look the oncoming nurse in the eye.

"Bed twelve's case is really sad," she said. It was the standard opening line for report on tragedies.

"Matthew N. is a twenty-two-year-old neuro patient who, six days ago, went for a walk out by McNulty's Beach. The girlfriend said he left just after midnight, but when she woke up at four A.M., he still hadn't returned home.

"She got worried and went out to see if maybe he'd fallen asleep on the beach. When she didn't find him, she called the sheriff's office. They found him in a steep ravine alongside the road with his head beaten in. The sheriff said it looked like his attackers used a tire iron on him."

Julie shrugged and answered a question I had not asked. "Who knows? Maybe the kid was drinking and said the wrong thing to the wrong people."

I nodded, silently hoping that he had been drunk enough or hit hard enough on the first blow not to have been conscious for what followed.

"Who are 'the wrong people'?"

Julie shrugged. "The sheriff thinks it might have been these three guys who were drinking out at Mick's Tavern. When they left at twelve-thirty, the bartender said they were drunk as skunks—maybe they saw the kid walking along the road and decided to take out their hostilities. Like one of those random, senseless killings that happen in the big cities."

Killing? But the patient isn't dead yet. . . .

"Anyway, whatever happened, the kid ran out of luck, you know?"

I did know. My only child, Joshua, was also a twenty-two-year-old, who had not all that long ago gone through his wild man stage of could-have-been-fatal car accidents, Evel Knievel motorcycle mishaps, and other Stupid Young Adult Stunts—those death-wish-granting-type activities that seem so attractive to fledgling adult males.

"Anyway, Mendoza did a crainy and evacuated a huge epidural hematoma."

I felt a brief flicker of hope—Louis Mendoza was the best neuro-surgeon in three counties. I'd seen him turn more than one potential Tragedy into a triumph.

"Unfortunately . . ." The nurse emphasized the word, drawing out each syllable. "The kid was down for six hours or more before he was found, and then there were transport problems and a bunch of screw ups in ER, so basically, he didn't get into the OR until about ten hours after the injury.

"Initially, Mendoza thought there was a chance the kid would come out of it after the swelling went down, but it's been five days since the surgery and he remains in a vegetative state—totally unresponsive. His EEGs are all grossly abnormal, and yesterday he started seizing—hasn't stopped."

The nurse tapped her forehead. "Nothing but mush up there, is my guess."

Unfolding the critical care flow sheet, Julie ran through the rest of the clinical details—vital signs, medications, results of neurological checks, lab procedures, and treatments. "He's not going to last long," she said, finally meeting my gaze. "So it isn't like you have to go all out. I mean, on paper he looks like a heavy patient, but we aren't really doing a whole lot. It's mostly comfort measures for appearance sake. Suctioning, turning, clean sheets—you know the routine."

I caught her gaze. "What do *you* think?" Early in nursing school, I learned that a nurse's intuition was more reliable than any test or expert physician's opinion. "Do you think there's any chance he'll . . ."

"No way," she said emphatically, then shrugged. "I mean, sure, I suppose he could come out of it, but there would have to be divine intervention. In my experience, these kids—some with less serious head injuries than him—rarely wake up. They either end up over at Deerpark Rehab for a few months until they die of respiratory problems, or they vegetate for months—until a family member comes to the conclusion Kevorkian has the right idea.

"Who knows?" she said flatly. "I've been an ICU nurse too long to be absolute about anything."

"What's the family situation?" Everybody knew the Tragedy patient was only half of any Tragedy story. Completing the cast were the walking wounded, otherwise known as the surviving family members.

Julie rolled her eyes. "Mom and the girlfriend—both in serious denial even though they've been told a hundred times exactly what the score is.

"I think they feed off each other. They keep insisting he's going to come out of it. Not only is the mother refusing to let us make him a no-code, but today she told Mendoza she wants everything done to keep him alive."

The nurse picked up her empty coffee cup and a sandwich bag holding a few carrot sticks. "Christ, it was awful this morning—the mother came running out to the station completely hysterical because she was sure he was trying to smile at her."

"What?"

"You know how head injuries make those weird grimaces when they seize? Well, she thought he was smiling. And then the girlfriend tried to tell me he squeezes her hand on command. I explained to them about involuntary reflexes, but they didn't want to hear it. It's ridiculous."

"No." I corrected. "It's desperate, blinding hope."

"Whatever." She waved away the subject and headed toward the time clock. "I'm just glad I've got some time off. Taking care of that kid for three days in a row is enough to depress God."

I regarded the Tragedy's info card and sighed. Considering the state of the world, it had always been my belief that if there really was a God, she was already pretty damned depressed.

It was not a conscious decision on my part to put the boy off until last. Actually, it wasn't until the moment I entered his room that I realized my level of reluctance was higher than if I'd been entering the room of a patient requiring an extensive bowel disimpaction.

His thin body was propped on its side, not with the usual single pillow tucked behind the low back—for this kid it took three to cover the distance. His six-foot-five-inch frame had further necessitated the removal of the footboard and the addition of a bed extender.

I inspected the urine in his drainage bag for quantity, clarity, odor, color, and viscosity before I briefly—surreptitiously—glanced at the face under the white bandage turban.

The eyelids, fluttering erratically, were opened just enough to reveal eyes aimlessly rolling from side to side, top to bottom.

Jesus, he's pale. Too pale. Poor baby. And that beautiful angular jaw— what a waste of . . .

Catching myself, I looked away, not wanting the face to become too real. If I allowed myself to see him as a real person, I might get involved and begin to hope.

"These kids rarely wake up."

The wall clock clicked behind me, reminding me that I had other high-acuity patients to tend to. Besides, there were miles to go before I could sit down and rest—I didn't have the time to invest in hope.

An instant later, the bed came alive as the young body contracted in a seizure. The eyes opened wide . . .

Hazel. The same shade. The same shape.

. . . and rolled back. The corners of his upper lip twitched, forming what would look to the untrained observer like a grin. His long thin arms rigidly extended and turned inward.

Shit. Decerebrate posturing—a sign of brain stem damage.

The cardiac monitor, interpreting the boy's frenetic muscle activity as a lethal rhythm, alarmed in harmony with the high-pitched blasts of the respirator alarm. I checked to make sure the bite block was securely wedged between his teeth. The last thing he needed was a crushed endotracheal tube—the piece of plastic tubing through which the ventilator fed him oxygen.

Pulling the suction catheter out from under his pillow, I suctioned the spittle which ran down his chin and onto his hospital gown. The skin of his neck and face turned a deep red as he bucked the respirator with his gagging. I was gratified to see he at least had a gag reflex. It wasn't much, but it was something.

But to what end? So he can linger as a zucchini that can cough?

I waited for the seizure to end, palpating his radial pulse—a thready, weak blip under the thin skin—and examined his three intravenous sites for signs of infiltration or infection. I had to squint in order to read the labels on each of the seven IV bags which hung from metal poles placed like sentinels around his bed. I made a mental list of the various medications going through the lines, contemplating actions, contraindications, side effects, and compatibilities.

According to the wall clock, his seizure had lasted a full minute.

How long can he last at this rate? Twenty-four hours? Less?

The ventilator alarm progressed from short blasts of warning to one long scream. Disconnecting him from the vent, I inserted the plastic nozzle of the ambu bag to the end of his endotracheal tube, waiting.

And then, as suddenly as it began, the seizure ended.

I forced several breaths into him and reconnected his ET tube to the respirator. His hospital gown had slipped away from his leg and hip. Something about the sight of that long, white, skinny leg made me stop. My throat tightened, and I quickly averted my eyes.

Don't look. Gotta hurry. Turn, suction, and give him a squirt of diazepam. But that leg—the way the hair grows to the ankle and stops. I know that leg. . . .

On the prowl for complications which might have arisen since his last assessment, I performed a physical exam, feeling for pulses with fingers trained to see, and listening to heart, lung, and abdomen for finite sounds my ears could translate into any of fifty different diagnoses. I separated his nasogastric feeding tube from the bag of thick formula . . .

Loaded with vitamins and minerals—like pumping fuel into a powerful car that has no steering wheel or tires.

. . . and aspirated the contents of his stomach for any residual lagging behind. Unpinning the grenade-shaped Jackson-Pratt drain from his turban, I measured and emptied its bloody contents, then calibrated the monitors, hung new IV bags, discarded the expired ones, and pushed myriad medications into his veins and down his feeding tube, using two sizes of syringes.

Exam completed, I searched for a place to spread out the flow sheet and chart the details of his clinical picture.

A living corpse?

In moving a sizable pile of martial arts magazines . . .

In case he should wake up and want to read?

. . . and odd assorted papers from his side table, a bag slid off and landed at my feet. A number of photographs spilled onto the floor. The angular, handsome face . . .

Don't look! Don't make him real. It's too close to home.

. . . smiled at me from the photo on top.

Beautiful teeth. Someone cared enough to give you a lovely set of braces, my friend. Those miserable braces days. I remember when Josh . . .

I smiled back and reached for another picture and then another, feeling like a snoop playing with fire.

He had been . . .

Slender and handsome . . . like Joshua.

. . . a karate instructor. In one photo he is in the process of executing a kick, the black cloth belt loosely tied about his waist. Close by, a group of awestruck young boys looks on, their eyes bright with admiration for their chosen hero.

In the next, he and a blond, slightly overweight girl kneel in front of a Christmas tree, holding hands. The Tao Ultimate Supreme symbol, Yin/Yang, is perched at the top of the tree instead of the usual star.

In another he is playing a guitar, his long spidery fingers pressing an A chord. His delicate mouth is opened wide—to let the song escape.

Toward the bottom I found a photo of a woman about my age wearing a Santa Claus hat and a smile that can only be described as joyous. With oven-mitted hands, she proudly offers a pumpkin pie to the camera to be forever preserved in its uneaten perfection.

At the last photo, I gasped, then whooped out a belly laugh. The face of a beautiful black Labrador filled the eight-by-ten glossy from border to border. In befuddled doggie manner, his huge head is cocked, ears floppy. The expressive brown eyes, wide under a slightly puzzled brow, are full of loving adoration and humor. His pink tongue hangs lopsided from a grinning muzzle, thus giving the canine an endearing buffoon quality.

Hurriedly I put all the photos, save one, back into the bag and began the routine neuro exam.

"Squeeze my fingers, Matthew."

No response.

I wiggled my fingers inside his, prompting him again to squeeze.

No response.

Holding open the wildly fluttering lids, I flashed my penlight into his eyes.

Right pupil was sluggish to respond. Left pupil remained fixed.

I ran the blunt end of my pen down the length of his soles. Predictably, the great toe pulled upward. The abnormal movement, known clinically as a positive Babinski's sign, was another indication of neurological damage.

The photo I'd put aside stared (barked?) at me from his bedside table. The idea instantly presented itself, and while it couldn't exactly be considered part of an orthodox neuro check, I figured a case like his gave license to use any means available to ascertain whether or not he was home. Not really expecting a reaction, I held the dog's photo directly in front of his eyes.

At once they stopped their chaotic dance as he focused on the image before him. A beautiful smile—the same one he wore in his photos—spread across his face. Unmistakably, recognition and joy registered in his eyes.

My heart was going like a jackhammer as I moved the picture to the left. His eyes tracked the photo to the left. The smile did not falter.

Holy bleeding Christ—he's actually in there!

The thought that I should contact Dr. Mendoza posthaste was still forming when Matthew disappeared inside another seizure.

I tended to the necessities—suctioning, giving oxygen, pushing more

Valium, protecting his limbs from sharp corners—while a variety of nagging, though completely logical, thoughts—

"Nothing but mush up there" . . . *"These kids rarely wake up"* . . . *six hours of lying in a ravine . . . plenty of time to cook up a whole batch of irreparable tissue damage. . . . a tire iron for Chrissake*—systematically attacked my newly born enthusiasm, eventually murdering it altogether. The notion that he was even slightly aware of what was happening to him, living—*trapped?*—forever in that distant twilight world and never knowing who or where or even what he was, horrified me to the point of feeling ill. Closing my eyes, I took five deep breaths, clearing my mind with thoughts of hiking in the mountains with my son.

Once he was still, I again held up the photo of the dog.

There was no sign of recognition this time—no response whatsoever. Whoever had briefly peered out from the attic window was no longer in evidence.

The wall clock clicked, reminding me that Mrs. Post's antibiotic was almost an hour late. Rapidly gathering my charting sheets together, I had turned to leave when the sight of the boy's bare leg and ankle made me stop again.

Exactly like Josh's leg . . . skinny and white with the fine dark hairs. Same eyes. Same smile. Same spidery fingers.

Softly, I laid my hand against his cheek, studying the young face.

Even the feel of his skin is right. It could so easily be Joshua. . . .

Taken by a sudden madness, I rearranged fate by pretending—believing—it was Josh who lay in bed 12. An indescribable anguish hit me with an impact as powerful as having been shot at close range with a .357 Magnum. The reality of losing Joshua from my life exploded inside my head and made my temples burn.

I began to weep, forcing the madness away.

Joshua is alive. Joshua is alive. Joshua is alive. . . .

It was while I was wiping away the tears that had run down my arms that someone touched my shoulder.

"Has something bad happened to Matt?" asked the woman in alarm.

Speechless, I stared into the tortured face. It was as if I was looking into a mirror.

She gripped my upper arm with such urgency I got the impression she was holding on for dear life. Understanding her concern, I shook my head in answer, unable to get my throat to work.

No, not bad—tragic.

Puzzled, she eased her grip, but did not move her hand. "Are you okay?"

Nodding, I sucked in a huge breath. When I spoke, my throat was so tight it hurt.

"I'm sorry. I'm Laura, Matthew's nurse."

Assured her son had not suffered any setback . . .

He's already set as far back as he can go.

. . . she nodded, though still confused by my tears. Her face was gaunt; it was the wasted look that came with grief and worry.

"I'm Matthew's mother." She extended her hand.

No name. She identifies herself only as his mother, afraid to make even that small separation.

"How is he?"

"Still having seizures about every"—I glanced at the wall clock—"ten to fifteen minutes."

She clucked her tongue in disappointment and laid her hand on his face exactly as I had done earlier. "Hello, honey. It's Mom." She bent close to him, a comical smile coming to her lips. "Are we still riding the same bus today, dear?"

The question came so far out of left field I started to laugh.

She turned around at the sound of my laughter, her mouth still holding the weird little smile, and immediately began to explain.

"When Matt turned seven, we took a Greyhound bus to my sister's in St. Louis. Well, he decided that he was too old to endure the mortification of having to sit with his mother like a baby. He wanted to be able to tell his cousins that he rode alone, so he sat waaaay in the back by himself and made me promise to act as though I didn't know him.

"Eventually the bus stopped for gas, and—unbeknownst to me—he got off to buy himself a soda pop. Fifty miles later, I turn around to offer the lone stranger a peanut butter sandwich and—whoa—Matt's disappeared."

She chuckled and as she did so, the strain faded from her face, transforming her into the perfect pumpkin pie woman—content, happy, safe from nightmares.

"We radioed the police, who found him sitting at the gas station, very calmly sipping his Mountain Dew. When the police asked why he didn't tell someone he'd been stranded, he answered, 'Oh, my mother'll come back for me as soon as she realizes we aren't riding the same bus.'

"After that, the phrase 'riding the same bus' came to mean that we were on the same wavelength, appreciative of each other's"—she frowned, the nightmare coming back—". . . presence."

When his presence is gone forever, memories like these will not bring laughter . . . they will instead bring her to her knees.

In a gesture of agitation bordering on desperation, she ran her fingers through her short-cropped hair and returned her attention to her son. "Can you hear me, Matty? Please, honey, squeeze my hand if you know it's me."

I stared at his hand lying still and felt her despair.

"He squeezed my hand this morning when I told him to," she said, not taking her eyes off his. "When Deb—that's his fiancée—called his name, he turned his head to—"

His back stiffened and the bed came alive with his convulsions. His mother scrutinized his face, intently watching the grimacing and the wildly rolling eyes.

How can she do that and not lose her mind? Isn't every tremor like a knife going into her heart?

I took care of the small tasks, my eyes continually drifting back to his legs and ankles. When I finally looked up, his mother was gripping the side rail with both hands, her head thrown back, her eyes shut tight. From deep within her throat came a sort of growl that turned into a strained moan of agony.

She shook her head from side to side, in rhythm with her groaning litany. "No. No. No. No. No. No. No."

I froze at the sound. It was the same one I made in my recurring nightmare of standing on a beach and watching Joshua drown offshore.

She is helpless . . . unable to stop the horror going on in front of her eyes.

"He's my only baby," she whispered. "My best friend. He loves life so much. I can't . . ." She held out her arms in a desperate plea for understanding. "I can't give up.

"He's stubborn. I know he's fighting like hell to get back. He'd be so pissed off if I gave up on him. If it were me lying there, you can bet he'd never give up."

She fixed me with a probing stare. "You know, don't you? You're the only one so far who doesn't look at him like he's a . . . a corpse and run out of the room the second I show up."

"My son . . ." I stopped because my voice strangled in my throat and my eyes welled up. I, the caregiver, the one supposedly in control, was breaking down on the job.

She reached out and touched my shoulders, then brought me into her arms, rocking ever so slightly.

We are both mothers—women. I know this woman's love and pain because we share the same heart.

"My son is the same age. When I saw Matthew, I thought of Joshua. I tried to imagine what it must be like, but I couldn't. I couldn't take the pain. It felt like I was going to die."

I pulled back to look at her, although I was afraid of seeing resentment in her eyes because it wasn't *my* son who lay dying instead of hers.

The lucky and the unlucky, the haves and the have-nots.

I was gratified to see nothing other than gentle compassion.

"How . . . how can you stand it?"

Releasing me, she wiped her tears with a yellow handkerchief she'd pulled from the sleeve of her sweater, then handed it to me.

"I stand it because I have to. I have to fight for Matthew."

"Matt drinking?" The zoftig blonde named Debbie raised her eyebrows, making her large blue eyes seem huge. Her voice was laced with annoyance. "He never drinks. Matt is totally into being healthy and fit—he'd never put anything into his body that wasn't pure, let alone a toxin like alcohol. Yeuck."

Always the present tense. As if he were only napping.

"Oh, yeah?" I tried for an offhanded, amused expression, though I more than likely just looked a little dopey; I was tired and it was way past the time I should have been finishing up my charting. But somehow I'd kept finding things to do for him.

Things I would do for Josh . . . small tasks beyond "comfort measures only."

"Then why was he out wandering around in the wee small hours of the morning?"

Debbie gave me a wry smile. "Well, he doesn't do drugs, but he *does* suffer from really bad insomnia. Whenever he can't sleep"—she rolled her eyes—"which is about two or three nights a week, he walks down to the beach and meditates. It's the main reason we decided to live out by McNulty."

She put down his left foot, picked up his right, and continued the passive range of motion exercises. ("He'd be pissed," she told me, "if he woke up and found himself unable to run at least a few miles right away.")

"We joke about moving our bed down to the beach so he doesn't have to walk. Actually, he loves walking at night because there's never anyone else around, so he gets to have the whole beach to himself."

Except for that night.

I watched her work over his feet for a minute, debating whether or not to ask her the question I could not bring myself to ask his mother. Her youth decided me.

"Neither you or Matt's mom have said a word about the people who mur—" I snapped my mouth shut, almost biting off my tongue. "Assaulted Matthew." The deep red blush of embarrassment spread upward from my neck. I examined the girl's round face to see if she had picked up on my miswording. If she had, she didn't show it.

"Matthew and I are Buddhists," she said gravely, as though the answer explained everything. Seeing my bewilderment, she smiled in a Zen-like, understanding manner. "We don't believe in violence or malice.

"As far as Mom goes, she just doesn't want to waste any energy on negative stuff."

She has made his mother her own. Just as well since they will be forever connected through his death.

"She wants to concentrate on the positive. The people who did this to Matt have their own karma to deal with."

Must be getting old. I believed all that karma everything-happens-for-a-reason bullshit too. Back in the sixties before reality sank in.

I dropped the subject and picked up the photo of the dog. "Who's this character?"

"Depot." She giggled. "Our babydog."

"Come here." I crooked my finger. When she was in perfect viewing position, I held the photo in front of him.

He again focused, recognized, and deliberately smiled. The reaction lasted all of two seconds, but at least I'd had a witness. To my surprise, Debbie only nodded and returned to exercising his foot. "Yeah, I know. He does that sometimes. That's why I know he's going to wake up."

"But—"

She held up a hand. "Save your breath—we've heard all the reasons why he isn't going to wake up." Shifting in her chair, she shook her head. "You guys don't know him. Matt's really special. Spiritually, he's totally connected. He doesn't have an enemy in the world."

Oh yes he does, Debbie. Waiting there, behind his left shoulder.

"Everyone who knows him loves him."

The cardiac monitor beeped once and went silent, as if to punctuate her statement with an audible exclamation point.

I spread a thin coat of Vaseline over his lips. The bottom lip was cracked and bleeding from the constant pressure of the ET tube. "Believe me when I tell you that I know exactly what kind of person Matt . . ."

Past tense, Laura.

". . . was."

A yellowish exudate was collecting in the corners of his eyes. I wrote a note on the palm of my hand to ask Dr. Mendoza for an ophthalmic antibiotic order. I'd post a warning on his info card, reminding—demanding—his nurses pay close attention to his susceptibility to infection.

The human petri dish—warm and moist, the perfect medium for any bacteria needing a place to hang out and grow.

"I honestly believe that Matt is aware on some level of what's going on here. But . . ." I held up my hand, feeling like Judas Iscariot. "It's not enough. Even if he was having moments of lucidity, what you must remember is that he will never again be the same person you knew before."

I blinked, ignoring the fact she had covered her ears and was rocking. "If he lives . . ."

Pray to whatever God you believe in, Deb, that he does not.

". . . he will be only a little better than he is now—and that's the best-case scenario."

I pulled her hands away from her ears and knelt down so that my eyes were level with hers. "Please hear me. We aren't the enemy. It's just that you and Matthew's mother are seeing only one tiny side of the picture. It's like you're in the forest and can't see the rest of the trees. If I were in your shoes . . ." I swallowed the lump forming in my throat.

Don't break down, Laura. Be true and strong . . . like an executioner doing a good job.

". . . I'd look at the quality of his life. Even if he eventually starts breathing on his own, do you think Matt would *want* to live if he knew he'd never be able to have another conscious thought . . . or talk . . . or brush his teeth . . . or go to the bathroom by himself or feed him—"

"Please . . . don't." Her chin quivered. "He isn't going to be like that. Matt's going to come out of this."

"No, Debbie. No, he isn't. That's why the nurses respond to him the way they do. They've seen this before—lots of times. They know what's in store for him and for his mother . . . and you."

A continuing nightmare from hell, Debbie. Pain every time you see his wasting arms and legs. Pain each time you wipe away the drool and spoon in the baby food.

"If Joshua . . ." I faltered, catching my slip. "I mean, if Matthew had a choice, would he really want that?"

Joshua would be furious at the very thought.

The young woman stared down at her lover's long narrow feet and did not answer.

I straightened out my knees and studied him a final time.

Goodbye, Matthew. I am so sorry. God rest your soul . . . wherever it may be.

From the expression she was wearing when I left his room . . .

Facing the demons?

. . . I thought she may have finally faced the shadows and had a glimpse of what horror was lurking there.

For the next two weeks I could not look at Josh without thinking of Matthew. I'd begun hugging him each time he came by and staring him directly in the eye when we spoke. For the first time since he was a young teen, I silently celebrated every accomplishment (mastering *"Stairway to Heaven"* on the guitar after three years of trial and error) and marveled over every word uttered ("Yo, Ma! What's ta eat?" Even: "Can ya do my laundry?").

Since it was shorts weather, I had to consciously force myself not to stare at his hairy white legs, or else be reduced to tears. A couple of times I started to call the ICU to see what had happened with Matt, decided against it, and took jobs at *other* ICUs until some three weeks later, when I was certain it would be safe to go back.

In hindsight, I should have known that as soon as one is sure of something, the fates will step in and arrange something a little different.

The automatic doors to the acute ICU swung open. I did not see this as a welcome like most people did—knowing what lay in wait on the other side, I instead saw those mechanical doors as a set of menacing jaws.

Heading for the refrigerator to deposit my lunch, I glanced into the first room and saw a woman sitting at the bedside, her head resting on the patient's chest. Although she lay as still as stone, she radiated such a deep sadness it could almost be seen.

In four yards, I realized who the woman was, stopped, and made myself hyperaware of my surroundings. The tension which permeated the unit and filled the faces of each person at the nurses' station was familiar. The peculiar silence that type of strain usually created wailed of failure, relief, and death. It all translated into the fact that somewhere on the unit, we'd lost one. I didn't need to think twice to know who.

Dropping my lunch and sweater on the nearest chair, I briefly explained to the night charge nurse where I would be. Not waiting to hear her protests, I walked briskly into Matthew's room and pulled the curtain across the glass door.

Close up, Matthew's mother looked terrible—like she'd fallen off a high-speed roller coaster. Tentatively, I touched her shoulder. Through the wreckage, a fragile quality had surfaced in her and a fleeting, irrational fear that she might shatter into a thousand pieces made me pull my hand back.

For a time I watched her watch her son fight for his final breaths. It was clear she had accepted that inconsiderate tenacious fate—ignoring his youth and the immeasurable value of his spirit—had chosen her son for death after all her valiant protests.

The war being over, she wept, her arms entangled with his.

All the IVs were gone save one. His breaths were shallow and irregular. The ventilator had been shoved into a corner, a white sheet had been thrown haphazardly over the top—perhaps in an attempt to hide the evidence of failure.

"He's going now," she said suddenly, never taking her eyes from his face. I didn't think she was talking to me—it seemed more likely she needed to hear the sound of her voice saying the words. It was an effort to ground herself and stay in touch with reality.

I looked over at the cardiac monitor, instantly thankful that someone had had the sense to silence the alarms. She was correct in her estimation—the complexes were now slow and wide, as usually happens when death is imminent.

"I love you, Matthew," she said in a battle-weary voice. "I always will."

Numbly, I backed toward the door, wanting to give them privacy, yet powerless to turn my eyes away—wanting to run away, yet anchored to that room.

She kissed him lightly on a mouth still swollen from the presence of the endotracheal tube, caressing his cheek with the palm of her hand. "Save a seat for me on that bus, honey," she whispered, smiling wanly. "You were too quick for me, hon. This time you left *me* behind, but I'll catch up with you before you know it."

The rhythm on his monitor went from eight complexes per screen to four.

"You are the heart of my life." She stroked his head, letting her fingers idle in the new growth of fine black hair that was less than an inch long. "You will be with me every . . ."

I turned and stumbled out of the room, unable to stand the pressure inside my chest. In the hallway, I collided with Debbie. I barely recognized the thin, pale woman who, on the outside, had aged ten years. Inside, I guessed, she had aged a hundred years or more.

Her huge frightened eyes stared into mine. The hope had been replaced by a reluctant acceptance and fear. "Is he . . ."

In answer, I stepped aside and gently pushed her into his room. "Hurry."

Head pressed against the coolness of the corridor wall, I waited until I heard the soft explosion of unrestrained weeping.

They had been released—finally free to begin healing through the process of mourning.

Ignoring the icy look of furious impatience on the face of the night shift nurse who waited to give me report, I called Joshua, and at the sound of my son's sleepy hello, I rejoiced at my good fortune.

"I love you, Josh," I whispered.

There was a confused, muffled pause as he pulled his head out from under the down quilt I'd given him for his birthday. Behind me, the sounds of the two women's grief grew louder.

How thin the lines between life and death, joy and sorrow. Chance . . . fate . . . the invisible forces which in split seconds change our lives forever.

"Love you too, Ma. You okay?"

"Yes."

The night nurse pointed to the wall clock over the nurses' station and frowned.

Please don't let there be a Tragedy assignment today.

"I just called to say . . ."

Matthew's mother and Debbie stepped into the corridor, weeping. They walked to the mechanical doors, using each other for support.

Survivors of a holocaust. What will be learned from such a hard lesson?

"I just called to say that I am very, very glad we're still riding the same bus."

Carol P.

Carol P. is a forty-one-year-old who, after fourteen years of working as a licensed vocational nurse in an acute neuro unit, is waiting to take her R.N. boards.

"I guess I wanted to become a nurse," she tells me, "because my grandmother was an army nurse during World War Two and I always thought she was a great person. Also, I'm the original caretaker personality. Very codependent. But I feel so good and so natural when I'm helping other people.

"When I used to work geriatrics on nights, I'd get to be with a lot of those folks who die in the early-morning hours. In the quiet of the night, when the rest of the world sleeps, a lot of scared or troubled souls open up and you can do a lot of good by just listening. There's something incredibly wonderful about sitting with some old soul watching the sun come up.

"It's such an amazing feeling, but when I try to explain this to non-nurses, they look at me like I'm nuts. And when the old ones die and you're there holding their hand, most of the time there's a pervading feeling of peaceful joy—like a miracle is taking place. The experience has helped me get through life because it has strengthened my own spirituality.

"A pitfall for me about being a nurse is that my whole identity gets wrapped up in it. Once when I couldn't work for a while, I went into a deep depression. I felt worthless. Even though I was raising three children and taking care of the household, it wasn't enough.

"Now that I'm finishing my R.N., I can see a light at the end of the tunnel—I just hope it isn't a train."

Her straightforward, no-nonsense manner led me to suspect Carol is streetwise and survival-oriented—one of those people who, in the worst of crises, resort to whatever works.

As her story unfolded, my suspicions were confirmed.

To walk around the deserted halls of a ninety-year-old hospital at 3:00 A.M. was spooky, the same way an old black-and-white Hitchcock film is spooky. But then again, since I was originally from Chicago, I thought Mobile was pretty scary in general—nighttime or broad daylight—much more violent and sinister than South Side Chicago.

Treading the acute-neurology-unit hallways each night, it was hard not to notice the cracked plaster and the peeling two-tone green paint (light on the top, dark on the bottom—isn't that always the way?). The only sound bouncing from wall to wall was the whoosh and click of the respirators and an occasional moan or scream.

We were full and I'd been busy with a lot of the postsurgical care for the craniotomies. We also had five motorcycle accidents with head injuries, and eight stroke-outs. These were people who needed full care, so I'd been running around turning everyone, doing tube feedings, adjusting the respirators, giving meds, changing dressings—the usual.

I'd been prepared for the worst since I walked into report and the charge nurse refused to look me in the eye. It was a sure sign of a lousy assignment load . . . and it was. Two of us for the ward.

Shouldering the responsibilities with me was a four-year R.N. who was also a new graduate. Marie was a sweet girl, who'd had lots of nursing theory pumped into her. Not that I had anything personal against them, but the four-year girls weren't exactly up to snuff when it came to clinical skills or common sense. It was the two- and three-year R.N.s who would always jump right in up to their necks before you could even say "Shit," and handle it right.

Comparing my assignment to hers, it didn't take a genius to see that I'd been given the patients who needed more than theory and eight pages of detailed charting.

The neuro unit was on the third floor and just happened to have the dubious distinction of being the only department which had a roof outside the windows. Because of this dubious distinction, we had the dubious privilege of receiving all the really whacked-out psych patients with head injuries who thought the only way out was through a window.

To this day I'll swear that every crazy, violent psychotic who ever existed in the state of Alabama has had, does have, or will have a head injury and has been, is now, or will be on the third floor of X——Memorial.

My most difficult patient had come in the night before from a prison in northern Alabama. Originally, Delbert had been in prison for

murdering two cops and three members of a drug dealer's family, including the mother, the grandmother, and a two-year-old niece.

Somehow (I never did quite get *that* story), he'd escaped maximum
security, gone to his home, forced his wife and their baby into the family
car, and led the police on a wild chase.

When things started getting hot at upwards of a hundred miles an
hour on open freeway, he'd tossed his sixteen-month-old baby girl out
the window as a way to shut her up. That also had the added benefits of
deterring the police. He was successful on both counts—the baby was at
another hospital nearby with burns, skin grafts, and head injuries and
was on a ventilator.

While he was waiting to go to trial for this, he'd gotten into a fight
with another prisoner at the jail and stabbed him with a pencil. He'd
sustained a concussion after the back of his skull got into a tangle with a
guard's nightstick, although the general consensus was that the nightstick got the worst of the deal.

Suffice it to say, Delbert was one big psychotic and scary guy. Restraining his six-foot-five, 340-pound body was a challenge which we
met with locked leather wrist and ankle cuffs, a canvas restraining jacket,
leather leg and torso straps, and around-the-clock sedation with three
different medications.

Marie pushed the med cart behind me as we finished giving
2:00 A.M. and 3:00 A.M. meds. In front of Delbert's room, I prepared his
3:00 A.M. vitamin H—Haldol—injection, uncapped the syringe, and entered his room as quietly as I could. If I could get away with giving him
the tranquilizer without waking him, I promised myself a nice cup of tea.

Forget the tea—if I lived to drink another cup of it, I'd consider myself lucky, for there, perched in the hole where the window once was—
with his gown open down the back and flapping in the breeze—stood a
wild-eyed Delbert arguing with enemies I couldn't see.

The window had been pulled out. I couldn't see how he'd managed
it, but the window wasn't just broken, the wood of the window frame
had been ripped out. The streetlight from across the street gave the
whole scene a surrealistic touch.

Actually, I'd begun feeling pretty surrealistic myself.

"Marie!" I screamed. "Call security stat and then get in here and
give me a hand!"

Behind me, I heard the door open and shut very quickly, but when I
turned around, no one was there. When I turned back, Delbert, the

unhappy and psychotic giant, was just noticing that someone was in his room.

The moment he saw me, the man with muscles like a bull and the stature of a bear growled like a dog.

What an animal, I thought.

I yelled out again to no avail, so I carefully backed to the door and looked down the hall in time to see Marie locking herself in the nurses' bathroom.

Because I knew Marie to be the lily-livered, yellow-bellied four-year (four-legged is more like it) girl that she was, it was a given she hadn't called security before she headed for sanctuary.

"I'm sorry," she said through the crack of the bathroom door as she flicked the locks into place, "Really, I'm sorry but I can't get involved with this."

Involved with what? I wondered. The death of a co-worker?

I glanced back at Delbert in time to see that he'd caught a glimpse of the needle in my hand, the sight of which seemed to trigger reactions of a circuslike nature.

Delbert actually took a flying leap from the window to the bed, bounced up, cracked his head on the ceiling, and then flew through the air with the greatest of ease and landed on his feet between me and the door.

I gotta tell you, the Flying Wallendas had nothing on this guy.

Delbert growled again and showed his teeth. King Kong did *not* die in New York City on the Empire State Building—he was right here in Mobile, Alabama.

My brain strained at the seams of its synapses.

Delbert took a threatening step toward me, his hand (the size of a five-pound ham) outstretched toward my throat. Somehow, I opened my mouth and my brain did the talking.

"Come on!" I commanded as gruffly as I could—which was pretty gruff since my throat was drier than Death Valley. "Let's get out of here!"

He raised his eyebrows. "Huh?"

The note of puzzlement in his voice encouraged my mind to reach into the dusty corners for something . . . anything.

"Your old lady paid me to break you out of this joint. I had to lock up the regular nurse, so we gotta hurry."

"You can't do nothin'," Delbert growled. "Where's your gun?"

"Ah man, quit wasting time and let's go before the cops get wise." I held up the uncapped syringe. "I got myself a three-fifty-eight-caliber spear needle with five thousand watts of electric juice. Stops their hearts from ten yards away."

God only knows where the hell I got this stuff, but I did enjoy science fiction comics as a kid. I'd assimilated the stories verbatim.

"Come on man, nobody's that stupid as to get in *our* way."

Did that really come out of my mouth?

"Time's a-wastin'. Your woman paid me a hundred bucks to do this job, now let's git."

Delbert's mouth was hanging open, and I could see he was on the fence about whether or not I was legitimate.

I handed him a gown. "You'd better put this on, 'cause it's real cold outside and we've got to run about two blocks to get where your old lady is waiting with the car."

"Lena don't drive," he said, eyeing me.

My brain didn't slow one beat. "That's why she hired my brother. He's the best getaway man in the business."

Things were looking up—Delbert put on the gown.

Yanking my nerve up off its face, I turned my back on him and rushed out the door. "We've gotta take the back stairs if you want to get to freedom without being seen," I said, heading toward the main stairwell.

I opened the door and started down those deserted three flights of stairs, feeling sick with panic. When the door clicked behind us, I felt his breathing on my head. All I could think during those few minutes was, *Well, this is it. They'll find my body here in this stairwell about six-thirty or so.* I sent up a prayer that my husband and kids wouldn't be watching the news when they showed pictures of me lying on the stairs in six or seven pieces.

"We gotta go over a wall. You can climb, can't you, Del?"

I didn't dare turn around, but I wanted to know where he was. For a big guy, he was quiet.

"I don't want to get no holes in my jammies," he said. "Lena don't like mendin' nothin'."

Somewhere in my mind, I knew that I'd find this hysterically funny someday—I even imagined myself relating the story from the stage of a stand-up comedy club—but at the moment, it sounded like a grave problem.

"It's okay, we got more jammies and some decent clothes waiting for you in the car. Lena's got plenty of clothes for you."

The ground-floor doorknob was under my hand. We sailed through, and took an immediate left-hand turn—right into the security guard's office.

Even if I'd had a film of the ensuing events, no one would have believed it had happened that way without a script and a director.

The two security guys—their feet up on the desk and leaned back in their chairs—looked up at the same time and saw me coming at them holding an uncapped syringe like I'm going to stab them with it. Behind me is the jolly black giant, sporting a couple of extra-large, sunny-side-up eggs for eyes.

I had to give it to them, though, because I've never seen two skinny runts move so fast in my life.

Both of them jumped up and grabbed ahold of Delbert, which, I saw right off, was going to be a problem because these guys were downright puny. (Ever notice how night security guards are always these ninety-pound-weakling types, and the guys on days—the ones who never have any problems—are always these three-hundred-pound bruisers?)

Moving like lightning, I jammed that needle into his butt right through the gowns.

Delbert started swinging and growling. Without taking time to consult with each other, the three of us decided we needed to wrestle him to the ground. We might as well have been three mosquitoes on an elephant's ass.

Old Delbert just kept swinging and walking around with us hanging off his neck and back like we were some kind of African art necklace.

It seemed like forever before the Haldol took hold and he slowed down a little. The guard who seemed more on the ball (a normal IQ status wasn't a requirement of the job) managed to get one of Delbert's hammy wrists handcuffed to the desk leg, which was bolted to the floor. If it had been a nonstationary desk, Delbert would have used it like a flyswatter to crush us.

I ran upstairs and got another two syringes full of dope. On my way back, I tried the bathroom door and found it still locked.

Now that the danger was past, I wanted Marie to suffer a little too. Forgive and forget wasn't going to do it for me on this one.

I violently jiggled the doorknob, then, when I heard the appropriate whimpering, banged and kicked the door with all the strength in my body. I growled in the lowest register I could find on my vocal cords and mimicked Delbert's monosyllabic way of speaking. I basically told her she had five minutes before I broke down the door.

After I assisted Delbert to attain the state of sedated Jell-O, and Marie had been coaxed out of the bathroom by one of the security guards, I was actually feeling relatively peaceful, knowing that I'd gotten "My Most Scary Experience" out of the way for the rest of my shift.

Hours later I was waiting for the elevator to take me to my car, when I began to chuckle, eager to share the humor of the experience with my husband. I was really getting into how I'd act out the whole scene— especially the dialogue—and how my husband would laugh over Delbert saying he didn't want to rip his jammies because Lena didn't like mending, when the elevator doors opened.

Inside was an armed security guard with a prisoner who I immediately recognized as Mr. X, a fifty-seven-year-old psychotic who had recently murdered and then decapitated his girlfriend, her twelve-year-old son, and the family dog. I couldn't remember what he'd done with the bodies, but I knew he'd stuffed their heads in a suitcase which he carried around in his car for a couple of weeks, until the smell attracted the attention of a traffic cop who'd stopped to write a ticket because the car was parked at an expired parking meter.

When he returned to his car, the Alabama State Police were waiting for him. He'd put up a struggle, and for his trouble was given a complimentary fractured neck and skull.

Right away, I noticed the guard was looking nervous. I didn't blame him—Mr. X was another huge, scary, psychotic guy on the order of Hannibal Lecter. This man was psychologically more scary than Delbert because he was clever and really evil. He always seemed to be laughing at you with a sneer and making signs at you behind the guard's back that were either sexual or threatening.

Someone—I really couldn't tell you who it was—made my legs move forward into the elevator. The doors closed behind me, and my nurse's sixth sense started kicking and screaming, calling me bad names and repeating, *What? Are you nuts?*

I was face-to-face with this guy as he stood there in his full regalia of straitjacket and the halo device for the stabilization of his neck injury.

The halo was really something to see. Rising up from the halter on his shoulders, two steel bars, pointed like antennas, were screwed into each side of his head—which had been shaved bald. Big stitches went across the top of his head like a Frankenstein look-alike, and a band of metal came down the front of his head and attached to a bar under his chin.

My upper lip had started to wet itself, when Mr. X, who was handcuffed to the guard by one hand, suddenly lowered his head and rammed the guard with his steel horns.

At that moment, I was a candidate for the third floor myself. I was convinced that either there was a conspiracy against me, or God was speaking to me, telling me I'd been a very, very bad girl.

Mr. X kept charging Barney Fife, who was running around the tiny box in circles, trying to get his gun out of his holster. As he rounded the control panel corner, he reached out to hit the emergency button. I didn't even need to watch to know he was going to hit the seventh-floor express button.

Great! Short of a direct atomic hit, there was no way we could stop until we reached the seventh floor.

I was jumping from corner to corner in order to avoid the steel horns and the guard, when I see good old Barney Fife reach into his pocket.

All right, I thought, he was going after the one bullet that Sheriff Taylor let him have, and he'd load his gun on the move, while getting his arm yanked out of its socket.

All I can think is that I *chose* to take the elevator. I didn't have to . . . I could have taken the stairs. It wasn't like I would've hurt anybody's feelings if I'd let the car go on without me.

I was starting to get short of breath, when Mr. X caught the edge of my sweater on one of his horns. In a panic, I untangled myself and dropped to the floor. It was the one place I figured he couldn't bend down low enough to stab me. Also, if old Barney ever did manage to get off a shot, I was sure the bullet would ricochet and make a beeline for my head.

Then a miracle happened. The doors opened. I looked up into the faces of about ten people who had heard the banging and figured we were trapped in the elevator.

Speed-crawling on hands and knees, I shot between people's legs, looking over my shoulder.

Mr. X had rammed his halo so hard into the side of the elevator he'd broken right through the cheap wood paneling and gotten stuck.

Everyone seemed to stand still—the ten people trying to process the sight before them; Mr. X, restricted from movement by his horns; and Barney Fife, who I think was just slow on the uptake. He was still handcuffed to the moose.

Then someone from another floor pushed the button for the elevator. The door closed and down the pair went. The elevator was sluggish in travel, but it was quick to depart.

Among the crowd there was a murmur of disappointment, then silence as they all stood watching the lighted floor markers as though hypnotized.

I don't know how long Barney and the psychotic moose rode the elevator, because I ran to the back stairwell and kept going until I was locked safely inside my car. I hoped that if the guard had been forced to finally shoot the guy, he'd remember to get the halo as a trophy for his wall.

I pulled out of the hospital parking lot, looked both ways, and headed for home, taking the long route. I had to have time to think of a way to tell my husband that I was going to pursue a career in Tupperware.

Linda Q.

Over the last ten years there has been an increasing incidence of violence in emergency rooms all over America. Twenty-nine-year-old Linda Q. worked in the emergency room of a small-town hospital in West Virginia. She'd convinced herself that the random killings of emergency personnel only happened in the big cities, to other nurses.

Right?

The culprit lima bean hit the steel kidney basin, bounced once, and came to rest in the lap of the injured party, a blue-eyed three-year-old named Rebecca.

Rebecca picked the bean from her lap and promptly inserted it for the second time that day into her right nostril. Without taking a nano-second to even groan, I firmly pinched the child's nose just below the bridge and yelled into the innocent little face, "Blow NOW!"

In the back of my mind, the thought *did* come up that I could be accused of unprofessional and child abuse–like behavior, but there was no way in hell any of us—the child, the mother, Dr. Milsap, or I—could repeat the tortures of searching for, and then removing, that wrinkled legume from the tiny recesses of Rebecca's nasal passages.

The child gave me a surprised, though somewhat blank, stare.

"NOW!" I screamed. "Blow like a . . . a . . . BEAR!"

Going one better than a bear, she blew like a nasal blowgun, shooting the bean across the ER's shiny puke-green tiles, never to be seen, or inserted into another nostril again.

While the mother tried to read the doctor's instructions about child supervision and childproofing a house, I stared at the wall in front of me in a sort of exhausted daze, wondering why I was able to continue in an upright position—smiling, no less. I felt battered.

The whole shift had been one freaky thing after another, which was the way full-moon nights often go. Having kicked off with day shift's leftovers of two drunks (lacerations and a broken nose) sleeping it off, one rape waiting for rape crisis, and a child with questionable meningitis waiting for a pedi ICU bed, things took a decided turn for the chaotic and peculiar about ten minutes into the shift.

Both paramedic units 12 and 18 called in at the same time with unassociated code three victims—one was an eleven-year-old drowning, and the other a sixty-nine-year-old suicide by exsanguination. We worked on them side by side, one patient not ten feet from the other. They died within forty seconds of each other.

An hour later a woman with a migraine was brought in by her husband. As I administered an intramuscular injection of Demerol, the husband, who'd gone outside for a smoke, had a cardiac arrest and could not be resuscitated.

Yawning, I retrieved Rebecca from under a patient's gurney, where she was diligently searching for the lima bean, and led her to her mother.

"Go and bean no more." I laughed, patting Rebecca's precious and beanless head. Protectively, she covered her nose.

With no recognition of my humor, her mother looked at me as though I had the brains of a titmouse, tore the instruction sheet out of my hand, and stormed off, her darling overindulged child in tow.

I sighed and turned to my next—and hopefully my last—chart: Mrs. Selby, a three-hundred-pound congestive heart failure who'd recently been on a three-day anchovy pizza binge.

She was so full of water, each time she moved, it was like watching the waves crash into the shores. I pumped her full of Lasix, handed her the call bell, and went on to my next three patients.

I was in the middle of moving a severed index and middle finger from a snot-encrusted handkerchief to a sterile gauze pad when Mrs. Selby's bell went off.

"Bring me the bedpan," she demanded.

Now I'd just happened to be near the registration desk when Mrs. Selby drove herself into the parking lot. The triage nurse and I made note that before she'd registered, she'd walked a good thirty yards to the candy machine at the other end of the lobby and purchased four Milky Ways, all of which were devoured by the time she covered the ninety feet back to the desk. It was kind of a bite, step, bite, step rhythm she'd gotten going.

"I'll get the commode," I said firmly. My back and shoulders were threatening me with a lawsuit if I so much as considered lifting her.

"No," the gargantuan said, "I want a bedpan. I'm too weak to get up on the commode."

Maybe it was wrong of me, maybe I should have been more compassionate and risked the last good vertebrae I owned and lifted her onto a bedpan, but the lateness of the hour, and the swelling of my ankles and feet, made me cranky.

I calmly pulled over the commode and set it at the end of the gurney. Then I got up in her face and pointed to her rather large posterior—that double-cheeked monstrosity that resembled a couple of hippopotamuses standing side by side. "You grew it—you move it! I'm not a lackey."

She moved it.

I ended the shift with the homeless old gomer with the lice between his toes. He'd walked in off the street and was immediately rendered unconscious. At first we'd thought he was simply seeking three hots and a cot, but when his blood tests showed a more than lethal potassium level, we'd filled his colon with Kayexalate, jammed in a plug, and rushed him up to acute CCU.

It was one in the morning by the time I started the quarter-mile trek to my car. I'd thought about asking the security guard to walk with me, but then again, I'd thought about it every time I'd left the hospital for the last five years. Plus, the security guard was about eighty years old and was not allowed to carry a firearm. With my luck, we'd be attacked and I'd end up trying to save him.

The sky was loaded with storm clouds, but it wasn't hard to see the moon was full. I rolled my eyes. I should have known it was the moon, especially after the angina patient who'd come in wearing a chicken suit, molting feathers everywhere.

I was walking with my head back and staring at the sky when I heard the crunch of a footstep behind me. I was already a good distance into the dark of the nurses' parking area behind the maintenance building. My car stood less than a hundred feet away.

The lot was made up of a three-sided chain-link fence, so there wasn't really anyplace to run, except to turn around and go in the direction I'd come, or to try and make it to my car. I manipulated my keys so the longest and thinnest could be used as a weapon.

The footsteps gathered momentum. Had I been Florence Griffith Joyner, I couldn't have made it to my car. Since I was cornered, I decided to look on the brighter side of things. What was the likelihood, really, that it would be bad news? If I'd been in New York City or New Orleans, sure—but a quiet suburb in West Virginia? It was a co-worker wanting to scare me—what else?

I spun around on my heel, twisting my features into the ugliest monster face I could make. If my boyfriend was to be believed, it was really scary.

"Boo!" I said, laughing.

The boo turned into a "boo woooo woooo hoooooshit!"

A small, round silver circle was what I focused on, even though it was situated between my eyes. The face behind the pistol was covered with a flowered scarf. I could smell the perfume Chloe coming from the delicate fabric.

"Are you a nurse?" A printed white flower over the mouth pushed in and out with each of the man's words. The effect was so weird I couldn't take my eyes off of it. Later, when I really sat down and thought about the whole thing, I decided it was that white flower that initially kept me from taking the situation seriously. All I could imagine was this poor guy stealing his mother's or his girlfriend's scarf so he could hide his face with it, and wishing it wasn't so sissy-looking.

"Yes, I'm a nurse, so you should know I don't have any money. I've got fifty-three cents left over from dinner. You're welcome to it, but I'd appreciate it if you'd leave the wallet—I work full-time, so I don't have time to go to the DMV for another driver's license." I dropped my purse to the ground and kicked it toward him.

The round circle jiggled a little, then lowered to about my aorta level. Great. He was going to blow a hole in my heart instead of my head so that I could think about it while I bled to death.

"I don't want money," the voice said hurriedly. "What kind of nurse are you?"

"A damned good one," I said, giving my stock answer.

The circle danced again. "What part of the hospital do you work?"

"Emergency room. Look, fella, I don't have any drugs in or on me, and I don't have any syringes or anything like—"

"Shut the fuck up and walk to the back of that building over there."

"What buil—"

The round circle, when shoved against the base of my skull, was cold. As it turned out, I didn't really need to ask what building he meant, since the pistol guided me quite adequately.

We headed toward the jumbo Dumpsters behind the maintenance building, and suddenly I went numb; this wasn't a mugging, it was going to be a rape. He was a patient who'd been kept in the waiting room a bit longer than he liked, and he was going to take his frustration and hostility out on me.

My thoughts jumped to the care packages (I'd come to know them as "scare packages") I received every blessed week from my mother, who lived in Washington, D.C.

Consistently included with the engagement announcements (always of my friends—never mine), obituaries (my unmarried classmates who overdosed or committed suicide or died from some horrible disease), articles on the relationship between breast cancer and breast implants (I had them), strokes from birth control pills (I took them), and sudden deaths from fad diets (I was always on them), was at least one article about nurses and/or doctors getting killed in or around emergency departments. I think she scanned the newsstands and police journals for them.

Nevertheless, her efforts hadn't been wasted—I had plenty of black-and-white photos ingrained in my memory of nurses' bodies lying under tarps (usually in parking lots), and bloody carnages of whole ER staffs blown away by automatic fire.

My mouth went dry as the panic crept into my throat and temples. In my ten years in ER, I'd cared for dozens of women and girls who had been sexually violated. In my mind's eye, I held a portrait of every one.

Through the filter of my upbringing, I'd always felt there was a sort of stigma that went with rape—a violence scar that never faded. I felt the cold muzzle of the gun and thought about death versus rape. For myself, it was six of one, half a dozen of the other.

I gasped for air as my throat tightened. The idea of running seemed out of the question, for I'd easily be overcome by my attacker. I supposed I could try and knee him or disable him in some other way, except I knew from working at the receiving end, the women who fought or tried to get away died, or at least wished they had.

But, I rationalized, I didn't have anything to lose. I decided to wait until he touched me and then I would try to knee him and then run. If I got a bullet lodged in the back of my brain for my efforts, well, that's the way it flopped.

I thanked God I didn't have any kids I *had* to survive for. My sister and brother didn't really know me that well since I was ten years older than they. My boyfriend would be sad for a few months, and when the novelty of wearing a mourning band over his Rollerblading outfit wore off, he'd be on to his next girl.

My mother would take it the worst, but only because she'd be tortured by guilty, secret thoughts that I'd somehow provoked the attack. Then she'd get to clean out my apartment and be shocked by my disregard for housekeeping skills. Before she'd given away the last of my treasures to Goodwill, her secret thoughts would be justified when she discovered my three-book collection of erotic writings by women.

We got to the Dumpsters and he told me to stop and turn around. I readied my knee. The right one would pack the most wallop since my right was my dominant side.

"Stay here," he said. "If you move or make a sound, I'll shoot your head off."

I waited. My cue was going to be the first touch.

Except the sound of a belt buckle being undone, followed by a zipper, didn't come. Instead, the sound of whispers reached through my panic. My heart froze for a beat. There were two men.

In a frantic, wild second, while the mental images of gang rape played garishly in my mind, I dropped my purse and flew.

Unfortunately, my hair—I'd grown it long for my boyfriend—trailed behind me like a rope. One of the men simply reached out and caught the tail end of the braid. That my head wasn't jerked clean off my shoulders was a miracle.

I was pushed to the ground and a boot held me there by the neck.

"Please don't do this. I'm three months pregnant." I started crying as my mind scrambled over the excuses I'd heard women used as a ploy to get out of being raped—pregnancy, HIV-positive, the clap, herpes, my husband is a special force detective, my husband is George Foreman. None of them ever worked.

Now I was really starting to wail, sobbing out of control. "I . . . I'll do anything, just please don't—"

A large hand which smelled of dirt and gasoline went over my mouth.

"Shut up!" hissed the other man, hidden in the shadows of the Dumpsters. "We ain't after pussy, you dumb bitch."

No money, no rape? Huh?

I stopped wailing immediately. After a second or two, the hand eased off my mouth. "What do you want?" I whispered hoarsely.

"You gotta fix her," said the white-flower mouth, pointing to a dark lump on the ground.

Hands grabbed the front of my scrub dress and yanked me to my feet. I was half dragged a few feet and then thrown to my knees again. I fell across the lump.

I stared into the face of a young girl who appeared to be dead. Even in the dark I could see the dusky ring around her lips—a definite sign her life was circling the drain, ready to go down. I reached out and felt her neck and arms. Every part of her was cold and clammy.

Automatically I switched into trauma nurse mode and grabbed for my stethoscope, which had fallen next to my purse. I pushed aside the girl's flimsy halter top and listened. Her breaths were slow and shallow, no more than five or six a minute. The heartbeat was irregular at about 38.

"Fentanyl," one of the men said.

I groaned, sinking in at the middle. Fentanyl was the anesthesiologist's favorite drug: a fast-acting narcotic which was about a hundred times stronger than morphine. It was a very pure and very addictive drug. It was supposed to give one of those instant, mellow highs which made it valuable to druggies.

"When and how much?" I barked. My manner and tone was exactly that of the emergency docs when in tight corners. Never again, I vowed, would I call one an asshole for it.

"Ten minutes ago. She did up a lot. Too much. Nobody was with her."

"She's going to die unless you get her inside stat!" Standing, I started for the entrance to the hospital. I yelped in pain when one of my arms was wrenched backward.

"What are you doing?" I asked in total bewilderment. "We've got to get her some help."

"She can't go in there," said the scarf.

"No cops," said the other man. "They'll bust her and then she'll talk."

I narrowed my eyes. "If she doesn't get some help, she's going to die of a respiratory arrest . . . like within the next few minutes. Nobody's going to call any cops." The cop part was a lie, but who cared?

The man in the shadows leaned toward me in a threatening way. "You go back inside and get what she needs and fix her up right here. She ain't going nowhere."

"I can't just go into the ER and get supplies and walk out without telling somebody what I'm doing."

I was actually wondering if I *could* get away with it. . . . All I'd need would be a flashlight, a syringe, and some Narcan. Maybe some oxygen.

I looked back at the girl. "How old is she?"

"Fifteen."

"Christ!" I said, painfully aware of the seconds ticking by. I stared at the taller of the two men, the one in the shadows. He was perhaps twenty. The resemblance to the girl was obviously familial.

"Look, she's going to die. I can't just let that happen. I'm going to go get a stretcher and another nurse to help me carry her inside." I picked up my purse and started at a jog toward the hospital. No one was going to hold me back this time, and by now I knew they wouldn't harm me.

"I'll be back in less than five minutes," I called back over my shoulder, "You can split if you want, but leave her here. You can call later and ask how she's doing."

Of course, when I came back with one of the docs and some Narcan, they were gone—all three of them.

That happened over five years ago. I've cut my hair, and I can barely remember anything about my then boyfriend or even if I loved him. I've married since then and had a baby. I got rid of the implants. My mother died two years ago of breast cancer. I think about her once in a while. Sometimes I even miss the weekly scare packages.

But not one day has gone by that I don't wonder what happened to that fifteen-year-old girl. Not one telling of the story rolls off my tongue that I don't agonize over whether or not I did the right thing.

And now that I have a daughter of my own, I imagine it will be that way every day for the rest of my life.

Charlie A.

Forty-eight-year-old Charlie A. was raised in Missouri. His introduction to the medical arena was an early one:

"I was diagnosed as an asthmatic when I was a baby. Back then, the primitive treatment for asthma was to give phenobarbital. I remember stumbling downstairs in grade school, half drugged. I was still wheezing and having trouble breathing of course, but I was so stoned I didn't care."

After being overdosed on theophylline, given Thorazine while in full respiratory distress, and placed on excessive doses of steroids, which stunted his growth, Charlie decided to say no to his doctors.

"By the age of ten the doctors labeled me a 'difficult' patient for being too inquisitive and argumentative. But I did develop a great appreciation for the nurses. They were the ones who listened and encouraged me. They were the ones who were at my bedside twenty-four hours a day."

Against his doctors' advice, he took himself off steroids at the age of fifteen and lived free of asthma.

"I still considered my life to be short, however, because that's what I'd been told by the doctors, so I compensated for time I'd spent being ill by indulging frequently and heavily in drugs.

"I perhaps approached my experimentation with a different slant than my peers. I always kept a PDR around to make sure my dosages were correct, and I never indulged in street drugs."

He began studying veterinary medicine, but slipped back into drugs and was subsequently arrested for burglary, possession of controlled substances, and carrying concealed weapons. The experience led to a new path with a job at the Red Cross.

"I stayed there five years, until it became apparent to me that the health-care industry was blatantly, grossly profit-driven. From 1980 to 1985, I witnessed firsthand the fact that certain organizations showed an overt disregard of HIV as being a potential threat. Testing was resisted at all cost because the organizations didn't want to incur the expense involved in keeping the blood supply safe."

From there, he went to nursing school, got married, and had a daughter.

"My first year of nursing was insane—a real baptism by fire. Of course, my marriage failed immediately. I don't think I was prepared for the emotional component of nursing. I sympathized too much with my patients and this was disastrous for me."

Not long after his divorce, Charlie met and married his present wife, also a nurse. At the time of this interview, he was building a bridge for her in their backyard. Of this experience he said:

"I found the building of this structure to be very enriching and rewarding. While I was building it, I realized the impermanence of all we do. Thus I've concluded that everything we do should be done with great care and as much love as possible."

I think the following two stories bring his meaning home.

The hospital was an ancient building, built back in the 1930s. The walls and floors were the original hospital-green tiles. The janitors, like their predecessors, still scrubbed those tiles with a strong germicidal detergent and hosed them down every Saturday. Only the uniforms had changed.

The beds were the old metal-framed kind, with the hand cranks at the bottom. Through the years, mattresses had come and gone, but the frames remained the same—hospital green and tall. So tall that the patients had to use step stools to get in and out of them, and the shorter nurses had to ask maintenance to remove the wheels just so they could tend to their patients.

My shoes squeaked and scrunched against the tiles as I walked down the corridor of wards. The medicine practiced in this small rural hospital was a good twenty years behind the times—like the equipment.

This particular floor had fifty-six beds, which were divided into rooms of either four, six, or eight. The floor was home to every type of patient: medical, surgical, pediatric, geriatric, acute, and long-term. As I glanced into the rooms, I saw two-year-olds lying next to octogenarians, fresh surgical patients lying next to infectious ones. Prisoners lying next to pastors.

I shook my head—in the one place where it would have been appropriate, there was a complete absence of segregation and discrimination.

My assignment was written on the clipboard tacked to the wall.

CHARLES A.:

Ward 21: Kaplan, Wilder, Fowler, McKeve

Ward 18: Kulish, Nielson, Arnst, Selinsky, Brown, Rafferty, Shooke, Morris.

Twelve patients. Five cancer, two cardiac, one fever of unknown origin, one gallbladder, one traumatic amputee, one burn, and one tonsillectomy.

For me, Ward 18 was the easier place to start. I wanted to put off Ward 21 as long as I could. Being a male nurse, maybe I found it easier because Ward 18 was the all-male ward, or maybe because hell would have been an easier place to work than Ward 21.

I made a quick detour into the kitchen to make an ice cream float, picked up two pitchers of fresh, cold water, and went to the ward, which resembled an army barracks. Four beds lined each long wall, the foot of each aligned with the foot of the bed against the opposite wall.

The bed closest to the door was my six-year-old tonsillectomy. The dark-haired child was awake, and staring intently at the bed catty-corner to his. His fascination lay with the sleeping prison guard's holstered gun.

"Hey champ," I whispered.

"Champ's" eyes left the gun long enough to search my person for the dreaded instruments of torture—a syringe, or a scalpel perhaps.

Instead, he saw the chocolate float.

Tentatively, he propped himself on one elbow and silently asked, "For me?"

I nodded, propped him up amongst the pillows—like a sultan—and pushed the bedside table over his lap.

"Drink it slow," I warned. "The ice cream will make your throat feel better."

"Why does that man have a gun?" he whispered, with a lot of effort. His curiosity was stronger than the pain of a raw throat.

"The man in the bed is a prisoner. The man with the gun is his guard. He's here to make sure the prisoner doesn't try to escape from the hospital."

The boy looked back at the guard, who was now awake and arranging his slouched bulk in a more dignified upright position.

Timidly, the boy waved. The guard grunted a gruff "Howdy" in return.

"Sip slow," I said once more as I passed down the rest of the row of sleeping men to the bed at the end—next to the windows.

It was obscured from view by three lead shields on rollers. I stepped between two of them. The seventy-two-year-old bladder cancer had radium implants.

Waking him, I handed over the urinal. "Pee," I said.

He grunted, wiped his mouth. "Jesus Christ," he muttered. His breath stunk of old blood and death.

While he peed, I poured him water and set out his dentures, mouthwash, and toothpaste.

He handed me his urinal, which I brought to the cramped bathroom. Standing over the toilet, I poured the dark yellow urine through a filter, looking for any implant which might have fallen out. That I was being exposed to radiation bothered me only when I thought about it, so I tried never to think of it, instead thinking about the more immediate chores to be done.

I usually referred to the prisoners only as Sir. This particular Sir was a relatively young guy, chock-full of bad temperament and coronary artery disease.

I approached the bed, and asked the guard to unshackle his feet from the metal frame. I counted the seconds it took for him to find his keys, select the right one, insert it, and work the shackles off Sir's feet.

Thirty-five. Thirty-five seconds too long. Nine out of ten of the prisoners we received from the county jail were there for coronary problems. There had been three incidents where the prisoner had coded and been defibrillated—before the shackles could be taken off. In essence, because the Sirs were grounded by the metal shackles attached to the metal bed frame, we actually ended up electrocuting them and causing horrendous burns. Not one of the three had survived.

"Hey sir, you need to sit up and take your meds."

"Fuck off, fairy boy."

I shook my head. I'd gotten so much negative feedback for being a male nurse—from the nursing school instructors who felt males did not belong in the profession, and other men who thought you had to be a sissy to be a nurse, to the gamut of professionals who looked down on

CHARLIE A.   39

the whole profession of nursing—that the comments no longer affected me or my steel hide.

"Yeah, well, you need to take your meds anyway."

"Stick them up your brownhole, queerboy."

"I'm done!" Champ cheerfully held out his float glass. All that remained was an inch or so of milky ginger ale.

The prisoner lifted his head long enough to see the child, groaned, and lay back, covering his face with his arm.

I cranked up the head of the bed and put the cup of pills on his bedside table. "Here's your pills," I said, hoping the child's presence would tone him down and make him act decent.

He uncovered his face, glanced over at the boy, and took his pills.

The boy waved at him. "Do you have a sore throat too?"

"Sure." The prisoner flopped back and tried to ignore the child. I took advantage of the situation to do a set of vital signs.

"Did you get ice cream too?"

The prisoner snorted. "Yeah, where's *my* ice cream, nursie?"

Champ hesitated. In his innocence, the child recognized the hurt inside the man, but did not know enough to interpret it as the kind of pain it was. Still holding his float glass, he climbed down the step stool and cautiously took a few steps toward the prisoner's bed.

"You can have the rest of mine. You can have my next one. It's gonna be chocolate!"

The prisoner's hard expression softened into one of tortured anguish. He reached out and took the offered glass. For one second, the callused, scarred hand touched the baby-smooth fingers. The prisoner seemed unwilling to break the contact, for he made a clumsy attempt at patting the back of Champ's hand.

"Okay, brother," he said softly. "You get back into bed now."

I looked away, not wanting him to know I'd glimpsed the human under the hardened shell. As sure as shit, I knew that somewhere there was a son, or a kid brother, who had seen a lot more of his human side than I, and probably loved him for it.

I helped the child into his bed, and gave him a supply of stories, coloring books, and crayons.

I looked around the ward. The rest of them I would let sleep while I did the daily weights next door.

Ward 21. The silent room. The denial room. Death row.

Four women lay dying of cancer. Breast, uterine, ovarian, and cervical. Their ages ran from thirty to sixty-seven.

I would not forget the occupants of this ward nor their effect upon the staff if I lived to be a hundred. It was as if denial, that all-powerful tool, was contagious.

And denial was working in Ward 21 like gangbusters.

The four women were all roughly in the last stages of their disease, each one wasting away a little at a time, keeping pace with her neighbors. As they were neighbors in death, so too they had been neighbors in life. Their children had gone to the same schools. Their husbands belonged to the Farmers' Lodge. These women had stood side by side at church and at bake sales, sharing kitchen and bedroom secrets, laughing over local gossip.

Yet from the beginning of their time in Ward 21, not one word had passed between them. They avoided looking at each other, even turned their backs to one another in sleep. In Ward 21 there was not one bit of laughter or any gesture of communication—only the severest, most unhappy denial and withdrawal.

It had a most unusual effect on the staff—as if we too were in denial of our own helplessness. We went into Ward 21 with a shield around our emotions as impenetrable as the lead shields we used on our radium-implant patients. We simply did our deathbed tasks, never speaking to the women or to each other. Report on the four women was always superficial and brief.

It was basic psychology for the patients of Ward 21: by not acknowledging each other, they denied the presence of the disease and death—like covering the mirror. For when the first one of them died, it would bring them all one-fourth closer to their own deaths.

For the staff, I could only guess: it was a quadruple defeat for the medical heroes—best not to mention it, lest our egos get hurt. This was one of those situations where medical personnel learned how to erect barriers and shut out certain things just so they could continue to work on a day-to-day basis.

For me, the main problem lay with Mrs. Fowler, the thirty-year-old cervical cancer. Halfway through the course of her illness, her husband had divorced her and taken the children to live in another state. Maybe it was her age, or maybe it was because not one visitor ever came for her—which is always a tragic thing in a hospital—that my lead shields always collapsed at the sight of her.

Daily weights were routine for all patients. No big deal. Except that for the women in Ward 21, the daily weights meant concentrated torture. The first day I was assigned to the ward, I couldn't help but notice how excruciatingly painful it was for Mrs. Fowler to get out of bed and stand on the machine. I'd actually had dreams about her bones crumbling through my fingers.

I weighed the other three women first, helping them stand, listening to their breath quicken with the pain. When I got to Mrs. Fowler, I saw the dread in those sunken eyes and knew I could not go through with the task.

The action was taken without much forethought. I pulled back her covers and slipped my arms under her body.

I was shocked by the lack of physical substance . . . to carry someone who is so fragile, knowing that if I were to tighten my grip by one small bit, her bones would snap and crumble like in my dream.

Gentle as a lover, I carried her in my arms to the scale and stood upon it. As I manipulated the balances, I wondered if she weighed anything at all.

With great delicacy and consideration afforded the dying, I placed her back in bed, staring at her eyes. Through the cloud came a look. She had been spared the pain.

At that moment, I was filled with the purest sense of love and caring that I had ever known. The words from a long-ago nursing school lecture drifted through my mind, making sense for perhaps the first time.

Caring is the most basic mode of being. It means people matter.

A murmur came from the cracked white lips lined with sores.

"Thank you."

"Yes," I said. "Thank you."

* * *

Nickie was three years old. Old enough to talk a blue streak and have developed a strong personality.

She was also the possessive overseer of a small stuffed, long-eared, and weathered rabbit named Binny. Binny was with Nickie at all times—like an extension of her body. When Nickie ate, Binny ate. When Nickie had her echocardiogram, Binny had his. When the lab came to draw blood, Binny had his drawn first. When Nickie went into the OR for her open-heart surgery, Binny went in for his—wrapped in a sterile plastic bag.

Nick never talked about death or the surgery. It was about the only thing she didn't talk about. She was brought to us prior to surgery for a tour of the unit and to meet the staff. That was supposed to lessen her anxiety.

It heightened ours. As we got to know these kids, and grew to like, maybe love them, they along with their families became emotional liabilities.

Like all the children we saw in that unit, Nickie was beautiful and innocent. Her parents were good people. Farming people. Caring people. Cruel as it sounds, there were times when I was convinced that it would be so much easier for everyone if children with congenital heart defects died at birth instead of after everyone was bonded and in love with one another.

I had to give these kids one thing, though: They were all fighters and survivors. Much more than adults. Their spirits were stronger— definitely more optimistic.

"Will you make me a paper rabbit?" she asked.

I looked at the clock. She had twenty minutes before they came to get her.

"Sure." I took a piece of paper from her chart—a blank progress note—and began folding. I didn't want to look at her too much, so I was glad for the task.

"Did I tell you I have a little girl just like you?"

"You do?"

I nodded.

"Where is she?"

"With her mommy. At home."

Nickie nodded in great understanding. "Does she have a Binny?"

"Uh-huh. Her Binny's name is Maggie. Maggie is a pink kitty."

"I'm sleepy," she said, rubbing her eyes. The preop was working.

"Do you want to go to sleep?"

She shook her head. "I have to take care of Binny. The doctor is giving him a new heart."

I handed her the paper toy, which she promptly showed to Binny for his approval.

"Binny wants one," she said in her tiny Binny voice. She held the stuffed toy in front of her face.

"Okay, but I have to take your and Nickie's blood pressure and pulse now. What kind of toy do you want?"

"I want a Nickie toy," Binny said, his voice getting more tired.

"Okay." I took their blood pressures and charted hers, then sat down again to make a Nickie paper doll.

Her large brown eyes watched in fascination as the paper began to take on the human form.

Binny watched from below her chin. Then he bobbed up to speak. "Give Nickie a good heart, please."

I stopped and swallowed. "Okay, but I'm going to need some help from Dr. Berg for that."

They stared at me glassy-eyed.

"Okay?"

They nodded.

"Charlie?"

I nodded, praying to God she would not ask me anything too hard.

"Will I ever see you again?"

"Sure." The odds were not good, but I made sure it didn't show in my face.

"Will you hug me?"

I hugged her . . . and then Binny.

As soon as she left the unit, I volunteered to work a double shift, to make sure I was the one to take care of her during those critical first twenty-four hours. The procedure of realigning all the blood vessels appropriately places stresses on the heart chambers that weren't previously there. Subsequently, ventricular failure is always a problem with the kids.

She came back surrounded not by the usual nervous concern, but by a thick air of panic. Nickie was circling the drain.

The parents were shooed off to the waiting room, and Dr. Berg and I ran like maniacs around her crib, adjusting IVs, titrating fluids and blood products, placing a dialysis catheter, giving medications, then more medications.

Dr. Berg was an older man, and in some ways had outlived his surgical skills. He'd been having a bad time of it as of late, because he'd had a string of deaths in his postsurgical kids.

Of course, the fact that his kids were all very sick to begin with did not help the options, but at the same time, he was a very caring physician—not like most of them, who rarely even knew their patients' names.

Dr. Berg worked with me, staying long into the night. He didn't regard me as an inferior because I had not become a doctor, nor did he push me too hard because I was a man. We worked hard and well together, as a team, talking and coming up with strategies to keep Nickie alive.

At 4:00 A.M., Nickie turned a corner and stabilized. Dr. Berg and I were beside ourselves with joy. Slapping me on the back, he left to go in search of the parents and hot coffee, while I sat down to chart all that had taken place in the preceding hellish hours.

As I turned to my second page of notes, the arterial monitor [the machine monitoring her blood pressure] alarmed. I looked up in time to see her systolic pressure drop: 100—90—66—40—

I felt for a pulse and got nothing, although the rhythm showing on the monitor was regular. Electrical mechanical dissociation. A death rhythm. I have never seen anyone—child or adult—come out of EMD alive.

But we tried. We did everything, including cracking her chest open.

Dr. Berg was crying as he did the cardiac massage. And when there wasn't any more to be done, when all the doors had been tried, he stopped.

He pronounced her, and I was left alone to clean up the aftermath of our efforts. Ten minutes was all I had before her parents would be led in—for that, I wanted to be as far away from the unit as I could get.

I leaned close to her to whisper my goodbye. Tears spilled into her, and forgetting that it no longer mattered, I had a momentary nurse's panic over mixing bodily fluids.

I looked down at the beautiful three-year-old, dark eyes half open, clouded over. And there she was, all small and innocent, her little fingers splattered with her own blood, her chest ripped open and her heart lying exposed and still.

Not still.

There, on the apex of her heart, was a tiny spot no larger than my little fingernail that was still trying to beat—still trying to pump blood. Survival. Even in death, her body fought overtime to stay alive.

It just about threw me over the edge. But just as I thought I'd start yelling, Binny, still wrapped in his sterile plastic chamber, peeped out from between the bed and the frame.

I freed him from his plastic bubble and held him out for examination. Not entirely sure of the status of my sanity, I would have sworn
that he *knew* his constant companion was dead. He'd never looked so
ragged or forlorn before.

I put him back into the plastic bag, placing him where her parents
would be certain to see him. Nickie would want to take him with her.

Melinda W.

Melinda W. uses her hands a lot when talking. The petite redhead's gestures and facial expressions, when combined with a quick wit and a sense of the dramatic, all go into making her extremely effective—and memorable—in her present role as an independent childbirth educator in Maine.

About the end of her twenty-eight-year career as a hospital nurse, she says: "I cried on the way home from work on a daily basis. I just couldn't give any more. There was nothing left of me. I had to get out of the hospital environment to save my sanity."

She has practiced in five different states in obstetrics, pediatrics, psych, medical-legal consulting, discharge planning, utilization review, union negotiations, union management, and case management. Despite the twenty-eight years of practice, the fifty-five-year-old mother of one says she did not choose the profession for herself.

"If I'd had my way, I'd have worked in a bookstore, been an actress, or done stand-up comedy," she says, laughing. "But my mother practically deified nurses, so she decided I was going to be a nurse before I was even born."

Melinda recalls that since the time she could walk, her father told her she was going to be a nurse so she wouldn't ever have to "depend on some man" for security. As it turned out, her career did just that by making it possible for her to raise her son alone after her first marriage failed.

"What bothers me now about this profession," Melinda says, "is the same thing that has bothered me for the last twenty-eight years—nurses' complacency about their lot in life. Nurses love to complain and bitch, but they really don't want to make waves. They don't mind if you do it for them, but when it comes right down to it, they won't back you up because they're afraid of losing what little they're being given."

———

It was all the ingredients for any number of disasters: The unit was loaded with chronic schizophrenics and respiratory patients age nineteen to eighty-five, it was a state hospital, I was green as a stick and naive not only as a new nurse but in the ways of life in general. I was a ticking bomb.

Making my 8:00 A.M. rounds down one of the back hallways where the majority of the TB patients were kept, I wondered if it was true that the longer I worked on the unit, the better my chances of contracting the disease. I had worked here a whole week, and I was getting worried.

The first patient at the top of my patient load was Mute Mary, a sixty-nine-year-old tubercular aphasic in total body failure. She also had the worst decubitus ulcer I'd ever seen in my years as a student or my short career. She had honest-to-God craters in her sacral area. Some of the bedsores were so deep it was difficult to see to the end of them.

The nurses had been telling the doctors about it for months, but it kept getting pushed off as a nonissue, even though she was obviously in pain and the sores were oozing with copious amounts of an odorless green slime. Two weeks before I started working, the nurses decided to take care of it themselves.

I greeted the perpetually silent woman and set about gathering all my ingredients for the nurses' recipe:

One cup granulated sugar.

One cup hydrogen peroxide.

I opened a package of instruments and began to scrape away the dead tissue. The peroxide went in first, followed by the cup of sugar. I set up the heat lamp over the areas.

It was very similar to baking a cake.

There were Polaroids of the original sores—taken the day before the "baker's cure" was begun—tacked up on the wall. Looking from those photos to the real thing, it was amazing to see how much the wounds had shrunk.

While listening to Mary's lungs, I heard a knocking sound.

Looking around, I saw there wasn't anyone at the door, so I walked out into the hall to see if perhaps there was some shy visitor timidly crouched in a corner close by.

No one was in the hall. The place was deserted.

I was taking her blood pressure when I heard the knocking again. Moving my head from side to side in the sonar imitation of a bat, I surmised the source of noise was coming from Mr. Sweeny's room next door.

Mr. Sweeny was an eighty-three-year-old schizophrenic with TB and epilepsy who, the night shift nurse said, hadn't been feeling so well during the night. Nothing concrete as an ache here or a pain there; it was more the same general malaise that affected older folks once they'd been deposited and forgotten about—loneliness, the leading cause of death in the elderly.

I stepped inside and immediately noticed that the bed was doing this *Exorcist* thing, shaking and banging against the wall so violently that it had actually moved several feet from its original location.

Amongst the jungle of bedclothes, I expected to find Mr. S. spewing forth pea soup and twisting his head around like a top. Instead, my untrained eye fell upon an old man having a whopper of a grand mal seizure.

I did what any new nurse might do—I ran into the hall and sounded the alarm by screaming at the top of my lungs: "Seizure! Seizure!" with all the urgency one might scream "Fire! Fire!" in a crowded store or movie theater.

"Help! Stat!" I continued to yell. "Mr. Sweeny's having a seizure!"

The thought that he might be choking on his tongue—look, I said I was new—suddenly panicked me further and I ran back into the room to make sure his airway wasn't obstructed.

The bed was rapidly making headway—it was headed toward the door. In the process of learning how to walk, the animated piece of furniture had bucked off all its covers, fully exposing a naked Mr. Sweeny.

I gawked. Mr. S. was not having a seizure at all. No, Mr. S. was masturbating like a fool.

In the split second before the crowds hit the door, I prayed to God as hard as I could that the floor might just open and let me fall out of sight. I didn't care where I landed—hell would have been fine. I wanted so badly to be invisible and then suddenly appear after the fray was over, casually denying that it was me who had called for help—stat no less. I would say I had been in Mary's room, thoroughly washing my hands before patient contact, just like the instructions on the towel dispenser read. I could say I had been involved with baking a cake inside Mary's sores and didn't hear a thing and that the screams must have come from one of the ambulatory crazy patients.

But that all sounded so lame. I looked around for an escape route.

Had the closet not been blocked by the bed, I would have slipped inside.

Immediately I realized God was not interested in helping me out, because the floor did not open, I didn't become invisible, and I distinctly heard the crowd's echoes coming down the hall.

Miserable, I looked at Mr. Sweeny, who was still going at it, staring at me with this sly I'm-the-cat-who-ate-the-mouse expression. His audacity pulled me from embarrassment to rage.

"Stop that right this minute!" I said, stamping my foot.

He kept right on going—like I said, the man had some gall.

Now I was presented with a rather immediate problem. I could grab his hand and stop him, but I really didn't want to touch him. Plus, it would be just my luck that the crowd I'd so desperately summoned would run in right at that moment and think I was assisting him in the activity.

Yet I couldn't let the hordes of healthcare professionals come rushing in to a patient who wasn't dying at all but instead having himself a bit of exercise.

Running back into the hall, I collided with two mental health techs and an R.N. Pushing them back from the door, I shook my head and attempted to smile.

"No, no. It's all right now. Don't go in there. Everything's okay. Mr. S. is just fine. Don't worry, just go back to work."

The R.N. pushed back. She had me halfway through the door before I managed to get a toehold on the doorjamb.

"I thought he was having a seizure," she said, straining to look over my shoulder. I was a good two inches taller, so she was having a devil of a time.

"Is the old guy having a seizure or what?" asked one of the med techs. You could tell his curiosity was up, because he was trying to sneak a peek under my other arm—the one that wasn't restraining the R.N.

"No, no," I said lightly. "He's just fine now. I . . . I made a mistake is all. He's fine."

"Well, why did you call for help if he wasn't having a seizure?" asked the R.N. "What's wrong with him?"

"Nothing. He's fine. He just . . . Well, he was just moving around and I thought he was having a seizure but he wasn't. He's . . . ah, fine."

The med tech started to push past me. "Let's check him out anyway. You never know with these old guys."

I grabbed him and pulled him back. "No, really," I said sternly. "He's okay now. I just made a goddamned mistake is all, now quit and go on with you."

"How could you mistake a seizure?" the R.N. said, knitting her brow into a suspicious frown. It was most unbecoming. "I think we should take a look anyway."

"No, really. He's . . . He was . . . I mean, he was, ah . . ."

You have to understand that one of the only words in the English language I am not comfortable vocalizing is the word "masturbate." I can barely read it in a book without some discomfort.

Now here I was, being forced into saying it in front of a group of people. And not only that, but that I had witnessed some old guy actually *doing* it? I wanted to barf and die at the same time.

I got around it the best way I knew how—I mumbled so that the word could barely be heard.

"He was ah, was, ah . . . mast-mumble-mumble-ing."

I felt weak in the knees. My face and neck were the color of a ripe tomato and there were perspiration rings under my armpits that met in the middle of my back and at my navel.

Everybody leaned toward me and said "What?" all at the same time—like a chorus.

I mumbled again, looking quickly over my shoulder to see if the old guy had finished yet. All I saw was the corner of the bed inching closer.

The mental health tech who was standing closest to me worked my mumble over in his mind like a crossword puzzle. A second later, a grin spread across his face, and then he began to howl like a hyena.

"Masturbating?" the tech repeated in what I thought was an unnecessarily booming voice. I mean, the word bounced off the walls for a full five seconds.

"The old guy was masturbating and you thought he was having a seizure?"

For ten minutes the miserable lot of them went as crazy as the patients with their lousy convulsions of laughter. If that weren't bad enough, within forty-five minutes the story had spread throughout the entire building.

For weeks afterwards the phone would ring and when I'd pick it up, people would ask if I was the nurse who didn't know the difference between a guy having a seizure or a good time.

A couple of the wise guy types made lewd comments about what a fun date I must be.

Let me tell you, I still hadn't lived that down by the time I was transferred a year later to the male admission unit of the hospital for the criminally insane on the other side of the compound.

The nurses referred to the unit as the male emission unit because all the patients there had committed violent sex crimes and were considered mentally disordered sex offenders. The majority of the offenses were rape-murders or child molestation–murders. The cream of society, so to speak.

The patients had either been judged insane at the time they committed the crime, or had gone insane shortly after imprisonment. Usually we got them straight from their crimes or from prison—when they were at their sickest.

Adding to the excitement was the fact that male emissions was a lock-in unit. That meant that the nurses were locked in with the prisoners.

The nurses' station had to remain open at all times so that they had access to us. I suppose you could say we had access to them too, but the simple fact remained that there were only four of us and anywhere between twenty and thirty-five of them. It seemed to me the odds were definitely in their favor.

It was while working in this unit that I had my eyes really opened as to what people could do to other people. Every intake I did, I read the prisoner's criminal and mental health history, which created within me an emotional roller coaster of horror, sadness, depression, and shock. The other staff, long since hardened to such atrocities, shook their heads as I gasped, cried, bit my fingernails, and made anguished verbal protestations. It was one of those things I never got used to, which was why I didn't stay long.

I suppose you could say I moved up in the world from there, because I next went to just a straight psych ward—no criminals or TB. But there were other things. . . .

It was the night I was in charge of the unit for the first time. We had a lot of manics, which meant the energy level was super high. We were also short-staffed.

Visiting hours were about to begin, and I was running around trying to get all my meds handed out, when I came to Mr. Pendelton's room. The sound of water splashing instantly put me on my guard.

"Mr. Pendelton?" I asked from outside the bathroom door. Mr. Pendelton was a fastidious older gentleman, always clean and smelling of aftershave. In that unit, it was something to appreciate.

"Say there, come on in," Mr. Pendelton shouted, sounding just a little too cheerful. "They're really biting today, I'll tell ya."

I knew it wasn't going to be good, so I opened the door very slowly and peeked in.

Mr. Pendelton was bending over the toilet, swishing around up to his elbows.

I sighed. I said it wasn't going to be good and it wasn't.

I must be psychic.

"What are you doing, Mr. Pendelton?" I asked. From the smell, I knew I didn't really want to know.

Mr. Pendelton threw back his distinguished white-haired head and laughed. "I caught me some speckled trout. They're thick as thieves today! Come on in and take a good look."

Like a fool—no, more like an insane woman—I went into the bathroom and took a look. Like I said, it wasn't good.

The "speckled trout" were of a particular brown variety that could be produced by the human body.

I backed up and, without meaning to, pushed the door shut. Mr. Pendelton had grabbed the largest of his catch and was, indeed, holding the piece of feces out to me as though it were a slippery, wriggling fish.

"No!" I screamed.

To my immense relief, Mr. Pendelton stopped advancing.

"You don't like fish? It's fresh! I just caught it here in this pool. Here, take a sniff."

I pushed against the door trying to think of something to yell. As the "trout" came closer to my face, I screamed at the top of my lungs.

"SHIT!"

I was scrambling to open the door—my hands kept slipping on the "trout" which had been smeared on the doorknob—when one of the med techs pulled it open and I went flying into the room.

The tech held his nose. I would have held mine, except my fingers weren't appropriate for holding much of anything, let alone my nose.

It wasn't until we were helping Mr. Pendelton into the shower that I noticed that the back of the bathroom door—the very one I'd leaned against—was literally painted with "speckled trout."

I had to finish the shift out like that. I cleaned up as best I could, but it didn't do a whole lot of good. And of course, that was the night that every visitor who came in wanted to talk to the charge nurse. Of course, they didn't talk long . . .

Needless to say, I didn't last there either, so my next stop was pediatrics. My rationale had been sound, I thought. After all, kids were so innocent, and it *had* to be better than working with the crazies.

And it was—for about the first eight weeks.

Then, one August night, the ER called to say they were sending up a four-month-old boy whose left hand had been traumatically amputated.

"How?" I asked the ER nurse.

There was a pause. "You know, I prefer you read the report. I don't want to go through it again. The only thing pertinent to his care is that he'll have to have rabies vaccine."

Pit bull or chow were the first animals that came to mind. I'd seen other kids who had been mauled by these two breeds, and I knew the damage they could cause.

Then it dawned on me that maybe it wasn't a dog.

I couldn't remember if raccoons were particularly ferocious, but I figured there was always a first time—especially if one was rabid.

I fell in love with Brian on sight. There are kids and there are kids, and he was one of the most loving babies I'd run into. Despite his injury, he didn't seem to be having much pain. He was such a good-natured baby that I instantly wanted to take him home with me . . . like under my uniform or inside my purse.

The mother did not come up to the unit, and I assumed she had been detained in the registration office filling out forms. But then again, the ER nurse had mentioned that the mother was extremely "slow" and seemed removed from the situation. Perhaps she was in shock, I thought. If the beautiful little boy had been my child, they would have been scraping me off the ceiling.

When I changed his sleeper and diaper, I noticed there were multiple deep scratches all over his body, including several to his neck and face. His eyes were untouched, and for that I was grateful. I also noticed signs of neglect. He was undersized for his age, and besides being dirty, his skin seemed dry and thin. The filthy sleeper and a bad case of diaper rash were enough to convince me his mother did not know much about mothering . . . or simply did not care.

I ran out to the nurses' station and found what there was of his chart. The plastic surgeon's scrawled notes were totally illegible, exactly as they were supposed to be, but the nurse's notes were another story. Reading the large, loopy handwriting—the kind where the *i*'s are all dotted with big O's—wasn't much easier, but I managed to make out the gist of what had taken place.

When I finished, I wished I hadn't read it at all. The lump in my throat and the lead ball in my stomach reminded me too closely of my intake days at the male emissions unit.

Brian and his mother lived in the "hollars"—a part of the mountain country renowned for its inbreeding. It seemed that when Brian awakened in the middle of the night screaming, the mother had propped a bottle in his mouth without turning on the lights, and had gone back to bed.

While she slept and Brian screamed, his small hand had been eaten by one of the many rats which infested their shack.

How was it, I wondered, incredulous, that a mother did not know the basics—like the difference between a cry of pain and a cry of hunger?

Horrible pictures went through my mind. A rat the size of a small cat, sniffing out the child's moist, milky hand. The first bite, then a ferocious attack.

My mind was merciless, for when it finished with that horror show, I began to think of another which I'd seen during my ER rotation as a student—a five-year-old girl who had been placed on a hot radiator and tied down. I recalled the burns covering her back and buttocks, scar tissue that looked like one of my grandma's old washboards.

But that had been an old injury. When I saw her, she was in for a fractured pelvis from when she'd "fallen" down the stairs.

As a student nurse, I did not understand a system that forced me to turn this young child back over to the very parents who were abusing her. It was the hardest thing I think I ever had to do.

I looked back at Brian resting in my arms, falling more and more in love with him, not really caring that I would most certainly go through the tortures of hell for allowing my emotions to take over. I knew as sure as I was standing there holding his warm body in my arms that not only would I go out the very next day and buy him a mobile for his crib, and some nice clothes, but I would also—in just a matter of days—hand him back to the same mother who allowed this to happen.

I started to cry, and decided that with the first nightmare, I would begin making plans to move on to another unit.

The first nightmare came that night.

A month later I headed for obstetrics—labor and delivery.

Other than women dying in childbirth or having monsters—both incidents, I was assured, were extremely rare—OB was a joyful and wonderful place to work. No more crazies, no more human horrors. I would be helping to usher in new life to parents who truly wanted these children.

My mentor, Miss Smith, was an OB nurse older than the hills. A no-nonsense type of nurse, she did her job with the efficiency of a German housewife during spring cleaning.

She'd been in labor and delivery a very long time. This I surmised the day she put one of our older, more arrogant doctors in his place with a stern reminder that she had been the one who had slapped his rosy, tiny bottom upon his own earthly entry. Other than a sheepish "Yes, Miss Smith," it shut him right up.

Miss Smith started me off with Women in Labor 101. I learned all about contractions, centimeter-by-centimeter dilation, water bags broken and unbroken, enemas, shaving patterns, breathing rhythms, and—most importantly—the mood changes of women as they went through the process.

Miss Smith taught me when to back off and leave them be—or risk having my nose bitten off—when to be encouraging, and when to be more commanding.

That was all fine and wonderful, except I was never allowed to view the products of my work. Never did I see the new mothers or the babies, since it was Miss Smith's belief that I needed to concentrate only on one part of the process at a time. Labor was labor was labor, and I had to know it backwards and forwards before I could move on.

My labor training however, went only as far as the delivery suite door. Although I was fairly certain that labor continued for some amount of time after the women got inside the delivery suite, never once had I been invited in beyond those swinging double doors—no exceptions.

Indeed, in my mind, the delivery suite began to take on the monumental proportions of something as mysterious and wondrous as the Gates of Heaven. Only the most privileged and divine were ever allowed to go there.

Miss Smith herself spoke of the delivery suite in hushed, awestruck tones—as though something truly miraculous took place there.

It made me wonder how women had ever delivered children without the delivery suite. I'd read accounts of women squatting in fields, popping out an infant, chewing through the cord, strapping the kid onto their bosoms, and going back to work. I myself was born on a kitchen table on a potato farm in Idaho. No doctor, no midwife, no divine delivery suite. And I turned out all right. Well, I thought I did. Now I was beginning to wonder.

Miss Smith would sometimes suggest, in that sacred time waaaaay in the future, that I too might be so graced as to attend as a handmaiden to the Almighty in the delivery suite.

But, she was always quick to assure, looking down her nose, that time would be long in the coming. I had many things to learn and many trials and tribulations to go through before that day might arrive.

The nature of L&D is such that when things were busy, it was pure insanity, but when no one was in labor, then there was nothing to do.

So it was one of those times when nothing was happening, and Miss Smith had us washing down the walls in the labor suites. Sometimes we'd wash them down about three times a shift. Like busywork.

I'd already washed down suites 1A and 2B twice, and was trying to decide what to do to avoid having to wash down the baby-pink-and-blue walls yet again. The paint was beginning to peel.

When my fingers resembled pieces of waterlogged bread sticks, I decided it was time for a recovery break.

In the back of the unit there was a small room which held surplus supplies, a ladder, and a mop and pail. I had never had occasion to go in there, but decided it might be a good place to daydream for a few minutes.

Closing the door after myself, I perched on top of what I thought was a worktable covered with black plastic. I was trying to imagine what Miss Smith might come up with next for me to do, when the worktable surged to life under me with a cough and a rattle.

Quickly overcoming gravity, I flew—as though flung—into the corner with the mop and pail. When the now humming worktable did not attack, produce noxious fumes, or shoot sparks, I reached over and peeked under the plastic.

I guessed it to be about a twenty-cubic-foot freezer. It was very much like the ones we kept on the farm while I was growing up.

I laughed, imagining a home video of myself flying off that freezer. My laughter stopped abruptly.

A freezer? In labor and delivery? No one packed a lunch that big—not even Betty, the evening shift nurse who weighed in close to two hundred pounds.

The hairs on the back of my neck prickled and I groaned. My days at the state hospital were coming back to haunt me with appalling clarity. I'd seen a horror—and horrible—movie once where the newborn child of some poor woman was spirited away from its crib and was discovered in a . . . freezer.

My curiosity about what was in the freezer tugged at my hand, making it reach for the handle. I prayed it would be locked.

But no. It released easily and began to spring upward.

I was being ridiculous, I thought. This was a modern hospital in a modern town in the twentieth century. This was obviously where surplus medications would be stored. It would be nothing more than—

My heart skipped a beat and I stopped breathing as I stared into the freezer. My eyes bugged out from my head and dried in their sockets from shock and lack of blinking.

Inside the box were fifteen or so plastic bags—closed with black twist ties, no less. Each contained a slab of what appeared to be a huge, sliced liver with umbilical cord. The outsides of the bags had notations in Magic Marker.

Frantically, my eyes went from one bag to another, reading the names—names of babies who had been born in the last two weeks. "Harrison—9/22 7lb 5oz," "Irussi—9/18 8lb 6oz," "Chrisman—9/17 6lb 10oz."

Of course, I thought. This was why I'd never been allowed to see the new mothers and their babies, or step inside the delivery suite—because it was all some sort of ghoulish plan. Miss Smith played some key part in it, like Bette Davis in *Dark Secret of Harvest Home.*

Armed with twenty-six years of watching horror pictures and reading scary stories, my mind raced ahead without me. The mothers were hypnotized and then implanted with demon monsters' sperm. Then they were forced to deliver these freaks of nature that were actually aliens who would grow into humanlike things and take over the bodies of real people. But until then, the monsters were kept in this very freezer and fed on . . . young, unsuspecting nurses?

My screams penetrated all the way down the corridor, past the double doors and into the delivery suite itself, where Miss Smith was restocking some of the demonic delivery equipment—things that most certainly had barbed spikes and razorlike edges.

It took a minute of concentrated effort on her part, but Miss Smith eventually managed to release the freezer handle from my grip.

"Mon . . . mon . . . monsters!" I managed to say, pointing to the freezer. "You're . . . growing monsters!"

The expression on Miss Smith's face was similar to the one I'd seen nurses wear in the mental hospital when they took care of a particularly crazy person—fear mixed with a few drops of compassion and mirth.

Miss Smith looked to the freezer and then back at me. She blinked a few times, frowned, and then the light broke.

I'd never seen Miss Smith smile before. It was weird.

"Gamma globulin, my dear," she said in a low, almost motherly tone.

Gamma globulin? The serum? No, she must have said goblin. They were incubating a bunch of goblins.

"The serum?" Miss Smith was saying. "Immune globulin? We take it from placentas. These placentas are picked up every week by the pharmaceutical company. The hospital gets twenty dollars apiece for them, and in turn, the mothers get free photographs of their babies."

I stayed with labor and delivery for quite a few years. I even made it into the delivery suite after Miss Smith retired. But you know, I never did get used to bagging those placentas for freezing.

Violet E.

Violet E. is a seventy-year-old single woman who has been a full-time labor and delivery nurse in the deep South for fifty years. In that time, she has taken one sick day—the day she was trapped inside the closet of a house that had been destroyed by a hurricane.

A self-proclaimed "down-home southern cracker," Violet was raised on a cotton plantation until she was seventeen, when she entered a three-year diploma program.

She has insisted on conducting our interview in the food court of a busy local mall. She expresses many fears about being interviewed, and insists her real name and the specific locality not be used.

I guess I became a nurse because I always looked up to the nurse in the doctor's office when I was a little girl. She became my heroine on a pedestal, the way she wore that white uniform and cap. I thought they were the most beautiful clothes I'd ever seen, all clean and white, and I meant to have me one of them uniforms no matter what.

My mother and father were wealthy, educated, and important people who traveled all over the world, so I was adopted out to some friends of the family who were of the same social standing as my own.

They tell me that I was a willful, mean-spirited child. I'm not sure where that streak came from, but maybe it was because my real parents didn't have time for me, and my adoptive parents left me to run wild with the coloreds in the cotton fields. I remember the housemaids used to take me home to their shacks at night, and not knowing any different, I'd play with the pickaninnies on them dirt floors. All I cared about was having a good time, and we sure did that. There was always somebody playing music, or doing some kind of conjuring tricks. . . . At that age, it was like going to a carnival.

Them colored women taught me how to sew and cook colored food real good too. I can still make a mighty good pot of fish and grits, and a Louisiana goochie, which is a wine made from rice that'll knock you down silly. To this day, I still make all my own clothes on account of them teaching me how to sew.

Then one day my real mother came to visit and found me eating supper in the kitchen with one of the maids. I was eating peas off my knife and scooping up the rest with a piece of corn bread. Well, let me tell you, that was the end of that right quick. After that, my adoptive parents, who were one of the old southern families, wouldn't let me associate with the niggers. [She pauses to gauge my reaction to the use of the word "nigger."] Now just hold on about that. That's what crackers call colored folk down here. I don't mean nothing bad by it, mind you. I know you northerners don't take kindly to that word, but us old crackers got different ways than you Yankees. The coloreds here don't mind it like the ones up north do. I'm too old to be learning all them fancy new names they call themselves like you see in the papers and on TV. African-Americans. [She rolls her eyes.] Lord. A colored is a colored or a nigger. I'm a white, or a cracker. Nothing wrong with that. I don't understand what all the fussing is about.

When I turned sixteen, I was already graduated from high school, and my adoptive mother started arranging dates with all these high-ranking government officials in order to get me married off. I didn't like the idea of getting married much because I knew that meant having babies, and I'd seen women go through childbirth on the plantation.

Now, remember that was in the days when women had their babies at home. There wasn't no such thing as going to the hospital just to have a baby. Anyway, I vowed never to go through that suffering—I was scared to death of it—so I went into nursing college instead.

That about mortified both sets of parents. First of all, young ladies of society did not work for a living, and to be a nurse was downright shameful because it meant that I would be seeing men's naked parts and having to touch them. That was the real shame behind becoming a nurse—only poor girls became nurses back then.

Nursing college was more like slave labor. We had to live in a nurses' residential home, where we were on call twenty-four hours a day. We had to be in our rooms by 7:00 P.M., seven nights a week, and be ready to get up at any hour of the night to go on duty—and that was besides our regular daytime nurses' training.

We were paid thirteen dollars a week, and it cost twenty-five dollars a month for room and board. I owned a car, and I liked new clothes, so it took me three years to save up a hundred dollars. When I graduated, my real mother said I wasn't no more than illiterate white trash because I'd only gone to college for nursing instead of being a doctor. She wouldn't even come to my graduation. Right then I decided not to go home but stay where I was. And that's what I did.

There was so much that was different in them days compared with now. Back then, it was the nurses that was expected to scrub the walls and boil the linens every day. We handled the switchboard and chipped ice and even made some of the meals. There wasn't no lab people either—the nurses drew the bloods and took the X rays.

Sterile technique was only for the operating room. I remember using the same razor from patient to patient, and washing off rubber gloves, drying them on a clothesline, and putting them back in boxes to be used again. Heck, right into the mid-seventies I was still delivering babies and doing vaginal exams with my bare hands.

You might think that sounds old-fashioned, but whatever we did back then, it worked pretty good anyway. I hated it when the fetal monitors came in. I still hate the damned things. Far as I'm concerned, the best way to judge when a baby is ready to get itself born is by the mother's screams: High-pitched screams come in the first part of labor. When they change to a guttural scream, they're ready to go. Or when you hear a colored gal cry out, "Oh dear Jesus help me," that's the time to get them into the delivery room.

I had a system for the preemies that worked pretty good too: I'd take those two-and-a-half-pounders and tie their ankles together with tape and loop it out the hole in the end of the incubator. Every time I'd walk by, I'd yank all the strings to make them breathe.

My first and only job started in a fifty-two-bed hospital. Behind the hospital was a two-room cabin called "the Backhouse." It was for the coloreds, you know. That was a terrible place; it was more like a fishing shack. There weren't no fans, and it stank to high heaven out there on account of the coloreds being all crowded in together—twelve beds in one of the rooms for the men and twelve in the other for the women and babies.

It was an awful place to be. The colored delivered their babies in the same bed and they always got their food brought out to them only after the whites had eaten; it was almost always cold and was covered with flies. Everything that went into the Backhouse was the whites' castoffs: used-up equipment that was mostly broke, and linens that had big holes or were too badly stained for the whites to use.

See now, most of them colored gals got themselves delivered by "Mother Mabel," who was a kind of self-appointed midwife for all the colored and the white trash over in Niggertown. When it got too busy for her, or if something went wrong, she'd send them over to us.

Of course, the white docs didn't want nothing to do with the colored on account of the colored wasn't paying customers, and the white patients didn't want the docs touching them after they had treated the niggers, so it was us nurses who did the whole thing.

Heck, I stopped counting the number of colored babies I delivered when I hit nine hundred, and that was early on in my career.

The colored got lots of strange superstitions and beliefs. I remember a lot of them women ate clay and Argo starch because they thought it made the baby more slippery on the way out. They believed the more vernix [an oily substance covering the baby's skin] on the baby, the better—it was a sign of a healthy baby.

Oh, they had so many old wives' tales. Like they believed if they squatted over a bucket of turpentine, it would draw the baby out sooner. And they used to come in saying, "I seen the sign," and I'd ask, "Well, did your water break?" or, "Did you see blood?" or, "Do you have contractions?" And they'd just shake their heads and say no, they just seen the sign. I never did find out what the heck that sign was.

Oh, and another one was they used to wear rags tied around their heads to keep them warm 'cause they believed if they got a chill, it would stop the blood to the baby. And we had to take all the rocking chairs out of the room, because if chairs moved during labor, it put an evil hex on the baby. Another one that we had to pay attention to was if any nurse, white or black, had her period, they couldn't go near them babies or else it would give the babies something called "the grannies." Never found out what the grannies was either.

We couldn't never place their shoes side by side under the bed. They had to be in pairs facing each other or it would be bad luck for the mother and child. Oh, and there always had to be a cat around. They said it was for good luck, but if you ask me, it had more to do with keeping rats away. I heard lots of stories about rats eating colored babies. If you ever seen them shacks, you'd know it was the truth too.

Another thing I remember was all the crazy, exotic-sounding names they gave their babies. Sometimes they'd ask us to name the babies for them, 'cause, see, it was good luck for a white person to name their babies. I always gave them the names of medications.

Oh, how they loved the sound of them names! I mean, I can't tell you how many colored folk are walking around today with names like Ergotrate, Morphine, Thialate, or Codeine. You know, I just give them the name of whatever drug was popular at the time.

Sometimes I'd be the only nurse on for three or four days in a row, and the way my luck ran, the worst things always happened during them stretches when I'd be all alone without no other help.

I recall one time when Mother Mabel sent me over this little brass-ankle gal? Brass-ankle gals were the colored girls who was only one-quarter colored. They got called that because they all had ankles that looked to be the color of brass. They were the most prized of all the colored women because they were the most beautiful women you ever seen in your life.

So, I remember this little gal was only ten years old, and she was carrying on hysterical because she didn't know what was happening. I knew the baby was in trouble right away, because she weren't no more than twenty-six weeks along.

Well, in the white hospital, I had four white mothers who were real socialite ladies—very rich women who were used to being waited on hand and foot—and that didn't lend me no time to give to this little brass-ankle girl. I mean, if a nurse was inside tending to a white woman when a colored gal was having her baby? Well, that was just too damned bad. At them times, the niggers were like an afterthought, really.

But this child was so scared that I tried real hard to talk to her whenever I could and explain that she was having a baby and it wasn't fully growed yet. Poor little thing asks me how the baby got inside her belly, so I ask her if any man had ever put his thing inside her where she peed. She tells me her uncle had done that, but told her he'd kill her if she ever told anybody.

So now she's scared double—about having this baby come out of her, and that this uncle of hers is gonna find out and come down and kill her.

So there I am trying to get this gal all calmed down, and before I can say "jump up," she delivers a baby boy with the blackest skin I ever seen on a colored child before or since. It couldn't have weighed no more than two pounds.

Back in those days, the colored preemies was put aside to die—especially the boys, 'cause the boys never made it anyway. So I wrapped him up and put him off to the side, the way I'd been taught, but then I noticed that his little hand was moving, and I opened up that there blanket, and said, "Lord God Almighty, this here baby is breathing!"

I wrapped him up real good, from head to toe, and covered every bit of black skin that I could see and tucked him up under my sweater and walked into the big white nursery where the air lock machine was.

The air lock was the only machine of its kind around at the time and it created a pressure lock that would help the preemies breathe. So I put that colored baby in the air lock and screwed down the hatch, and that baby started breathing right and I fed it with the special formula kept for the white babies and everything was fine.

I went on about my business for about an hour, and I felt so good knowing that little baby boy was going to live, I was almost in tears. Except then Dr. Paul, one of the pediatricians, came in and saw that baby in the air lock and asked me what the hell that nigger was doing in there.

I was so proud of myself that I says to him, "He wasn't breathing very well, so I put him in there, and see for yourself . . . he's breathing just fine now."

"Well," he says, "you better get that nigger out of here or you're going to be fired."

"Why?" I asked, "It's just a baby. There ain't no white babies who need that machine, so why not? A baby is a baby, isn't it?"

Dr. Paul told me again to get the baby out of there and not to let nobody see it in the hospital. Well, I couldn't hardly believe that this doctor who takes care of babies and children would really want this innocent baby to die, and I looked at that little baby breathing just fine and I just couldn't bring myself to do it, so I went about my business taking care of them white ladies and all, and then came the visiting hours.

I pulled back the curtain to let the fathers see their new babies, and they was out there oohing and aahing, and it must have been then that that there colored baby started moving around, and an arm or a leg got outside the blanket.

One of them white men saw it, and they started knocking at the viewing window and pointing to the air lock machine. They were yelling and a-fussing, so I went outside to see what the matter was, and as soon as I opened the door, they went off screaming at me to get that nigger out of the same room as their children. They were swearing and saying they didn't want no sick nigger baby's breath fouling up their babies' air. When I didn't say anything back, they started hollering that they were going to ruin me and I would never work anywhere again.

I told them I'd take the baby out and closed the curtain. But I still let that baby stay in the machine, until one of the white mothers heard about what the commotion was and got out of bed and walked herself down to the nursery to see if that nigger boy was out of there.

Next thing I know, the head pediatrician of the whole county came in and grabbed me by the uniform and picked me right up off my feet. He slapped me upside the head and went off hollering to get that nigger child out of his machine right NOW!

Well, I begged that man to let the baby stay in there. I tried to reason with him about that the baby wasn't breathing the same air, but that doctor, he just kept yelling, "It don't matter. Get that damned nigger out of there now!" He didn't even want to touch it with his own hands, especially with them white folk—who was the paying customers—watching him.

Pretty soon there was a crowd outside in the viewing area of about ten men. Some of them was Klan members, I could see, and they were all hollering and pounding on the window and the door, saying they were going to break in and break that colored boy's neck like a chicken if I didn't get it away from their babies.

I tried to stall, telling them I'd take the baby out as soon as I got the right blankets and equipment to carry him in. I used all these crazy excuses because, see, I was trying to let that baby have as many good breaths as possible, but then I got real scared because they finally broke in the door and started running for that air lock machine.

Well, I picked the baby up right quick and wrapped him up real good while I was running to the Backhouse. On the way, I dropped him in a trash barrel and covered him up real good, because them white men was hell-bent on killing that little infant who had dared to breathe the same air as their babies.

I know to put him in the trash sounds terrible, but see, them was Klan people and they woulda wrung that child's neck sure as I'm sitting here. I know, because I seen things they done like that before.

Anyway, them men go running on out to the Backhouse, and as soon as the colored women seen them coming, they start up hollering and hiding under the beds with their babies all tucked up inside their clothes. I swear it was like something you seen in a movie about the Civil War days.

Anyway, I hollered over all that commotion and told them that I gave the baby to the grandma and she run away with it. I pointed in the opposite direction as Niggertown and sent them on their way.

As soon as they was gone, I went back and got that colored baby out of the trash and gave him more of the good formula. I gave the boy to the mama and put hot-water bottles all around it and showed her how to stimulate the bottom of his feet to keep him breathing.

But that baby died anyway. I gave him to the grandma to bury and she was real bitter, but they didn't say nothing to me because I was a white woman and back then they wouldn't never talk back to a white— not like now.

After that, the white patients wouldn't let me touch them, and people I worked with started calling me a nigger lover. My supervisor threatened to report me to the state board of nursing, and I can tell you that nobody let me forget that colored baby in the air lock for about six years after that.

Now we got reverse discrimination. Now I see all the new colored doctors—pediatricians and obstetricians both—taking really good care of their own, but treating their white patients and the white nurses like trash under their feet.

I had one colored female doctor come up to me her first day in the nursery and say right to my face, "I hate whites, especially white crackers."

What could I say? I was afraid that she'd come after me with a knife if I talked back. But it's sad, you know. I mean, when the hell is the god-damned Civil War going to end down here?

Susan L.

Susan L. is a fifty-year-old R.N. from Philadelphia. She is divorced with three sons. As she puts it, she's had a "gnarly and twisted career."

I started out in nursing at the tender age of eight. I'd always wanted to take care of people, and one day, my brother was hit by a car while playing on a sidewalk in front of our house. My mother had three other kids to take care of and a part-time job at the local slaughterhouse, so I was the one who lifted him on and off the bedpan, did his physical therapy, and gave him his baths and his medicines.

Officially, I didn't start out as a nurse. I married my high school sweetheart and over the course of ten years had three sons. But after they were all in school, I decided I needed to work, so I took one of those hokey medical-assistant training courses you see advertised on TV in the wee hours of the morning.

Then—and this is the really scary part—I went to work in a sort of general walk-in clinic with a slant toward weight loss. This was back in the sixties, so it was all very far out and groovy and laid back.

I had my own caseload of patients and I did everything . . . and I do mean everything. I was writing prescriptions for speed and giving it out like it was candy. I did all the lab work and gave out results, wrote prescriptions for all sorts of things from minor procedures to major drugs.

We were insane at that clinic. There were two doctors who ran the place, and they were as crazy as we were. I loved playing practical jokes on them. I remember taking a urine sample from a patient and pouring off what we needed for the real test. The rest, I placed in a fresh container.

Then I went to the pet store and bought some brine shrimp and added those to the urine. When I ran the analysis, I put on a very concerned expression and hailed one of the doctors to come in and give his opinion of the sample.

He looked through the scope and after a few hums and ohs, said, "Hmmm. This patient has a pretty bad case of brine shrimp disease. Make sure he stays away from aquariums."

About three years later, I got too big for my britches when I brought my husband into the clinic, took some X rays, did some blood work, and diagnosed him with pneumonia. I treated him with IV fluids and IV Keflex, then wrote a prescription for the follow-up drugs.

The weird part was that I was doing this every day for strangers, and had never gotten into trouble. Well, one of the doctors happened to come in and found me there with my husband all hooked up to an IV. The doc asked what I was doing, so I told him. Hell, I even showed him the X rays I'd taken and shared with him my diagnosis and treatment plan.

That was the end of that career.

I decided to do it the right way and go to nursing school. Those weren't very happy days for anybody. About halfway through, my marriage began to fall apart, and of course, there were those days when I'd get up at 4:00 A.M. and ask the haggard image in the mirror, *Do I really want to do this?*

I remember the day I walked into the training hospital's emergency room and there was a PCP overdose who was going wild—he was throwing people around and then pulled his IV bag down and ate it. I mean, he chewed it up and swallowed it—like it was a tenderloin steak. All I could think of was, *Sweet Jesus save me! What the hell have I gotten myself into here?*

For my final clinical experience, we were assigned to work full-time for a month in various parts of the hospital, just like regular staff, only of course, we weren't paid for our time.

Maybe because of my previous medical experience, or maybe because I was a major wiseass mouth-off, but I was given a "special" assignment in ICU. What that translated into was a nineteen-year-old male with motorcycle-versus-concrete-wall accident whose brains were brought in in a bucket. I mean literally—the highway patrolman brought them into the ER in a plastic paint bucket.

This kid was basically dead, but that was back in the days when we filed the burrs off needles with emery boards, had one-on-one assignments, and kept corpses alive for months.

Of course there were a thousand details to attend to in his care, so it was the perfect patient for a nursing student. He was perfect for me, because my own boys were approaching his age, and I just made believe I was taking care of one of my own kids.

I'd talk to him all the time I took care of him. I'd tell him about the news in the world and the weather and whatever was on my mind at the time. The other nurses used to make fun of me, saying he didn't have any brain, and that he couldn't possibly hear me.

I took care of him every day for a month, and on the last day, in the last hour of my shift, I went in to him and put my hand in his and begged him to give me a sign that he'd heard me. I told him it was my last day with him and I wanted him to say goodbye.

Who knows what it was? A reflex? A response? But for the first time, he moved his little finger in a purposeful motion. From then on, I've talked to every comatose patient I've ever had, and encourage families to do so as well.

Little did I know that less than a year later, my youngest son would be badly injured in a car accident when his friend fell asleep behind the wheel. Every bone had been fractured, and his brain stem was contused. He lay in a coma for three weeks and we were told there wasn't any chance in hell he would make it.

The day does not go by that I don't wake up and the first thing I do is bless the two paramedics who made the choice to bring him to a private hospital that had the best neurosurgeon in the region. The other choice—the closer facility—was a big HMO. One of the paramedics confided to me that they'd taken a vote as they were loading my son into the back of the ambulance about whether or not to break the rules and bypass the HMO. They knew the HMO would let him die, and they decided he was too young to have his chances taken away.

Those nurses who took care of my son taught me how to treat a family. They were my lifeline and made all the difference in the world. They always were straight with me about what was going on, even if it was bad news, which it was most of the time.

As it was coming to the point where even I was beginning to lose hope that my son would ever wake up, one of his former elementary teachers came to me and asked if she could do a laying on of hands.

I didn't really believe in that New Age religious stuff, but I gave her permission, and she and a group of her church people came in and did this laying on of hands. Three hours later I got a call at the hotel that my son was awake.

Hey, what can I say? I don't discount anything anymore when it comes to healing, whether it be laying on of hands, or religion, acupuncture, dried herbs, or cow droppings in tablet form . . . Whatever works—that's my motto.

After my son was home and back to normal, I went to work on an ortho-med-surg ward where I was responsible for about twenty-six patients. Working with me were one aide and one LVN, and sometimes I had to do it without one or both of them.

It was on this job that I first started hating management. Every single time I ever applied for a day off or vacation time, I was told I couldn't have the time off. And when I'd ask for a reason why, they'd always say, "Because it isn't convenient for us." So I used to call in sick a lot.

When I got sick of that bullshit, I took a critical care course. Thank God it was before hospitals made them mandatory and then demanded twenty-five hundred dollars to take the course.

Right out of that course I got a job in ICU. That lasted a year. First I realized that the personalities of the physicians who admitted there were really something else. Prima donnas all the way.

Like the little weasel of a doctor who came in once and wrote an order for a huge amount of pain medication to be given IV to a patient. It was obviously an error, so first I called him and pointed the error out and asked for a correct dosage, because the patient was in pain.

The guy went into a rage—an honest-to-God rage—over the fact that I had the nerve to question his orders, even though they were incorrect.

Then the head nurse called and tried her best to be diplomatic and pointed out again that the order was unsafe and needed to be changed. He threatened her with having her fired and told her to give the drug as it was—which, of course, would have killed a horse, let alone a human being.

We eventually called the chief of medicine—at home—and told him the situation. But the good-old-boy system is strong here, so he wouldn't change the error, but rather put a hold on it and then refused to give us another pain medication order.

As a result, the patient went unmedicated for his pain for over twenty-four hours because some asshole of a physician couldn't admit he was wrong until the chart review board got to him and made him change it.

My decision to leave was made the day I stopped in the middle of the unit and looked around. There were ten patients, all very sick—the kind that had been there for weeks and months and would be there for more weeks and more months. Then I realized that out of those ten people, there were only two who had any chance of ever seeing the sun again, or who had any hope of life beyond the respirators and the drips.

Goodbye ICU, hello emergency room, where the pace was fast and every second counted. Patch and run. No time to think about what you were doing.

Actually, it wasn't so much the rough patients as it was a rough place. My first night on duty, I had an irate patient jump into my car as I was going home and threaten to kill me.

It was the cops that got to me at that hospital—the way they'd slam those patients around? Sometimes they'd just stand there and keep punching the patients while I was trying to get some kind of history. When I'd complain or tell them to stop, they'd say, "Hey, don't you care that this guy just murdered two people?"

In response, I'd always say, "Not right now. All I know is he's my patient, and I can't take care of him while you're doing that."

I remember this one cop—notoriously lazy and indifferent—who brought in a drunk driver one night who had driven across six lanes of traffic on the freeway—going in the wrong direction.

Now this patient was a chronic alcoholic, so his blood alcohol level wasn't that far off the charts, but he was totally, one hundred percent drunk off his ass. He couldn't walk, talk, or see, he was so drunk.

But the cop decided to let the guy go. That meant the drunk would go find his car, get behind the wheel, and drive to the nearest bar, maybe killing a few people on the way.

The nurses all argued with him, but he was one of those charming grunting types of cops who had to have the final control, so he proceeded to walk out.

As he was going, Bertha Jackson, one of our more outspoken nurses, yelled at him, "Hey sugar, you got a mama round here?"

The cop stopped, turned around, and gave Bertha one very hairy look-over. Then he says, "Yeah, I got my mama here. What's it to you, girl?"

"Well," she says, "I sure hope yo' mama is gonna be out drivin' tonight when this here drunk gets himself back on that road. Matter of fact, if you tell us where yo' mama lives, we'll make sure we point him in the right direction."

Oh, that was such a wild place. We had an inmate who came in to have a bullet dug out of his back, and while the doc was doing the procedure, the guard kind of slacked off his duty, because the inmate just flew off the surgical table and went flying out the window. He thought it was a ground-floor ER, when in fact it was on the fourth floor. That guy ended up in surgical ICU for five weeks before he died of injuries from the fall.

Then we had a repeater who was a really nice American Indian guy. This poor man was so young and so bright, but he was just tortured by alcohol—I mean, his DTs started when his blood alcohol level was at .25.

One of the ER docs fell in love with him, and one night she just took him home with her. She did everything to reform him, sent him to clinics and everything else, but it didn't work. The guy ended up dying at the age of thirty-four from alcohol.

My last night in ER was what every hospital administrator has nightmares about. Every healthcare professional and administrator in every hospital in this country knew of and feared the JCAHO [Joint Commission on Accreditation of Healthcare Organizations—an investigative committee which examines hospitals to make sure that certain standards are met].

Back then, the way the JCAHO worked was to pay surprise visits to hospitals—not like now where everything is set up months in advance with an exact time and day for the visit.

So, for me, this particular nightmare started in the parking lot of the hospital. As soon as I drove in, I knew we were in trouble—the parking lot was full, the halls were full, the lobby was full, the moon was full, and there wasn't one available bed in the whole house. I thought maybe we'd had a national disaster while I was sleeping.

The ER was a scene—we had a child with epiglottitis, ten gang war casualties, random-gunshot wounds, two trauma codes, and one medical code going on all at the same time. It was such a horrific mess that I didn't even bother to get report.

I took a PCP overdose patient—we have a lot of those—who was going even more crazy with all the stimulation, down to a room at the end of the hall that we never used for anything but storage of extra equipment. I put him in five-point leather restraints, locked the brakes on the gurney, and put up the side rails.

I walked out of there and into a female cop who had a thirty-six-year-old woman and her five-year-old daughter in tow. She barked at me that she needed a place to park them. I put them in a surgical room, thinking that because the daughter was hysterical and holding her belly, maybe she had a hot appendix.

I quickly asked the mother when her daughter's symptoms began, when the cop literally grabs ahold of my scrub top and pulls me out into the hallway, where she explains that both mom and kid are in on a 261 [rape]. I was so stunned that I couldn't quite grasp the idea—until I heard all the details.

They were middle-class people from a nice section of town. While the husband was out of town on business, two psychos walked into their home, terrorized the mother and child for five hours and raped them repeatedly.

As I'm heading back to the mother and daughter, one of the other nurses pulls me into a treatment room where she shows me a patient who has gone through some kind of window—ass first—and has hundreds upon hundreds of glass splinters embedded in his butt. She asked me to help her tweeze them out, but I declined.

Knowing that we were swamped and his problem could wait, I told her to put the guy on his stomach and explain that we'd be able to tweeze the glass from his ass—in volleys. The nurse made up some wild excuse about if she did it all at once, he'd pass out.

Meanwhile, we had a three-hundred-pound woman come in for an infected earlobe. She'd been seen by the doctor, who'd incised and drained it and was waiting for one of us to put on some ointment and give her her discharge orders. Well, she decides to use the ER bathroom—which was right in the middle of the unit. When, an hour later, she hadn't come out and she didn't respond to our knocking or our questions, I went in and found her dead as a doornail sitting on—actually, stuck to—the pot.

As it turned out, we couldn't get her out of there because the morgue was really busy, and nobody could lift her without a Hoyer lift. Plus, we knew it would be a scene with all the patients watching, so we decided to wait until we cleared out a little, which actually didn't happen until the end of the shift.

At 6:30, I remembered about the PCP patient in the storage room, so I went flying down there only to find that he'd gotten out of the five-point leathers, broken the window, slithered under the gurney and slashed both his wrists.

With his blood he'd written across the walls, "I AM IN HELL!"

I was crawling under the gurney, trying to see if the patient even had a pulse, when the door opens behind me and the head nurse leads in three JCAHO investigators who have chosen this particular time and this particular unit for a surprise inspection. They'd already seen the bathroom, complete with dead patient. The totally depleted crash carts had also been a big hit.

I found a pulse and crawled back out. I made believe the group of investigators—who were now furiously writing in their notebooks—were invisible. I didn't even blink at my head nurse, who was very silent and very flushed.

By the time I left the room, they'd just entered the treatment room next door. The investigators had stopped writing and stood in tremendous awe.

I peeked over their shoulders.

Inside, three of the night nurses and one volunteer—all working pairs of tweezers—were huddled around Mr. B.'s bare ass, which was sticking up in the air. Two of the nurses were blowing air across the area, at the behest of the patient.

If I ever want to laugh, all I have to do is remember his impassioned cries of "Oh that's it! Blow on it, girls, blow on it."

Mildred M.

Mildred M. is an eighty-year-old retired med-surg nurse. She grew up on a farm in Manitoba as the third-youngest of thirteen children.

She lives alone in a senior citizen apartment house on the outskirts of St. Paul. Her hobbies are music and reading and taking walks early in the morning. She says she never gets lonely because she always has one good friend she can share things with.

She tells me she doesn't know why she became a nurse, but that she could not imagine being anything else.

From time to time during our interview, she would pause to search my face. Then she'd say, "Oh for goodness' sakes, dear, I'm not interesting at all. I don't have anything to say . . ."

Right out of nurse's training—that was back in the late thirties, dear—I went to a thousand-bed hospital in St. Louis, Missouri, and applied for a job on the medical wards. I was hired on the spot.

During that first year I worked in Missouri, I made friends with another of the nurses, who wanted in the worst way to go to Hawaii. I'd always dreamed about going there, so we decided to save our money and go over.

The funny thing about this is that I walked into the first hospital I saw when I arrived in Honolulu, and again, I was hired on the spot.

It was a dream of a job. I worked on a very classy, private medical ward. Besides "the girls," I took care of all sorts of famous and infamous people. Oh honey, I don't remember all their names . . . No, wait—I remember now. I took care of the guy who wrote the Tarzan series? [She starts laughing.] Do you know, in his sleep he would start yelling just like the Tarzan in his stories, honest to God.

The girls? Well, let me tell you, these were some of the most beautiful women I'd ever seen. Oh! That skin and hair! Some of them had the most beautiful faces. I mean, some of them were just gorgeous enough to knock your eyes out. What did I know about that sort of thing? I had my training with the nuns, and I was still pretty young.

All I knew was that these gorgeous women would come in for what the doctors referred to as a "rest cure." Those girls were so wonderful and nice, and they really took care of each other if one of them ever got really sick with . . . uhn, with an occupational-hazard disease, I suppose you could call it.

I worked with the girls for a full year before I finally asked one of the other nurses why they were called "the girls," and don't you know, when she told me, I was really shocked. Here all this time I'd been working with prostitutes and never knew it. It didn't change my attitude about them, though, because they really were just lovely people.

The place was full of servicemen. It was a girl's paradise, I want to tell you. Why, any girl could have a different date for breakfast, lunch, and dinner.

I recall that on Saturday nights the boys would get a little wild sometimes and go out and really tie one on. So, on that Sunday morning, December seventh nineteen forty-one, I was bathing one of the girls. We heard the planes going over, and I started laughing and I turned to one of the other nurses and said, "My, those boys must still be a little drunk to be up there flying around *this* early in the morning."

I remember later going out into the hall and one of the Japanese nurses told me that Pearl Harbor had just been bombed.

My fiancé was stationed at Schofield Barracks at the time, and he told me that he'd been playing cards and when they heard the planes, he pretty much thought the same thing I had. A lot of the men were joking about what those crazy guys were doing flying around at that hour of the morning.

When more and more planes came, the men started running out onto the field. My husband said they got mowed down like grass. His best friend was killed less than fifty feet away from where he stood.

The Japs wanted to cripple the planes. They could have done so much more damage if they'd wanted. If they'd have followed up with warships, we would have been done in.

Well, as soon as it was over, all us civilian nurses piled into trucks and went out to Schofield Hospital, Tripler Army Hospital, and Hickam Field to help. It was strange, but the service nurses didn't exactly welcome us civilians. They really didn't want us working. Nobody was ever sure why that was, but it was.

The head nurse at the hospital I went to locked herself in her little glass office and didn't come out. She had the corpsmen doing all the work. We were the only nurses around.

Most of the men who survived were badly burned. They had to swim through the oil, you see. I always worked with the burned boys. Oh God, that was horrible. Those men hurt so bad I'd be afraid to turn them.

At that time they were using tannic acid spray on the burns that would take a little of the pain away and leave a thin, leathery covering. And oh, how those men appreciated every little thing you did for them. You'd go up to do something for them and they'd always say, "Oh, don't do me—go help my buddy over there. He's worse than I am." They always wanted to make sure somebody else was taken care of before them.

Even though we weren't wanted, we hung in there and really did good basic nursing care. Of course we didn't do anything like start IVs or any of that. Critical care didn't really exist then. The only thing close to critical care would have been the emergency room.

After Pearl Harbor, we were always afraid of another attack. We had so many Japanese nurses working in the hospital, and we were afraid of them after that, God forgive me. That was terrible of us now that I think back on it, but we wouldn't even go to the bathroom without two or three other people.

Then I got married, and after the war, we moved to New York City. My husband was old-fashioned about my working, so I left nursing and went ahead and had my four children. When my youngest was ten, I was eager to go back. I loved bedside nursing with my whole heart.

So, one day I was walking home with my groceries, and I saw this hospital and kind of stood there and just stared at it. Then I saw a doctor get out of his car, so I asked him if he knew whether or not they needed nurses.

Well, that man took me by the elbow and personally led me to the director of nurses—groceries and all. I told them I hadn't worked in about fifteen years, but she said she didn't care, God bless her, and I was hired that day.

Two weeks into work, I got down on my knees and thanked the nuns for giving me such wonderful training, because even though I hadn't worked in all those years, it all came back to me.

When the supervisor changed me over from patient care to working the medications cart, I was so nervous I'd count those drugs over and over again with tears running down my face. I'd swear I was going to quit, I'd get so upset.

I stayed for five years.

Then my husband got transferred and we moved to California.

One day, I left the house to buy a pair of shoes. I was walking toward the store, when my feet just went into this convalescent hospital. I was hired that day and worked there for five years.

My poor husband never did understand my love for nursing. It frustrated him more than anything. He thought my job was like a job in an office; at 3:30, he thought, I should be done and just walk out. Poor man never learned that nurses can't do that.

When I was nursing, the nurses did everything—bed baths, back rubs. We had time to listen. I'd walk into a ward and I'd be given twenty patients. This was basic nursing care, so every one of them would have to have a bath, so I'd have all my buckets of water, and I'd start on one row of patients one day, then do the second row of patients the next day, and so on.

I don't think there's any more nursing now. The days of real nursing are over. I'm glad I'm out of the business, because nurses nowadays are really more mechanics than nurses. There isn't any hands-on kind of get-in-there-and-touch-the-patient care anymore. That seems wrong to me.

In the old days, you got to really know those patients. You talked to them and got to know about who they were and their families.

I never wanted to get out of nursing. I never felt this thing you girls call burning up. No, wait—what do you call it? Oh yes, burning out. Maybe you girls get tired because nowadays it's a whole different ball game. I only got rewards from it. I really felt good. I never got tired of being a nurse. Actually, I think I'm a much better person for having been a nurse. I'm a good listener and compassionate. Even though my mind was on all the things I had to do, I always had time to listen.

The crazy thing is that I'll still do anything for anybody that I can. When you're a nurse, you're naturally that way, I guess.

Crystal G.

The moment forty-year-old Crystal stepped into a labor and delivery ward during her student nursing obstetrics rotation, she knew she was home. A divorced mother of three, she presently works labor and delivery in central California.

"I have wanted to be a nurse since I was a little kid. I've only been in labor and delivery for seven years, and I love what I do, but I hate the way nurses conduct themselves in their profession. When I got out of school at the age of thirty-three, I had all these wonderful ideals, and then all of a sudden reality set in. Management is bad enough, but the nurses themselves are so negative about each other. It's viciousness at its worst."—Crystal G.

There are two universalities that I have found in labor and delivery.

One is that women in labor always want their doctors there the entire time, from the moment their water breaks until they're ready to go home. The second is that the moment the baby's feet clear the birth canal, the mom wants to know how much that baby weighs.

The sounds of labor differ from culture to culture. It is a very specific thing—a very cultural thing.

For instance, Hispanic women—the ones who are new from Mexico—aren't very loud, but they are very vocal. Usually they say the same thing over and over: *Madre de Dios*, or *Oh mi madre*.

When I have Asian patients who are fairly new to this country, they don't say a word. They don't give any indication that anything at all is going on. If you hear a small, soft grunt? It's too late—you know they've delivered the baby and you've missed the whole thing.

Young African-American girls are pretty vocal during the labor and delivery. When I say they're vocal, I mean just that—they don't yell much, but there's a lot of verbal communication going on. They are either talking to any number of the hundred or so family members who have gathered around the bed, or they're on the phone to their friends and family from beginning to end.

Then you have the yuppies. They come in loaded down with forty-two pieces of luggage, the tripod, the movie camera, the still camera, and six sizes of floodlights.

These women walk in, not even in contractions yet, and the first thing out of their mouths is: "I want an epidural." Yuppies do not tolerate pain well. They scream a lot and they want pain medication and they want it *now*!

The more down-to-earth Caucasians cope with it better. The old hippies or the blue-collar workers are really great. They'll be into going the natural way, or trying new things that are more in tune with some natural spiritual path.

Philippine families usually have great support for the patients. They're also very vocal but usually they'll call out for a family member to help them. In turn, the family member will come to us. The families are quite supportive before, during, and after the delivery. In this culture, women who've just delivered stay in bed for two to three weeks and don't do anything at all. They don't move. One family member will hold the baby to the breast while another family member guides the breast to the baby's mouth, and another will burp the baby after.

Middle Eastern patients are very modest and protective of their bodies. They don't want anything left open to view. Rarely is a man allowed to be in the labor room. Middle Eastern women tend to be demeaning and demanding. They will literally snap their fingers in the nurses' faces and treat them like subservient scum.

Probably my favorite cultural group to work with are the rural Hispanic families—the migrant farm workers. They are so appreciative of everything you do for them. They inspire me and fuel me to get through some of my other patients.

Of all the groups, however, the women—girls—who have the worst time with labor are adolescents. Teenagers do *not* do well with labor, which is why I think they should have a film of a teen in labor and then delivering. I guarantee you it would be the best birth control method in the world, because those girls would never have sex again!

Leah I.

"Emergency room nursing was my first love and it remains my first love. It's a part of my life" is how Leah I., a forty-six-year-old R.N. from Washington, D.C., describes the first seventeen years of her twenty-six-year career.

"It's hard to tell laypersons about what happens in ER nursing," she says, "because they have to look at all these horrible, emotional issues they don't normally face, whereas a nurse faces those upheavals every day. When I tell people stories like the one I've told you, they think I'm exaggerating.

"I don't have any reason to exaggerate, because these things really happen every day. Real life is more terrible, more funny, and weirder than any story you can make up.

"Regular people ask me why I wanted to become a nurse at all. To be honest, I really wanted to be a ballet dancer. I studied ballet until I was sixteen, at which time my mother took me aside and said I needed to become a nurse because I would always have a job to fall back on.

"Sometimes I think about what my life would have been like if I'd stuck to ballet. I figure I'd be retired, living in Paris, running my own ballet school, have fabulous legs, and never once would I have ever been peed, vomited, or pooped on."

It has turned out to be one of those shifts that happen once every thousand years. Usually there are definite warning signs that a nurse recognizes early on to let her know the shift from hell is on its way—a full moon, the first of July, temperatures that stay at the 100 degrees plus mark for over a week. None of those red flags are in evidence now.

If I'd had any idea how it was going to turn out, I'd never have volunteered to work a double shift—7:00 A.M. to midnight. But then again, even after all my years in St. A.'s ER, I didn't want to miss anything either.

I just wish the patients hadn't come in one right after the other. Then again, I have to look on the bright side—I mean, they could have come in all at once. So far, we've had more than our fair share of those patients who abuse the services of "the Pit," using it as a clinic. They come in wielding their Medicaid cards like lifetime free ride vouchers, sure that they are entitled to some kind of hop-to priority service. The winner of the Medicaid Abuser of the Year Award went to the patient who came in via ambulance at 7:15 A.M., complaining of a sore throat.

At 7:55, one of our frequent flyers, an alcoholic by the name of Dobbs, comes in drunk and angry. It's Thursday, so her visit is not a surprise to the staff. Dobbs is head chef at one of the fancy local restaurants, and Thursday is her only day off. Thursday is also the only day any of the house staff will eat at her restaurant.

Usually Dobbs starts drinking late Wednesday afternoon, and sometime between 3:00 and 7:00 A.M., she gets pissed off and finds someone she can unleash on. After a dozen or more arrests for giving various unlucky citizens a taste of her wrath, Dobbs has smartened up—now she goes where she knows she can vent at will and not be incarcerated. The bonus is that we are bound to take what she has to dish out without complaint—we refuse no one.

Phyllis, Michael, and I, the three "old-timer" R.N.'s on duty, are prepared. Each of us dressed head to toe in protective gear, we set about getting the cantankerous old crone undressed and assessed, treated, and streeted. I kept a verbal running score of the battle:

In the first five minutes of the game, the nurses score one blood pressure and a pulse.

In center court, Dobbs scores two bites to Michael's arm, then a triple-whammy full-contact kick to my knees, chest, and arms.

Phyllis gets temperature with instant ear probe.

Lab scores a couple of tubes of blood.

Dobbs breaks one of them. . . .

The extremely colorful verbal abuse doesn't faze Phyllis or me in the least—we've both grown up believing in the old taunt "Sticks and stones will break my bones, but names will never hurt me." Only Michael, a strict Catholic, blushes at each malediction.

As soon as Dobbs realizes she has failed to make any lasting impressions, she resorts to her old bag of tricks (no pun intended), also known by the emergency room nurses as Dobbs Colostomy Throw Event.

If we aren't quick enough (and we rarely are), Dobbs can have her colostomy bag unhooked and ready to hurl in less than a second. She then swings it directly at the offenders, splattering everyone in her path. Michael's face shield ends up looking like the mudguard on a semi rolling through Iowa on a rainy spring day.

At 9:05, we shove Dobbs (a pound or two lighter) out the door and on her way to outpatient psych, that wonderful unit providing Band-Aid psychiatry for the outgoing.

Kevin and Karen arrive at 9:08. The complaint written on the chart is made by the school nurse who brings the ten- and eight-year-old siblings in for treatment and evaluation. A cursory glance, and all I see are the words "school nurse" and "treatment and evaluation," so I shuffle into room 2, thinking of head lice and Kwell. What I see are two kids with the sweetest round faces, crying, desperately clinging to each other. A hundred or more fresh burns cover every inch of their pale, undernourished bodies, except the areas which can't be hidden—the hands, necks, and faces.

I recognize the wounds as cigarette burns and instantly I feel like I have been kicked in the heart—my daughters are close in age to these two. Looking down at the names again, I now recognize them—Kevin and Karen S., repeaters of the worst kind.

". . . I don't think anyone would have noticed," the woman who'd introduced herself as the school nurse is saying, "except that the wounds started oozing through their clothes. The mother always dresses them in long-sleeved shirts and pants no matter how hot it is."

Smiling, I step toward the gurney with the intention of inspecting the burns. Kevin screams.

"You can't take her without me!" he sobs, clinging to his golden-haired sister for dear life. In one long, hurried, hysterical plea, he continues: "We have to be together oh please please we have to go together because Karen's littler and I can I can protect her and do all the work don't break us apart we'll go back home if we can't go together we'll take it because we can be together."

He pauses to breathe, and I notice how dark the circles are under both sets of eyes. The circles of purple gray look garishly unnatural in these sweet faces.

I hold up my hand. "It's okay. It's okay. You can stay together, I prom—"

I shut my mouth, because I can't promise. I don't know if they can stay together, and the worst sin I can commit besides sending them back to their tormentors will be to make a promise that might be broken.

The other person in the room, a rail-thin man in a flannel shirt, rubs Kevin's head, murmuring a soothing stream of words. He turns to me and whispers, "I'm Carl Robinson, the school psychologist. Susan called me to come in with them today. I'm familiar with their case."

I nod, glad that he is present and rooting for the right side.

"Okay. Just let me go look at the old charts."

I leave the room knowing there isn't much I can do. I refuse to prod and poke them with thermometers and blood pressure cuffs. They've been assaulted enough.

The day clerk hands me a thick stack of old charts, which I skim through, trying not to cry or scream in rage. It has been only two weeks since Kevin and Karen's last visit to ER.

Official-looking reports, too numerous to count, describe the "suspicious" injuries—soft-tissue wounds, burns, strangulation marks, concussions, starvation, rope burns, and on and on for pages.

There are copies of reports from social workers, school psychologists, psychiatrists, and nurses about suspicious injuries and the results of psychological tests indicating that physical, emotional, and mental damage is being perpetrated upon the children by the mother and various boyfriends on a routine basis. There are hundreds of social service referrals and documents of how the children have been removed from the home, separated, placed for a few days, and then . . . sent back to the same mother to be beaten and tortured by her and whatever boyfriend is currently in residence.

"Do you have a minute?"

I turn to see a distraught-looking school psychologist.

I nod, not really sure if I do.

"Do you know the story on these kids?"

"I think I'm getting the idea." I point to the stack of charts. "I don't understand. Why do they keep getting sent back to the home?"

"It's the pediatrician."

The look of dumb wonder on my face asks the question for me.

"He won't sign the reports saying that the kids are being abused. No matter how badly the kids get hurt, he denies the fact that the mother is abusing them."

I blink and look around the busy room. One of the paramedic rigs has pulled up outside. From the speed with which they've come in, I know it's going to be bad.

"Why?"

The young man sighs. "I've talked to this clown a dozen times before he started refusing my calls. But I got enough from him to know that the mother threatened to ruin his practice if he ever turned her in for child abuse. He's afraid she'll spread it around that he routinely turns parents in."

"Jesus," I whisper. "How can he sleep at night knowing what's happening?"

"I don't know, but he's not the only pediatrician in this county who does this. There are at least three I know of who won't sign the reports or turn the parents in. . . . I'm wondering if you could call in a different pediatrician this time?"

Over the psychologist's shoulder I see the back doors of the rig fly open. "If this turkey has been named on the chart as the regular physician, I don't know if we can do that. I . . ."

The stretcher is pulled out of the rig and the legs snap down to meet the ground. Blood is everywhere. CPR is in progress, a line of Ringer's is running, but I'm stunned that there is no endotracheal tube in place.

The paramedics run past us, giving me a glimpse of a young face with blood pouring out of both nostrils and mouth. My nurse's eye says the boy is two minutes away from a DOA status.

The bloody sheets and the lifeless face seem to paralyze Dr. Robinson. His mouth has fallen open and his eyes are glassy.

"We'll try calling someone else," I shout over the noise, falling in behind the gurney. "We'll lie if we have to."

The second the door of the trauma-surgical room closes, the paramedic begins giving report. His voice is loud and urgent over the controlled confusion going on around the body.

A resident wrestles with the laryngoscope, passes the ET tube, once . . . twice . . . in! Interns do CPR, while fourth-year med students do what they're supposed to do—stand off to the side and wait to be used as scut monkeys. The nurses are on automatic pilot, checking the line, inserting another. The crash cart sits near the boy's head, its drawers opened and violated. Vital signs and labs are gathered simultaneously.

". . . sixteen-year-old shot at close range through the heart in a fight over a girl. The shooting took place in the corridor outside the principal's office. Nine-one-one was activated immediately.

"Upon our arrival, the victim had been down approximately six minutes and was in asystole with a BP of zero. Pupils were dilated and fixed.

"CPR was initiated. . . ."

"Mistake number one," Phyllis says, cutting off the teen's clothes. She is very pissed off at having to take time out from the other patients to tend to a corpse. "Why didn't you call for authorization to pronounce him at the scene? This kid is—"

The paramedic throws her a look that says if he had a gun he'd shoot *her*. She shrugs and shuts up, probably thinking the same thing I am, which is: *Prime learning-experience meat*. After all, we are a teaching hospital.

"There was too much blood to intubate. I tried four or five times. We got an oral airway in and started a sixteen-gauge line with wide-open Ringer's. Epinephrine was given. He remained unresponsive. . . ."

"No shit, Einstein," says Phyllis, unable to keep quiet. She has a real thing about dealing with overzealous Eagle Scout rescuers who should know better.

There are scores of residents and interns running around ordering labs and directing the meds given, but it's clear they know the score. It will be only a matter of minutes before the attending will come and call off our efforts.

The chief surgical resident struts in, eyes ablaze with self-importance gone rampant. He demands to know what is going on.

Dr. Marchones, a second-year resident, begins to recite the facts of the case, while Phyllis, Michael, and I fidget uncomfortably in apprehension.

The current chief surgical resident perfectly fills the usual profile of a chief surgical resident down to the last ugly detail: arrogant, rude, brash, and so full of himself he can't see beyond the end of his own nose. He fits the well-established definition of a hot-shit blade—often wrong, but never in doubt.

For five minutes, all of us endure the man's insults and verbal abuses while he directs useless courses of action to be carried out on the dead boy's body.

Finally a voice rises above his.

"Why are we flogging this kid?" asks Dr. Marchones. "He was dead when he came in."

"I suppose you think we should call the code, Marchones?" The chief blade's voice is full of condescension.

"Yes I do. He's obviously—"

It is all the chief blade needs. As if announcing his candidacy for public office, he says: "I'm gonna crack his chest."

The room goes silent as we all stop what we're doing and look at each other. Michael's mouth opens in disbelief.

"You're *not* serious?"

The blade barely looks in Michael's direction. "When I want a nurse telling me how to practice medicine, I'll ask. Get the equipment!"

Michael, his neck held stiff, goes over to the cabinet containing the surgical packs. Dr. Marchones leaves, rolling her eyes. Two residents and an intern crowd in closer. Phyllis declares she will not have any part of the butchery, and follows Dr. Marchones.

As for myself, I try to believe he really thinks cracking this boy's chest is going to make a difference—or, at the very least, that he is doing it for the benefit of the interns and residents . . . a sort of teaching experience. But he cracks the kid's chest quickly and without taking the time or care to show the others what he's doing.

And the blood flows. I mean, it *pours*, literally spilling over the sides of the table and onto the floor. We all watch as the blade does cardiac massage on a heart that has been sheared into three separate pieces. I don't know what he's thinking, except maybe what a great story it'll make for his girlfriend and some of the underling interns and residents who are still too green not to admire him.

When I get disgusted enough, I leave the room. It is 11:00 A.M.—only thirteen more hours to go.

The charts are backed up, so I grab two and head for the waiting room, reading the complaints as I go. Monica is a twenty-three-year-old with all the symptoms of a urinary tract infection, and sixty-five-year-old Louise is complaining of vaginal discharge and "a growth."

I always feel sorry for the patients who come in for GYN problems; first they have a pelvic by a med student, and then by the intern and finally by the resident. To top it off, the resident runs a continuous commentary, giving detailed explanations and descriptions about what things are and where they're *supposed* to be, and how they function. The whole time, the poor patient is spread-eagled and having to listen to it all.

I lead the pair to the exam room and divide the room in half by drawing a thick curtain between them. Standing outside the linen wall, I give them instructions on what to take off and what to leave on and how to provide me with a midstream urine specimen.

I know getting the specimen won't be a problem for Monica, a petite brunette who blushes when she explains she is on her honeymoon and hopes it won't take too long to be seen. As for Louise . . .

Louise tips the scales at 250 pounds, and seems to walk gingerly. I ask if walking is painful, thinking in terms of sore feet, arthritis, or a severe vaginitis, but she answers that she doesn't have pain, she's being careful of her "growth."

After sending off the urine specs, I get their vitals and brief GYN histories, set up two vaginal exam trays, and return the charts to the doctor's pickup box.

Monica is clearly a case of honeymooner's UTI (having intercourse upwards of four times a night left no question of it being anything else). To her I give the usual advice about drinking plenty of fluids, and urinating after making love. I am going on about the medication she'll most likely be taking, when Louise's voice comes through the curtain.

"You got to take some slippery elm, bearberry, yarrow, and cornsilk tea, girl. Three times a day. Clear you right up." She cackles. "And make that man drink some valerian root, girl. He sounds like he need to sleep more before he wear hisself out."

Monica grabs a pencil and writes down the names of the herbs.

I notice she has underlined the valerian root.

The med student, intern, and resident enter the room, discussing the details of Monica's charted information. While I position her and the exam light, the three men continue to talk about her in the third person.

"'Like hellllloooo?" she says, waving at them. "I'm right here, breathing and having mental activity, so don't talk about me like I'm a corpse or something, okay?"

Her outspokenness delights me. She, like most women of her generation, is liberated—on equal footing with everybody, including physicians, celebrities, and, I suspect, even God.

The three men chuckle nervously and apologize, then go on talking about her *with* her, in third person—like they are talking about a corpse, but with the corpse included.

I go out to the desk for the urinalyses reports, and when I return, the intern and the resident have the fourth-year med student cornered and are giving him a pep talk.

The med student is obviously nervous. His hands are shaking and red splotches are starting to appear on his neck. He has every right to be nervous; not only is it his first pelvic exam, but he is approximately the same age as the patient. Worse yet, the patient is an extremely attractive woman.

I overhear the intern saying something like, "Don't be such a pussy," when Monica, tired of waiting, gets up on her elbows and looks the perspiring student in the eye.

"Look," she says matter-of-factly. "I know this is your first time, and I promise I'll be gentle, but please just get it over with, write the prescription, and let me out of here, okay?"

The resident pats the student on the back. "Go on," he coaxes. "You've watched me do this fifty times. You can do it."

The student sits on the rolling stool of honor and Monica expertly places herself in position.

"Okay, Mrs. . . ." The student looks around for the chart, which the intern holds out to him, pointing to the last name. ". . . Aubrey. I'm going to be as gentle as I can, but I want you to tell me if I hurt you at all and I'll stop."

He lifts the drape, and his neck splotches go into hyperspread to his hairline. I hand him a pair of exam gloves, which he puts on with some trouble due to his hands being so sweaty and shaky.

The resident, I notice, is rubbing his chin, wearing a doubtful expression.

The student speaks in a hushed, quivery voice. It is so low, in fact, we all have to lean forward to hear him.

"Okay, the first thing I want you to do is take a big deep breath and relax."

At once, all five of us take a deep breath and let it out.

"That's right. Now, I'm going to . . ."

I hold the speculum out toward him.

". . . very , very gently . . ."

He takes the speculum, studying it with a puzzled expression, and it dawns on me that he isn't sure which end to insert. I squirt lubrication on the correct end and give an encouraging nod.

He stares at the two openings before him, looking from one to the other. After a moment, he places the tip of his finger at the base of the woman's vaginal opening. He shifts his gaze to the ceiling and, as if in prayer, closes his eyes and takes another deep breath. He resembles a man who is about to enter the gas chamber.

I hold my breath, waiting.

". . . very gently . . ."

He looks at me again.

I nod.

". . . slip my foot into your rectum."

His statement hangs heavily on the very still and silent air for approximately two seconds before the collective "WHAT!?" hits the airwaves.

Startled, Monica flies into a sitting position, half laughing.

The intern is bent at the waist, the resident hangs off the counter with one hand. His knees are on the floor.

From Louise's side of the curtain comes a rich chuckling and the simple comment: "Somebody give that boy a beer."

Utterly mortified, the student excuses himself and leaves the room—speculum still in hand—while the rest of us finish laughing. When he returns, his mortification seems to have put him in a state of command, for he proceeds to do a thorough and professional pelvic exam without so much as one splotch.

With Monica prescribed for and further advised on the merits of cranberry juice and postcoital urination, we move on to Louise.

The woman listens intently to the resident reciting all her vital statistics to his colleagues. Every so often she nods in approval and adds, "That's right. Uh-huh. Yassir, that's right."

"Can you tell me a little more about this growth?" the resident asks.

"Uh-huh, yassir, I can."

We wait.

The intern decides on a more direct line of questioning. "When did you notice it?"

"It shot up last week."

"And where is it, exactly?"

"Down there, between my legs. It's about five inches long now."

The resident raises his eyebrows. "The growth started growing last week and it's already five inches long?"

"When did the discharge start?" asks the med student.

"That came on me 'bout a month ago, right after my man left for sea. But see, the growth's on account of the drippins. The drippins is what makes it grow good."

The resident pats her shoulder and smiles. He doesn't have a clue what she's talking about and probably doesn't really care.

"Well, I think we need to have a look-see," he says.

Louise smiles and pats his shoulder right back. "You go right ahead and have yourself a look-see, but keep your foots to yourselfs."

The resident laughs in spite of himself and helps Louise put her feet in the stirrups. The intern helps her scoot down to the end of the table.

"No feet, I promise," he says as he sits down and rolls closer to the exam site. "Okay, now what I want you to . . ."

He flips off the drape and spreads the woman's huge thighs in one smooth motion. "Relax and take a big . . ."

"Jesus." The med student initially takes a step back. "What is that?"

We all crowd in for a good "look-see."

I don't know what thoughts went through the others' minds, but I am instantly transported back to my fifth-grade science project.

One of my exhibits was a fifty-foot-long sweet potato vine I'd managed to grow simply by placing one end of the potato in a jelly jar of water. I found it to be the hardiest of plants; they grew anywhere, under almost any condition.

Obviously.

"Sweet potato, isn't it?" I ask so casually the resident looks at me like I'm in cahoots on some kind of practical joke.

He checks the corners of the ceiling for *Candid Camera*.

"Yas ma'am." She studies me thoughtfully. "You know 'bout them?"

I nod, recalling from my Cultural Diversities class in nursing school that sweet potatoes had once been used in certain cultures as a treatment for minor vaginal infections.

The resident shakes his head. "Well I don't know, so why don't you tell me why you've got one growing down there."

"Well see, I got the itching fever after my man gone?"

I translate for the resident and intern, who are both in awe of the conversation. "She had a yeast infection."

"Mama said if I put in a sweet tater, it draws out the itching and make it sweet in there."

"Did it work?"

The woman nods. "Yas ma'am, it sure did, but now I got the drippins and the growth."

The resident shakes his head to clear it and returns to the foliage at hand.

"You want scissors or pruning shears?" I ask.

No one else except Louise thinks this is funny.

Now before I go on here, I have to explain about the Quirks.

Each group of residents who rotate through the ER always have a quirk. My guess is that they're taught these various idiosyncrasies of technique by the attendings as a joke: "Hey, I know—let's teach all the residents in *this* group to twirl their stethoscope three times in the air before they listen to the lungs of an emphysema patient!"

This particular resident was in a group who, when checking GYN patients with discharge, all had the strange habit of sniffing the discharge. Instead of placing the matter on a slide, or smelling a swab of the stuff, they had been taught by some ho-ho attending to actually bring their nose close to the patient's private parts and take in a good whiff.

No matter how hard the nurses tried to break them of the unorthodox practice, nothing would make them stop.

With all the gentleness due an exotic plant, the resident removes what is left of the sweet potato. Then, bringing his nose within an inch or two of the vital source of "drippins," he begins sniffing.

As if on command from some perverse higher power, Louise immediately has a grand mal seizure.

Her back arches and her arms go stiff as boards. In horror, I see her legs clamp together in a death grip around the resident's head. The top of his head is bobbing up and down as Louise rocks.

I know that unless we release his head from that fleshy vise grip, he is going to suffocate. I try to imagine how we would explain his death to his wife or mother, and to the attending, and I start to laugh.

The resident manages a muffled "Help!" and my laughter turns to out-and-out howls. None of us can help. The intern and med student are both on the floor, and I am doing my best to keep Louise from falling off the table and myself from wetting my pants. Each time I turn my head, all I can see is the top of the resident's head bobbing like a crab trap marker in rough waters.

Just as he starts looking bluish, the intern manages to pull himself off the floor and pries Louise's legs open enough for extrication.

By the time I leave the exam room, it is almost 2:00 P.M. From the looks of the backed-up charts—I estimate fifty—I kiss the idea of lunch good-bye. The steady flow of patients—chest pains, lacerations, a chemical burn, a gallbladder attack, motor vehicle accidents, abdominal pains, and asthma attacks—escalates the level of chaos. Each barrage of patients has enough of the offbeat or the tragic to keep us on our toes.

It seems to be a day of "inserters"—those people who find it necessary to insert things into the various orifices of their bodies. At 5:05 a fifty-year-old inserter who is also a hospital hopper comes in complaining of rectal pain. His history of putting glass objects up his rectum and getting them broken is enough of a tip to call the attending blade, who recognizes him immediately, having been the surgeon who performed his fifth temporary colostomy just six months ago.

The attending relates to us that the man started years ago with the glass tubes from TV sets, then went on to wine bottles. He is presently working his way through the various liquor bottles, a scotch bottle being the immediate problem.

He is followed by a thirty-two-year-old woman complaining of not being able to urinate. We gather around the X-ray view box as Dr. Marchones puts up the woman's film. The outline of a ballpoint pen which has been inserted into her urethra is quite clear.

"I don't want to hear one 'Flick my Bic' joke," Dr. Marchones jokes.

Dr. Marchones is a hot, whoa-babe kind of resident—the type who is able to spend thirty-six hours on and then go and party for the next twenty-four. She is also someone who wears her scrub dresses halfway to the moon, so that whenever she bends over or sits down, it's easy to see she doesn't believe in underwear.

She reaches into her scrub dress pocket for her pen—to use as a pointer on the X ray. Out flips her diaphragm. The flesh-colored disk rolls across the floor, does a neat pirouette over Michael's foot, and comes to rest—still on its edge—in the middle of the department floor.

Completely mute, everyone stares at the thing as though it is an alien being.

One by one, we drift away, the Bic inserter's film blotted from our recent memories by embarrassment. The device sits there, undisturbed, for another few seconds until Dr. Marchones rescues it.

Before I take a new chart, I search for Kevin and Karen's discharge notes. At first glance, I see that they are signed by the same pediatrician who has allowed the abuse to continue. My heart sinks, but as I read through the notes, a cry of surprise and exhilaration escapes me—brother and sister have been placed in a temporary foster home by Child Protective Services pending further investigation.

I briefly wonder what changed the pediatrician's mind and guess that he got tired of not being able to sleep at night.

At 6:30 we get report by radio that ambulance 12 is coming in code three, bringing us a woman in full arrest.

Now, there are ambulance companies and there are ambulance companies—some of the EMTs are sharper than others. In my experience, the private ambulance companies employ emergency personnel who are a cut above, while the "free" ambulances are magnets for paramedic wannabes—those cowboys and -girls who, if given a smidgen of medical knowledge, could be dangerous people in the field.

Ambulance 12 is of the cowboy variety.

Sure enough, the rig comes to a brake-burning halt, almost running down an older man in a walker. CPR is, indeed, in progress, albeit the patient is sitting up, so that the chest compressions are being delivered at a sideways angle. In reverse of the gunshot patient, this woman is intubated but has no IV line.

The patient is clutching a bodice-ripper paperback in one hand. *Love's Delight*.

"Sixty-eight-year-old female was seen by her neighbor at ten this morning in her yard sunning herself," begins the EMT who is bagging.

The sunburn can be seen through the grayish blue hue of the patient's skin. It is strange-looking.

"At six the neighbor realized that she was still in the lounger, sitting in the same position. He went over and found the patient unresponsive and called nine-one-one."

As we move the patient off the gurney and onto the trauma room exam table, Dr. Marchones and I notice the livor mortis—the discoloration of dependent parts of the body which takes place some time after death—on the woman's thighs and buttocks.

We attempt to lay her on her back—her legs remain at right angles to her torso.

Dr. Marchones pushes on her knees to straighten out the legs, and the torso springs up into the sitting position.

I hold down the torso, and the legs spring back into chaise lounge position.

"Ah, guys?" I throw a killing glance at the EMT giving report. He falters under my gaze.

"This woman has been dead for a very long time."

"Actually"—Dr. Marchones holds up the rectal thermometer and lays a commanding hand on the EMT doing chest compressions—"she probably died before noon. We're looking at some pretty advanced rigor mortis here."

This piece of information throws the charge EMT into the defensive mode and he begins to defend his decision to begin CPR.

I decide the live patients need me more and go back to the mountain of charts. I can tell the rest of the world outside those double doors is having a big happy hour, as the parade of crackheads, drunks, and bleeding gang members coming through the Pit increases in number and hostility.

At 8:30 P.M., Michael and I are hailed out to the waiting room by a group of very excited, hand-fluttering nuns. The head nun, who Michael reverently calls "Sister Superior," speaks in a flustery, rapid whisper.

"You must bring a wheelchair to our car." She points through the double entrance doors at a new four-door station wagon. "One of the sisters is very ill. I think she is hemorrhaging."

Michael runs for a gurney—I run behind the penguin brigade.

In the back seat, a nun lies flat on her back with her knees bent. She is cold and clammy, and beyond pale. Gripped tightly in her icy fingers is a giant black rosary.

Michael carefully slides her over the seat and lifts her onto the gurney. I make note of the thick smear of fresh blood which contrasts sharply with the blue upholstery.

We fly to the first open room, calling for the GYN staff as we go.

Her BP is barely palpable at 70, and her heart rate is 134.

Michael starts a line while I undress her, removing layer after layer of medieval-habit getup. The thing must weigh a ton. Wearing these clothes in this heat strikes me as such a primitive concept that I fully expect to see a hair shirt underneath.

I carefully examine the three soaked sanitary pads and the hand towel which I remove from between her legs, and look at Michael. "My God, this looks like the tissue and clots women pass after delivery!"

Michael's eyes narrow. "She's a nun. It's not even within the realm of possibility. Don't even think such a thing."

"Okay, okay, I'm just making an observation."

We both try to extract some kind of history from the thirty-two-year-old, but she ignores our questions about the date of her last menstrual period, and did she take any kind of hormones for regulation, and how long has the bleeding been going on?

Neither Michael or I think it is strange that she doesn't answer. She is in shock, after all. What I do think is strange, however, is the long dark brown stripe down the center of her abdomen—*striae gravidarum*—which I'd seen in some pregnant women. Michael sees it too, but acts like he doesn't.

The GYN resident—the sniffer—comes in, takes one look, and before I can say "Nun's the word," asks, "Are you pregnant? Have you recently delivered?"

At the sacrilege, Michael places himself between the patient and the resident. It is a gesture of protection and anger.

"This woman is a nun, Doctor. I suggest you show her the respect due her station in the church."

The resident studies Michael's expression and then the chart. Without another word he writes a list of orders for labs and asks Michael to bring them to the clerk. As soon as Michael is gone, he does a quick-look pelvic exam, during which he delivers a piece of placenta.

"How long ago did you deliver?" he asks quietly.

The nun begins to cry. The resident puts a hand on her arm and repeats his question. His voice is less quiet, more demanding.

Begging God for his divine forgiveness, she answers, "A few hours ago. In my room at the convent."

"Where's the baby?" I ask on my way out the door.

The nun refuses to answer my question, again crying out for God's forgiveness.

The nuns in the waiting room answer my direct questions with their heads bowed. Yes, Sister Luke Marie was pregnant, but they don't know anything about a baby.

I am furious with their pretended ignorance, but keep my rage under control. I recall other newborns I've tried to save—ones who had been abandoned in trash bins and ditches. A cavalcade of tiny faces runs through my mind while I tell the skeptical policeman who has been called to go to the convent stat, and search for the newborn infant. It will need medical attention, so I tell him to have an ambulance on hand.

As I get the nun ready to go upstairs, I am barely civil.

She cries out to her God to forgive her.

Michael coos and hushes her. I tell her to get over herself and get real.

Michael doesn't talk to me for the rest of the shift.

I sit down for the first time since 5:00 A.M. and lay my head on the nurses' charting desk. I watch the clock to see how long I can stay like this.

Three minutes and twenty seconds later, I feel a presence standing over me. From the overpowering smell of Chanel No. 5, I know it is Mercedes, our evening intake clerk.

I groan and look up. The older woman is standing behind an occupied wheelchair, her mouth set in a pink pucker that looks for all the world like my dog's bunghole.

No one likes Mercedes. She doesn't belong in the emergency department; she belongs at the art and garden club, nibbling on tea cakes. She is wealthy and doesn't really need to work. None of us can figure out why she does—we all wish she wouldn't.

She is also cold, slow, and methodical. She speaks in a harsh monotone, enunciating each syllable so that she sounds very much like a robot from *Deep Space Nine*. The most important strike against her, however, is that she hasn't got one ounce of the street smarts and common sense needed to be an intake clerk in the emergency department. Intake clerks are the front line. They need to be able to roll with the punches. Mercedes couldn't deal with a mouse fart.

If someone was out in front having a coronary, they might very well have a birthday before Mercedes got done asking them the information and making up the chart. Sometimes we got the charts of really sick patients two or three hours after they'd checked in.

"I've got a problem," she says, giving a curt nod of her head to the wizened person sitting in the wheelchair. I can't see the patient's face because it is mostly hidden by a blanket which has been wrapped around the head like a cowl.

"Someone rolled this patient into the reception area when I was busy, and just left him sitting there. He refuses to answer any questions.

"The security guard said he walked in off the street complaining of chest pain, so he put him in the chair and—"

Adrenaline surges through me like a tidal wave. I am up and jumping over the counter like someone at an Olympic event. I throw back the blanket and see the dusky, mottled skin and the trail of vomit down the front of his otherwise neat sweater. I know he has been dead for at least an hour.

Mercedes—I know it as well as I know I am standing on swollen, sore feet—will never work in the Pit again. She won't even be allowed near it unless she herself is on a stretcher.

I have just given report to the night shift nurse when a cop comes in. He has his hat off and is holding it respectfully in his hands.

"Are you Leah?"

I say that I am and my stomach tightens in fear. I think like an emergency department nurse: My husband has been hit by a drunk driver and is dead. My daughters have been abducted and raped or shot.

"We went to the convent."

"Uh-huh?" I say casually to hide my relief. I start to call Michael over, but change my mind—I don't want to take on the karma of vindictiveness.

I move the policeman to the side of the room where no one else can hear what he is going to say.

"She cut the baby's cord with a pair of nail scissors," he continues, uncomfortable with the words. "Then she wrapped the cord from the venetian blinds around the little boy's neck and strangled him. The baby was in her wastepaper basket."

The cop has to stop because he's starting to choke up. I put my hand on his arm, trying to feel shocked or sad or something, but I can't, so I end up feeling guilty instead.

"The other nuns said they didn't know about the baby," he said after a minute or two. "But I don't believe them."

I thank him and walk out to my car on legs and feet which feel like blocks of concrete. A hollow feeling which I have never been able to identify begins in my chest and spreads to my throat and temples.

I feel more tired than I ever have in my life. Maybe, if luck is on my side, just maybe I'll be able to sleep tonight.

Ellen N.

Among themselves, nurses readily agree that of all the branches of nursing, one of the most difficult places to work is in the burn unit.

Not everyone can work in a burn unit. It takes a very special kind of person. Thirty-three-year-old Ellen N. of San Diego, California, is one of those people.

March 26, 1972, was the day that changed my life forever and sealed my destiny as a burn nurse.

I was seven years old the morning that my oldest sister and I woke up early and decided we were going to surprise everyone by cooking breakfast. We were camping at the time, so it was going to be quite an undertaking.

We put about two weeks' worth of newspaper in one of those cement-ring fire pits, and we grabbed this unmarked can that we thought had lighter fluid in it.

Except it was gasoline. We didn't know any better, so my sister poured it on the papers. I was standing right next to her when the fire went back into the can and exploded.

My sister knew to stop, drop, and roll, but I did the thing you are never supposed to do, which was run around the campground screaming. Everybody came out of their tents and smothered our bodies with sleeping bags. All I remember thinking was *Oh my God, they're trying to kill me!*

My whole family was crying. My mother, who is a very nonemotional person, was putting a wet washcloth on my face with tears streaming down her face. As soon as I saw her crying, I knew something really bad had happened, but I didn't know what.

I was the only one who wasn't crying, even though my face was swelling and felt like plastic. As I went into shock, I asked my mother, "Am I going to die?"

She said, "Absolutely not! I am not going to let you die!"

That was what saved me. Those two statements stuck with me for all those months of torture.

My father drove like a madman to the nearest medical facility, which was a small community hospital. The ER staff was completely blown away as these two major-burn kids come strolling into their ER.

Of course we were immediately transported to a larger medical facility, where they commenced cutting off my clothes. That was when I finally got hysterical, because I didn't want them to cut my new Snoopy sweatshirt. What I didn't know at that point was that it had completely melted into my chest.

My sister had bilateral legs burns, which was about thirty percent of her body. I was sixty percent: bilateral legs, hands, face, neck, chest, and scatter areas. I was very fortunate. My eyesight was still intact, I didn't have any inhalation damage to my lungs, and I didn't lose any digits.

There weren't really any burn centers back then, so I stayed at the medical facility until I was discharged at the end of August. "Discharged" isn't really a good word to use because I basically went in and out of the hospital for years—every vacation, every holiday break, I would go back in for more grafting and reconstructive surgery.

I learned at an early age that the hospital is a little city of its own. I liked the environment and I liked what went on there. I knew that no matter what, I wanted to be a part of that and do something in the medical profession. I was always inspired by the nurses who cared for me, so I thought that if I could give back one tenth of what those nurses gave to me, it would be the right decision. And I'd have to say that going into nursing is the best decision I have ever made in my life.

My mother is a nurse, but she was adamant about my not becoming a nurse. She did everything she could to discourage me by pushing me into other majors, because she thought there were so many other—better—options for women.

I was about to graduate with a psych degree, when I finally said, "No! This is NOT what I want to do. I really want to do nursing, and I want to do burn nursing."

So I switched my major, knowing that my mother would be furious. She was very burnt out at this point in her own career, and sure enough—

she was upset. She refused to talk to me for two weeks. Of course, my father was supportive of anything I wanted to do for a living, so that was fine with him.

For my last semester of nursing school, I chose the burn unit as my clinical practice unit. I was terrified. I kept thinking, *What if I can't handle it? What if the patients can't handle it? What if the staff can't handle it?* I didn't want to be viewed as having a negative effect or causing negative outcomes in the patients or the staff.

My very first night there, they had a couple of eighty-percenters and a seventy-percenter, so they were totally involved in some very, very sick patients. It was decided that I would help the nurses change dressings. I did a lot of mental preparation for that because I didn't want to get into the tub room and flip out and have flashbacks. So, as I walked into the tub room, I thought I was prepared.

The first dressing was on this eighty-percenter who had set herself on fire. She was septic, and the only part of her that wasn't burned was the bottoms of her feet and her face. I handled the wounds and I handled the sepsis and the woman's anguish, but the one thing I had not prepared myself for was the smell of the drainage from the wounds. It caused me to flash back in the strongest way.

It's funny how smell can trigger your memory. For most burn nurses, the smell is hard to deal with; you go home and you can't get the smells of burned hair and flesh, or Pseudomonas [a type of bacterial infection], out of your nose. It sticks to your hair and skin. To this day, it still kind of gets me.

But I got through it. I loved the semester and was well received by patients and staff. The nurse manager of that unit asked me to come work there. At first I thought I should probably go out and get some basic nursing experience, but I took the job and ended up in the burn unit fresh out of school.

In retrospect, I wouldn't recommend a new grad to go right into ICU/burn unit. During that first year, I had to learn all the burn stuff, the pediatric ICU stuff, the wound care stuff, the nutritional issues, the regular ICU stuff, and even basic nursing stuff, like how to start an IV and draw bloods. And then there were all the psychosocial aspects and all the teaching and learning how to deal with the associated trauma due to the mechanism of injury.

Also, you have to remember that no one is immune to getting

burned, so we deal with every age, every economic level, every disease process including HIV, every race, every religion, every culture, pregnant women, the homeless, the wealthy—you name it, the burn unit has it.

There are so many difficult areas of burn nursing. By definition, the skin is the largest organ of the body, so that when it's damaged or destroyed, the body is open to infection, which is the primary killer of burn patients. It throws the circulation, fluid balances, coagulation, and body temperature into critical states, which puts a burden on the heart, kidneys, liver, bone marrow, the gastrointestinal system, and the immune system.

With the serious burns, there is always the trauma of the surgical process. First there's the removal of the dead skin, which is full of bacteria. On deep burns, the skin is literally sliced off the body right down to the capillary openings, so there's a huge loss of blood that must be replaced.

If the patient survives that, the doctors cover the wounds temporarily with cadaver skin—an allograft. Once the wound bed is ready and healthy, we then do an autograft, using the patient's own skin.

For me, the most difficult part of burn nursing was and is pain control. A burn injury is the most excruciatingly painful, life-altering injury that a human being can possibly go through and still survive. Everything the nurse does is painful: changing the linen, moving the body, moving the bed. Sometimes they're screaming and crying and swearing at you and yet they're helpless. The burn survivor's life has been turned upside down and a lot of them can't take it.

We give fentanyl and morphine like it's water. Giving huge doses of narcotics and still not being able to take away someone's pain is the most difficult thing, because you know you have to do the wound care and you know you are going to hurt them.

It's very difficult to hurt someone for eight hours a day and go home and feel good about it. When we have patients with severe burns and there are high-level-pain issues, you can feel the tension on the unit.

Emotionally, pediatric burns are the hardest for me—they're the hardest for every nurse. I do love taking care of kids, and having to hurt a kid is not fun, let me tell you. Hurting an adult isn't any easier, but at least they can understand the process and why it has to be done. I mean, imagine a child who is staring at you while you're peeling away the dead skin, or taking out the skin staples, and they're screaming? God, it's so hard.

The staff gets tired. There have been so many times where I've held it together on the unit and the minute I get into the car I start crying. It makes me wonder sometimes if I'm doing the right thing.

But then something happens which is a reinforcement of why I'm there. It's happened my whole life like that. I really believe that things happen for a reason. Not that I think I was burned for a reason, but that I survived for a reason. While those bad things are happening, you don't always know what the reason could possibly be for it, but over time, you find out.

Let's face it—in burn unit nursing, you either love it or hate it. If you love it, you make your whole career there. If you don't love it, you get out very quickly. I really haven't been a nurse that long—only since 1989—but considering what I do, it really is a monumental amount of time.

When I'm on the unit, I'm a nurse and it's important for me to stay focused on the nursing part. I have always made a point never—*ever*— to go into a patient's room and talk about my injury, because I'm not there for my injury. If the patient has questions, they can ask by all means, but I tell them right out that I'm only an expert on my own experience, and not theirs.

It's true. No two burns are alike. Every burn patient has his own experience. I try to be sensitive to the families and the patients about that.

When I have a patient who has facial burns, I'm especially careful because I know that when I walk in, they think: *Oh my God, am I going to look like that?*

From the standpoint of a burn survivor, it's funny, but there are all these issues that come up that are different for pediatric patients and adult patients. I've talked to so many burn survivors and the adults say, "I couldn't have done it as a kid."

As a pediatric burn, I think, *I couldn't have done it as an adult.* I mean, I got to grow with it and I don't know anything else. At seven years old, you have no idea of how important looks are in society. Looking back, I had a wonderful childhood with two very supportive parents. If it hadn't been for them, I wouldn't be here today, because they never gave up on me. Other than being in and out of the hospital, they really tried to give me a very normal childhood. They didn't cut me more slack than the other kids because I was burned.

I had a lot of friends and a lot of love. You see a difference in the burn kids who have nonsupportive families and those who have a lot of support. A burn patient has to believe in their own rehabilitation—they need the support of the staff and the family for that.

I was seventeen before I went through a grieving process. I was suddenly aware of how important looks were, and the dating scene, and everybody was obsessed with "thin." So I became obsessed with my weight, stopped eating, and went down to ninety-five pounds. My thought process was: *Well, if I'm thin enough, people won't notice my burns.*

My grades went down and I grew suicidal. Finally I was sent to a psychologist, and he immediately told me my weight wasn't the problem—it was my burns.

I was irate with him, but it was really a turning point because it was the first time I'd ever looked at the fact I was burned. That was when I quit acting like a burn victim and started being a burn survivor.

Now I say being burned creates this natural screening process: anyone who has a problem with me isn't going to deal with me. I've been very fortunate to meet some incredible people who see Ellen and not the scars.

There have been so many patients who've touched my heart and made an impact on me. That can't help but happen to everyone. I mean, you really develop an incredible relationship with burn patients because you're with them for so long.

Plus, you have to look at the nature of the injury. These people's whole lives are so disrupted, and they are so vulnerable. Everything is out in the open . . . their bodies, their family. And there you are at the lowest, worst point, when their lives are turned upside down in an instant.

They go through all those critical stages where they try to die on you, and then you get them better, and then they get septic and try to die again. You get them through and you don't give up on them, and because of that, they don't give up.

Then comes the rehab stage, where they start to walk and feed themselves, and then one day, you get to see them walk out. It's such an emotional connection for everyone. There have been so many times when patients have walked out of here crying tears of joy.

The staff is crying too, because they've worked so hard, and this person you've become so close to is about to start life again. Oh God, it's a joyful time. You carry these people with you for the rest of your life, you know.

I remember when I was in nursing school, I was in the hospital cafeteria and this doctor walked past me, stopped, and looked at me for a long time. Finally, he said, "Are you Ellen?"

I told him yes, and he started talking a mile a minute, saying how he couldn't believe that it was me, and how, right after I was burned, I'd been so sick they never thought I would live, and now here I was a nursing student, and on and on. Then, finally, he broke down and started to cry and walked away.

I stood there with my mouth hanging open. He made it to the elevators, where he turned around and came back and put his arms around me and gave me a big hug. Then I started crying and he cried harder. Then he said, "I've thought of you so often, wondering what kind of life you'd have. I'm so happy to see you are well and prospering."

Then, still crying, he walked away. A social worker from the unit I was rotating through had seen the whole thing, came over and asked what was going on.

When I told her, she responded by thanking me for allowing this doctor to experience all those wonderful emotions of being a human being.

You know, it's true. We get so much from the patients—they touch us deep down. I wonder if patients know how much of an impact they have on those who care for them. They break our hearts, change our lives.

It really is the success stories—the ones who walk out and go on in life stronger than ever—that keep me going back every day.

There are two patients who stand out in my mind, I guess, because I had such a difficult time controlling their pain.

Sandy was a gorgeous girl. Twenty-three, blond hair and blue eyes, creamy skin. She had been in a master's program, and her life was really going great until the day she and her stepmother were hit by a drunk driver. The stepmother was killed instantly. Sandy, who had been driving, was trapped inside the car, which caught on fire. She'd been burned on her upper back, buttocks, and legs, though the legs were so severely burned a bilateral amputation was done immediately.

We didn't get her until ten days after the accident, mainly because she had a severe head injury and her neuro status had to be addressed first. In a way, the head injury was a blessing because she was so out of it.

As she became more awake, so did her awareness of the pain.

Sandy's dressing changes were always traumatic. Controlling burn pain is hard enough, but controlling pain with amputees is the worst. Through it all, she and I got very close. That was when I realized how full of life and spirit she was.

At one point, she started losing weight because her nutritional status was bad, so of course her grafts weren't healing very well. Then she got methicillin-resistant staphylococcus aureus [MRSA] in all her wounds, so she had to be in isolation.

There was a nurse on our unit who Sandy was terrified of. This man had been on the burn unit forever, and had lost his compassion. As a result, he was very rough with the patients. Worse than that, he was really into playing power and control games with them too.

Every time he was assigned to do her dressing change, she'd go crazy. "Please don't let him touch me," she'd beg. "Don't let him near me, and if he has to . . . please don't leave me alone with him. Promise you won't let him hurt me."

This one time when he was going to do her dressing change, I stayed in there the whole time. Sandy was still a little confused from the head injury, but she was joking around with him, trying to be nice, asking him about his kids and his wife, and he was being totally antagonistic.

He kept telling me that he thought she didn't know what she was saying, that she was completely insane. I told him right out that she knew exactly what she was saying, and that she was trying to be nice.

Well, he didn't buy that, and at one point, he stepped out of the dressing change to get something and Sandy whispered, "You know why I'm being so nice to him? I'm brownnosing him so he won't hurt me so bad this time."

Hearing that remark, I lost it. I went out and pulled him aside and I told him he was going to do the dressing exactly as she wanted and he was going to be gentle and he was going to be nice to her.

Sandy was finally discharged to a hospital closer to where she lived. I got a postcard from her mom a few months later saying that Sandy had gotten her wheelchair and was doing okay.

It must have been almost a year later that I took care of a thirty-three-year-old man whose plane had crashed. Andrew had been badly burned, and as it turned out, he had to have his left leg amputated. We did everything to save that leg. Nothing worked. Eight weeks into his admission, it came off.

He was having horrible phantom-leg and -stump pain, which was extremely difficult to control. Then his white count went up, and he began having fevers. His stump looked like it had a pocket of infection brewing.

One day I was with him in the tub room, and he'd been in so much pain and I'd given him so much medication that I was worried about his respiratory status because he wasn't intubated.

Just about then, a resident came in and told me that he wanted to drain the pus pocket and maybe take a look around in there.

My first thought was that this should be done in the OR, where Andrew could be completely put out, but the doctor turned to me and told me what size scalpel he wanted to use, and I realized he meant to do it right there.

So, while he was telling Andrew that he was just going to "take a look," I found the scalpel and put it on the table, and had begun to push more fentanyl into Andrew's IV, when this doctor—without so much as a word of warning or a thought to the pain he would cause—takes the scalpel and literally slits open the raw stump with all these exposed nerve endings.

Andrew hit the ceiling. His screams went through every bone in my body. I felt it, literally, in my bones. He didn't stop screaming. It went on and on, and you could hear him throughout the unit. I can't tell you what it was like to be in that tub room with a patient in that much pain, who wasn't intubated, and not be able to do anything for him.

That was the cruelest, most inhumane thing I have ever seen done to a human. It was one of the worst experiences I'd ever had as a nurse. I have never seen a human being in that much pain.

Consequently, for Andrew every subsequent dressing change from that moment on was a traumatic experience. Andrew never forgot that doctor, and neither have I. To this day, Andrew still says it was his worst experience out of everything—the crash, the burn, the amputation.

When I got Andrew back to his room, and after I'd given the resident a piece of my mind, I felt emotionally drained—like I'd failed as a nurse. One of the staff developers pulled me aside, made me sit down, and simply said, "Are you okay?"

I sat there for an hour and sobbed. I'd never lost it that bad before. I was so beat up. All I kept thinking was that I couldn't take the pain of dealing with people's pain anymore.

I left early that day, and when I got home, I found a letter from Sandy. It was such perfect timing it was amazing.

I've kept the letter, and I want to read it to you:

> *Dear Ellen—How is the sunshine of the burn unit? I think of you so often and always with such admiration and gratitude for what you do.*
>
> *I don't remember much about those early days, but I do remember you. There is no doubt in my mind that I am alive today because of the expert care I received from you. You will always have a special place in my heart.*
>
> *I'm adjusting, doing the fake-leg thing. It takes so long. It isn't fun. I am back in school and have met a beautiful light. His name is Michael. You will meet him soon.*
>
> *I know this sounds strange, but the burn unit is exactly what I needed. I was so lucky to be surrounded by such wonderful people. I have decided I am the luckiest and the unluckiest girl in the world.*
>
> *Thank you for being such a special part of my life and heart*
>
> *—Sandy*

After reading the letter, I started sobbing. I needed to hear that so much. Like I said, things really do happen for a reason.

I introduced Sandy and Andrew about a year after Andrew's discharge. They hit it off immediately, and remain good friends to this day, and probably for the rest of their lives.

Regular, everyday people don't understand at all what nurses have to do on a daily basis. Go home and try to explain to your friends or family what took place during your day, about the pain and the trauma, and they look at you like you're from another planet . . . or: "Oh yeah, right."

Sometimes I see nurses who are burned out and it just kills me. I see how they lose their compassion and get hard, and I think if I *ever* get to that point, I'm going to get out because it doesn't do anybody any good.

With managed care, our area is getting hit really hard with having less and less experienced people in the burn ICU—I can't tell you how scary that is. Upper administration is so far from the bedside that there is a lack of understanding as to what is going on there. Sometimes I think if they could only walk in our shoes for one day . . . I don't think they could do it, but if they could, they'd have a better understanding of what's going on.

A nurse takes her satisfaction and reward by being at the bedside and connecting with the patients. When you get away from the bedside, your perspective as to what is doable and isn't doable becomes warped as to staffing.

There is so much nurses can do. I expanded my role and began teaching ABLS—advanced burn life support—and doing community outreach. I teach the paramedics and the schoolkids from kindergarten to high school to nursing students. I worked extensively on the World Burn Conference, and I do a lot of lecturing on burn injuries all over the country.

Whether it's burn camp for kids, support groups for burned women, or peer counseling, it's important for me to do this work because twenty-four years ago there wasn't a lot of support for burn survivors.

You know, people think I'm crazy when I say this, but if I had my life to live all over again and I could change anything I wanted, I'd want to have it all happen exactly as it has.

My life is full and rich. I've met the most incredible people, and made the best friends. I've had so much love in my life I wouldn't change a thing.

Diane C.

Diane C. is a thirty-three-year-old Mexican American who received her licensed practical nurse degree thirteen years ago. She began her career in hospital pediatric nursing, then changed to prison nursing—a transition she wouldn't recommend. On the day she found herself drawing simple anatomical pictures for an inmate caught smuggling in birth control pills because he was convinced he could get pregnant by the other male inmates, she decided to return to pediatrics via the home healthcare route.

Unable to have children of her own, Diane now channels all her maternal instincts into taking care of other people's kids—kids who have special needs.

When asked why she became a nurse, she explains:

"I like to say I became a nurse because it was on my bus line. Actually, that isn't far from the truth. It was my mother's goal to have one of her children be in the church and another be in the medical profession. I entered a convent at the age of thirteen to become a nun because the idea of nursing was offensive to me.

"Six years later I knew being a nun wasn't for me. Much to the Holy Sisters' relief and joy, I left the convent and told my mother I was going to run my own life and make my own decisions from then on.

"She said, 'Sure, fine, okay—but first you have to become a nurse.'

"So—I became a nurse."

The scuffed and dented dashboard of my 1975 VW bug held a collection of practical objects. I'd Krazy Glued them to every available inch of space. The tiny Mickey Mouse travel clock read 5:30 P.M. The indoor-outdoor thermometer with happy faces on it held at 100 degrees even.

I licked the sweat from my upper lip and thanked God it was cooling off. Sometimes the families could afford air-conditioning, sometimes not. From the looks of the dingy apartment set over a garage and the general look of the neighborhood, I guessed these people would not.

It was one of the poorest neighborhoods in Houston—a high-risk area. Okay, so no big deal; I almost always worked in the high-crime areas, taking care of kids whose medical problems usually stemmed from the dysfunction of the parents. I'd had my share of children who were brain-damaged because the parents were too drunk to care when they fell into the pool, or babies who had multisystem failures because the mother took drugs during her pregnancy. Occasionally, my patients had been beaten, smothered, or shaken to near death or mental retardation.

In my opinion, working with these kinds of families was far more rewarding than working with the upper-middle-class yuppies.

I worked only once with a yuppie couple's child. I remember the first day I walked into the child's playroom in this mansion of a house and tried to introduce myself to the little girl. The child, who was suffering from a common cold and overprotective parents, was sitting in front of a TV, singing along with Big Bird.

As soon as I said, "Hello, my name is—" the mother turned on me in a rage. "Shhhhhhh!" she practically spit. "Not now! Can't you see the child is *interfacing*!"

It was the last time I went there.

The high-crime factor was the only reason I endured the constant teasing from my friends about my wreckage of a vehicle. Had I driven a newer car, it would either be stolen outright or stripped down to its bare bones. As it was, the old VW had long since lost its bumpers, VW emblem, and cabin-light cover to thieves.

On the passenger seat lay my purse—an oversized gray canvas bag. I sighed. It suddenly took on the status of a dangerous liability. I'd forgotten to leave it at home, which meant I'd have to worry about it for the whole shift. Carrying it to and from the apartment unconcealed was an open invitation for a mugging.

I searched under the seats until I found one of my husband's old sweatshirts, wrapped it around the purse, then craned my neck to make sure the number crudely painted on the orange door of the apartment matched the address on my assignment sheet.

Gathering the rest of my things—a grocery bag holding two melting TV dinners, two Cokes, and my med kit—I crammed the stuffed sweatshirt on top of my dinner, and let my eyes rest momentarily on the plastic portrait of Virgin Mary glued next to the thermometer.

Her expression seemed to be one of perpetual worry. Saluting, I left the car unlocked with direct orders that she protect the vehicle from harm.

My apprehensions mounted as I made my way toward the flight of half-rotted wooden stairs going up the side of the garage. When the agency director called earlier in the day to ask if I would schedule an additional hour for "case orientation," I knew I was letting myself in for something especially heinous. Orientation was rarely requested by the agency and was usually a signal that there were "special"—meaning traumatic—circumstances involved.

Orientation gave the nurse time to observe the family's particular—"peculiar" is a more accurate word here—routine needs. In my last orientation case, I'd been escorted in and out of the apartment by a police officer, then spent the night crouched on the floor of a back bedroom doing what I could for the patient. I had been told by the officers to stay down below the level of the windows or risk bullet spray from automatic weapons. My five-year-old patient's sibling, age fourteen, had been shot to death while watching TV in the same apartment only a week before. The five-year-old was lucky—he'd been hit by the same series of automatic fire but had only a couple of flesh wounds.

For a second I thought perhaps it might be the pediatrician on this case who was the problem, and searched my memory for the doctor's name.

Some of the pediatricians could make our jobs more difficult than they needed to be—either in withholding orders for necessary treatments and drugs, or by being temperamental when it came to the nurse's judgment. I recalled the first case I ever had. The child was an anencephalic baby—she had only a brain stem and no cranial vault. The child had constant seizures and was very spastic.

Of course, the doctor had been predicting the child's death every day since she was born, and thus there was a great deal of indifference on his part. The battle—which lasted a full year—had centered around my wanting to get some Valium to ease some of her seizures, but this doctor simply refused to give it to me on the grounds that the child would become addicted.

Every time I'd talk to this idiot on the phone, I'd say, "My God, diazepam is only palliative for the seizures and spasms—it's not like we're going to check her into the Betty Ford Clinic or anything, Doctor. She's going to die."

But he continued to refuse, and that child—due to his arrogance and his ignorance—died one very ugly, unnecessarily painful death.

I glanced once more at my assignment sheet and sighed. The pediatrician was Dr. Flores. Very nurse/patient-friendly. Letting my eyes once more skim the standing report, I reviewed the case history: Roberto had been born premature, with a cleft palate. The surgeons waited three months before they dared repair the defect, due to his failure to thrive. His present weight of ten pounds was a red flag that this child was still failing to thrive at home.

At the bottom of the steps, I realized that the noise I'd thought was someone's boom box cranked to full volume was coming from a TV inside the apartment. It was tuned to a Spanish station.

I prayed someone in the family spoke some English. With the child, it wouldn't make a difference—children understood the primary language: a gentle touch, a kind smile. Even though I was a Latina, I did not speak Spanish. *No hablo español, sí, no comprendo,* and *dónde baño?* was the extent of my vocabulary.

It never ceased to amuse our friends that my WASP husband spoke the language fluently. It was inevitable that every time I tried to speak the language, I somehow managed to say exactly the wrong thing. Once, during an interview with a Mexican family who spoke no English and who did not understand why their Latina nurse couldn't speak Spanish, we had managed, by way of crude sign language, to get across the basics. At one point the mother pointed to my wedding ring and asked, *"Esposo español?"*

"Oh no," I'd answered proudly. *"Mi esposo es amaricón."*

My answer sent the entire family first into shocked silence, and then into excited, rapid conversation among themselves. By the time I returned to the agency, the family was already on the line with the supervisor—another WASP who also spoke fluent Spanish.

She was laughing so hard she was purple in the face. Eventually she said the family wanted to know when I was going to be on *Oprah* to talk about my marriage.

Confused, I cocked my head in question.

She asked if I had by any chance told the family I was married to an American. When I told her I had, she informed me that the word for American was *americano—maricón* was the Spanish word for homosexual. . . .

I had been pounding on the door for a while when it was opened by a young Latino wearing a pair of tattered boxer shorts. From the sparseness of his mustache and goatee, I guessed him to be in his early twenties.

He barked a few words of Spanish which I interpreted as "Who the hell are you?" and pointed to my uniform and med kit.

"Hi. I'm the night nurse for the baby? Um, *bambino nana? Efirmera?*"

I peered over his shoulder into the darkness behind him. There were ragged curtains, some of which were drawn against the sun, but what took my breath away—literally—was that every window in the place was shut tight. The day shift nurse was nowhere to be seen. Perhaps, I thought, I would find her backed into a corner.

From under a snarl, the man asked another question in Spanish.

I shrugged. *"No hablo español. Habla inglese?"*

He gave me the same skeptical look I'd seen from other Latinos. It said, *What? Are you kidding me?*

"You the nurse?"

I nodded. "Is the day nurse here?"

Slowly he shook his head. "She's gone."

I gasped; my hand started fluttering upward toward my open mouth. I stopped it before it could get to my chin. "The nurse left? Are you sure?"

With a shrug, he left me at the door and flopped down on a badly soiled orange couch. Holding out a remote control, he turned down the volume on the TV. It did not surprise me that the set was brand-new, and one of the ones with a screen that was so many feet by so many feet instead of inches.

"Yeah." He motioned for me to enter. "My wife, she's pissed. We don't want her comin' back here no more."

I took one step inside, hesitated, then forced myself to take another. It was hot, the way an oven at 400 degrees is hot, and the smell was putrid. As soon as my eyes grew accustomed to the dark, I could see a fair number of adults and children crowded into the living room.

The word "clutter" came to the forefront of my mind. Actually, clutter was a charitable description; filth was more accurate. Dirty dishes and cups littered the floor and every available flat surface. Piles of dirty clothes, broken toys, and plastic garbage bags filled to bursting lay about the room haphazardly. One woman was using one of the garbage bags as a sitting cushion, while a child of about six was asleep in one of the piles of laundry.

In a small, cramped eating area off the main room, an Anglo

woman was talking on a mobile phone. She was petite, but she looked tough; maybe it was the stringy blond hair pulled tightly back from her face, or perhaps it was the tattoo of a dagger inside a bleeding heart on her upper arm. Whatever it was, I didn't want to cross her.

She jerked her chin toward me. "You the nurse?" It seemed incongruous that such a soft voice would come from so hard a mouth.

I nodded, trying to breathe around the heat and the smell, wondering how the hell I was going to make it through the night.

"The other nurse split at three," she said after she hung up the phone. "The bitch just left the baby sittin' here, like I'm supposed to do all that fuckin' nursing shit by myself? She said she didn't wanna be here after dark." She looked me over. Her eyes were dark and had a worn-out look about them.

"What kinda shit are you people trying to hand us here, anyway? I thought you were supposed to be responsible."

I started to answer that I didn't know what kind of shit it was but I sure was going to find out, when she cut me off.

"I tried putting one of them sucking tubes down the kid's breathing hole?" She made a waving motion with her cigarette. The trail of smoke looked like a question mark. "I got some snot stuff out, but I don't know what I'm doing. I got two other kids. I don't have time to be doin' this shit."

It was rude, but I couldn't stop my mouth. "How old are you?"

"Nineteen last month."

Not wanting to show my shock, I put on a poker face—the teenager looked not a day under forty-five. "May I use your phone? I need to notify my supervisor."

As she handed me the phone, the young man, who I now assumed was the father, jumped off the couch and none too gently slapped the face of a naked child who was about to put her hand on the side of the television set. He shoved her backward so that she stumbled and landed on her buttocks.

Thinking a game was being played, the toddler scrambled to her feet and ran to touch the side of the set again.

As I dialed the agency's number, Dad once more slapped the child and pushed her down—harder than before.

"Seems the day shift nurse left at three," I managed to say through clenched teeth when Inez, the supervisor, came on the line. "The family isn't happy."

"Oh, not again," Inez groaned. "This is the second time she's left early on this case. I'll try to locate her and have her call you with report. Sorry about that."

The young man slapped the little girl again so hard that her head jerked backward and then rolled side to side. She was not as quick to get up as she had been before. Standing over her, he yelled above her sobs and the TV, first in Spanish, then ended in English. "I told you no touch the TV!"

In response, the child wailed, which served only to further infuriate him. The noise was deafening.

"I *dare* you touch the TV!" he taunted. "Go on, I dare you!"

I turned my back on the scene, stuck my finger in my free ear, and returned to the supervisor. "Don't bother getting her. Just give me a basic report to tide me over until you find her."

"Okay, basic report is that Roberto was born six weeks premature with cleft palate. They had to wait until now to repair it because of low weight and failure to thrive. He has a gastric button, a tracheostomy, and a mist mask. He's got dressings that—"

I lowered my voice. "Skip the clinical stuff, I can get that from the chart. Just give me the psychosocial picture. I'm not sure I understand who all these people are here." I cringed at the sound of another loud slap and renewed wails.

Inez snickered. "I'm not sure anybody understands who all is living there, but the way we've got it down here is that the apartment is the father's parents'. The parents live in one of the bedrooms. Two of Dad's sisters and three of their children live in another, and the other is for Mom and Dad and their three kids, including the patient."

Inez stopped, and I sensed she was listening to the pandemonium going on in the background. "Try to hang in there," she said. "These people need some continuity of personnel. Three nurses have refused night assignments there."

"Well, other than the obvious, do you know why that might be?" I asked, ever the innocent.

"Not entirely sure," Inez hedged, "but I don't think you're in any personal danger."

"What aren't you telling me, Inez?"

There was a pause. "Don't worry about it, Diane. You can handle whatever it is. My phone's ringing. Gotta go."

I mumbled my goodbye to a dead line and hung up. The heavy arms of depression wrapped themselves around me. Without asking permission, I deposited my dinner and two Cokes in the refrigerator. I tried like hell to ignore the stacks of dirty dishes and pans piled everywhere, but found myself studying them instead. All the pans were crusted with food that had to be months old. Some of the dishes were growing mold.

From the living room came the sound of another slap, and then another. Peering around the corner, I saw red welts rising on the child's cheeks and buttocks. As a home health nurse working for an agency, I'd been taught not to interfere with the family dynamics. I also had to keep in mind that the family was my boss. Frustrating as it was, whether or not I worked for this family again did not depend on my skills—after all, what did most laypeople know about trach care or sterile dressing changes? Mostly, the families we worked for judged us on things such as whether we were skinny or overweight, the color of our skin—even the bumper stickers on our cars could evoke hostile reports. I'd had one family make me a DNS (do not send) solely on the complaint that I wore a gold crucifix on a chain.

It didn't matter how attached the nurse had grown to the child or the family, you simply never went back. The worst part, though, was that the nurse was never allowed to say one word in defense of herself no matter what allegation had been leveled against her.

There was another slap followed by a piercing scream.

One of the ways I got to be a top-rated nurse was by ignoring the rules. If the family requested I not be sent back, so be it, but I wasn't going to stand by and watch a child be physically abused.

"Excuse me?" I approached the young man, smiling in a way that said I wasn't really smiling. "Please don't hit her again. She's too young to understand why you're punishing her. Your hitting her isn't going to do anything." I held my breath while he sneered at me. It seemed to be the only expression his face knew.

The four other adults in the room glanced at him, then at me. It was as if a challenge had been thrown into the ring.

"If you explain to her—"

"I'm the father." He thumped his hairless chest and stuck it out. "I know what's good for my kid."

"I'm sure you do." I let the smile fade. "But you can't keep hitting her. You have to teach her gently, with words and examples, not—"

"You comin' in *my*"—he hit his chest again—"house and tellin' me how to raise *my* kids?"

I stepped back. He was in my face, his hands balled into fists. From behind there was a quick tug at my uniform. When I turned, the mother was fixing me with a wide-eyed warning look.

"You don't want to be pissin' José off, lady. What he does here's his business, so don't go messin' with him."

I wanted to ask just what José's business was other than abusing children, sensed the violence potential, and stepped back. The mother was pulling me into the hallway.

"Okay," I said, walking backward out of the room. I may have actually been rubbing my hands together—as if I were accepting the challenge of my life. "So, take me to my patient."

The first thing that shocked me about the baby was his size. Fussing unhappily in his crib, Roberto looked like a newborn infant instead of a twelve-week-old baby. Then there were his eyes: dark, large, and endlessly sad. They conveyed a definite message that he already knew about the downside of the world he'd been thrust into.

The mask, which was supposed to be over his trach providing a fine, humidifying mist, lay useless at the foot of the crib. It wouldn't have mattered even if it were in the right place, as the reservoir had run dry of water. His gastric button was crusted with old feedings, indicating it hadn't been cleaned in a while.

I rolled up my sleeves and began at the top of the list. Bathe him and tend to the diaper rash which had turned his groin and buttocks into one scarlet wound, clean the gastric button, do a feeding, clean the button again and replace it, fill the mist reservoir, and give the ordered medications. His nebulizer and suctioning treatments weren't due until midnight, which gave us a window of time.

Wrapping him in one of the agency's soft cotton blankets, I picked him up. He stopped fussing instantly. I cradled the tiny child in my arms, reminded for the thousandth time of why I gravitated toward pediatrics. With kids there was so much hope. They were so resilient. Up to a point, they could go through all sorts of pain and trauma and bounce back.

I cooed and smiled until the sadness in his eyes seemed to fade away. The infant was starved for nurturing and love. This didn't surprise me. In the hour I'd been there, I'd gotten a full dose of the family's dynamics. The adults, including the grandparents, did not interact with any of the children other than to hit or yell. There was no physical affection displayed whatsoever.

Even in the poorest and most violent of homes, I couldn't think of one where *some* affection—even if just holding a child on a lap—was not shown. What I was seeing in this family structure was complete indifference.

Gently, I stroked Roberto's tiny legs, and then his arms, cooing to him the entire time. Like a little brown sponge, he seemed to soak up my touch. As if mesmerized, his breathing grew less erratic, and the tiny legs stopped jerking altogether. Until the light of day had faded into night, I sat with him in my arms, stroking his head and his cheeks, singing my repertoire of nursery rhymes.

Roberto had been asleep for about two hours when I began to worry about where I would be expected to take care of the baby once the family decided to go to bed. Surely they wouldn't want me in the room where they all slept. No sooner had the worry-thought crossed my mind than the door burst open and the father strutted into the room in a way which told me I was going to find out.

He flipped on the overhead lights, which were bright enough to double for spotlights, and stood over my chair, jerking his thumb in the direction of the hall.

"Move to the other room. I don't want you and him here when I sleep."

I opened my mouth to ask where I was supposed to go, when he switched on the portable TV in the corner and turned the volume to maximum level.

Roberto awoke with a grimace. At once, his tiny arms began to flail.

The night progressed strangely. The family's routine was not at all unlike the routine in a prison system: as soon as the father announced he and his family were going to bed, the other adults immediately gathered up their children and belongings, and retired to their individual rooms.

But instead of the peace and quiet most people required for rest, each room became ablaze with the lights and noise that seemed to be a necessity in this home. Three individual television sets blared out three different programs.

I'd lugged the crib and all Roberto's equipment to the alcove next to the kitchen. No one offered to help.

A little after midnight, I lowered the lights in the living room and quietly opened the windows as much as I dared. There wasn't a breeze to be had for love or money, but I couldn't help sticking my head out anyway in hopes of finding a few breaths of fresh air.

I sat trying to think of positive aspects of Roberto's situation, and found I could only come up with one—pitiful as it was. Usually in families with a "special needs" child, that child gets all the attention while the siblings are ignored. This often creates such deep-seated jealousies in the other children, all the nurses know good and well that if the sibling could push the wheelchair off the balcony, or hold a pillow over the face of the sick child and get away with it, they would in a hot second.

I pulled my head back inside. No problem of special-child jealousy here, I thought as I made my way back to the crib. Barely halfway across the living room, I stopped.

The hairs on the back of my arms stood up and I blinked, uncertain at first what I was seeing.

The place had come alive!

Thousands—not hundreds, thousands—of cockroaches swarmed over every object standing. The walls, the ceiling, undulated.

No wonder these people slept in well-lighted, noisy rooms; both were tactics to keep the roaches at bay. I remembered Inez saying that the day shift nurse had left this assignment early before. Sure—made perfect sense, putting that together with the mother's account of how the nurse had told her she needed to be out of there before dark, and that three other nurses refused night shifts here. After all, *didn't roaches only come out at night?*

Now, I'm no babe in the woods. I had taken assignments in places where the filth was so bad it killed your appetite for a week. I've worked in homes where rats larger than my dog have chased me around a kitchen. I've worked among myriad bugs, once a boa constrictor, maggots, roaches, and all *sorts* of critters human and otherwise, but never, ever before had I seen anything like what I was looking at. Stephen King and David Lynch would have loved this place.

I rushed to the crib in time to see several roaches scurry over the crib mattress and drop to the floor. A thought of what I might find inside the infant's diaper caused me to rip open the fastening tabs. I sighed in relief when I found nothing other than a dry, roachless cotton lining.

Not wanting to leave the child alone for more than a few seconds, I rolled the crib closer to me. I felt the NPH insulin I'd given myself earlier in the day beginning to kick in. A lifelong diabetic, I had learned the hard way never to go anywhere without having a Coke or two on hand. I needed to get the sodas out of the fridge, but the kitchen had transformed into a roachophobe's worst nightmare.

The refrigerator was covered. I swatted them away, stepping on the ones I could, and, constantly stamping my feet to keep them from crawling up my legs, opened the door.

Never again would I believe that a refrigerator is a sealed compartment. I was thankful that the Cokes were in recappable bottles, and even more thankful that the bottles were in *front*.

I unscrewed one and drank enough to keep me from getting shaky, then turned my attention to the tasks of warming the formula and preparing for the nebulizer and suctioning treatments.

I found a non-stick pan, deroached it, washed it as best I could, and took a bottle of formula from my kit. I ran to check the crib, crunching and slipping my way back to the sink.

Reaching for the faucet, I wrote, directed, and starred in my own instant *Creepshow* episode. I could hear the screams of the audience as I turned the cold-water tap and imagined the faucet spewing forth a steady stream of roaches and rats.

Five minutes later, I stood skimming dead roaches out of the water while they fell in a steady stream from the nonfunctional hood fan above. One of Roberto's aunts came into the kitchen and took a pan of crusted-over refried beans and onions off the counter. I didn't really want to, but unable to help myself, I turned to watch.

Shaking a roach from the spoon, the woman waved her hand over the pan. The slower, larger roaches crawled down the handle of the pan onto her arm, down her clothes to the floor. The roaches that had gotten stuck in the food and drowned, she picked out with her fingers, dropped them on the floor—next to the crib—and commenced to eat with relish, and I don't mean the kind you put on hot dogs.

My stomach lurched and swayed. Inside my head I screamed. I busied myself with gathering the equipment needed for the treatments. As soon as the aunt left, I set about cleaning off the dinette table with alcohol and disposable towels from my med kit. I spread out a couple of sterile towels, on which I laid the nebulizer and the suction catheter. Twice I had to stop and, using the casing from a used syringe, push out roaches that were attempting to crawl inside my shoes. I added snug-topped athletic socks to my list of things to be grateful for.

After the nebulizer treatment, I turned on the suction, checked overhead to make sure the ceiling was clear, and donned sterile gloves.

Slowly threading the catheter into the tracheostomy tube, I went as far as I dared and applied the suction. I pulled back the catheter, vacuuming the insides of the tube for the mucus which had accumulated there and in his lungs.

Several dark specks went through the catheter and into the canister. Old blood. The report had said the infant's intubation had been traumatic and there had been a problem in the past with blood clots. I gave Roberto a few puffs of extra oxygen with the ambu bag before I went down with the catheter a second time. When it came to kids' lungs, I was a fastidious housekeeper, so this time I pushed the tube a littler further than before, wanting to get a good, deep suction.

I was rewarded with a large amount of mucus and a few more specks of old blood. As I was just about to pull the catheter all the way out, a clot that appeared to be larger than the rest shot by.

Suddenly I was furious. I wanted to lash out at someone: at the day nurse for having left four hours early, and for not having done a thorough deep suctioning, at the adults for allowing such filth, at the parents for having and then not loving this child. Didn't they know—as human beings—that children could not thrive without nurturing? Couldn't someone see that this infant was dying from lack of love?

I closed my eyes and took a long, slow breath. When the anger passed into sadness and the sadness passed once again into resignation, I disconnected the catheter and cleared the tubing with sterile water.

In my notes I would have to describe the clot in detail, and knowing the pediatrician on the case as well as I did, I knew she would insist on a specimen. I opened the canister and started to unscrew the top off the specimen cup, when, out of the corner of my eye, I saw the clot unfold like a tiny, blossoming flower. I swore at the dim overhead light, and pulled out my penlight which I shined directly on the clot. Using a tongue blade, I fished around until I got ahold of it and slipped it into the specimen cup.

With the aid of my reading glasses and penlight, I made myself study the baby roach carefully. It was complete—all legs and antennae accounted for. As much as I wanted to, I could not convince myself it was anything else.

I broke into a cold sweat, debating whether or not to just dump the specimen down the john and forget about it. At the same time, I wanted to call the agency and tell someone—some veteran home health nurse who would know how to handle the situation.

I vacillated between being appalled and furious. When I was furious, I didn't know if I could wait until morning to march into the pediatrician's office and personally show her the specimen, demanding the child be removed permanently from the home.

I drank off the rest of the Coke and opened the second bottle. The soft drink was my survival food. Briefly I toyed with the idea of sending the Coca-Cola Company a testimonial about how the beverage had saved my life. I imagined explaining the details of my situation: *Dear Sirs . . . Due to cockroaches and my diabetes, your delicious, tightly capped beverage saved my . . .* Naw, the customer service people definitely wouldn't get it.

I went back to the canister, where I fished out a couple of the other "specks" that I'd seen in the tubing earlier. One was a small blood clot; the other was part of a roach leg.

I asked myself a number of questions, none of which I had answers for, and blocked out visions of what atrocities might be taking place inside the infant's chest at that very moment.

Part of me wanted to pack up my stuff and run, screaming, out the door. Collecting myself, I picked up Roberto and gazed into his huge dark eyes. I couldn't fall apart; I had to keep it together. This child was depending on me for at least that much.

Whispering in his ear, I made him a promise.

Then, I reached for the phone.

At dawn I decided I would tell only the mother. She was smaller than I: if she got violent and went off on me, I'd have a good chance at defending myself. Hopefully she would be reasonable when the medical transport crew showed up at the front door to take her son back to the hospital.

The father was another story. I was banking on the fact that he didn't care much for the child and would welcome the chance to be rid of him.

I switched Roberto to my other arm—I had not let him out of my arms all night except once to go to the bathroom. That I had managed to keep my balance and accurately aim while crouched high over the rim on which I stood, I supposed, could have been considered a blessing.

As the sun began to show itself, and the roaches began their general retreat, I started to laugh the laugh of the exhausted. I tried to imagine what a person off the street might think if they were to see me: a woman and baby in a chair that was surrounded by double loops of packing tape.

That necessity is the mother of invention is true. I had created my own Roach Motel from strips of packing tape someone had left in the box of supplies the agency sent over. Whenever a strip would fill up with roaches, I'd throw it to the side and lay down another. Only once did my plan fail—when a pair of mating cockroaches, obviously in the throes of roach passion, had fallen from the ceiling and landed on the toe of my shoe. I simply flipped them onto the nearest piece of unoccupied tape.

By the time the mother came into the kitchen, I was packed and waiting for the day shift nurse, who would assist with the medical transport. Without so much as a glance in the direction of the infant or me, she prepared a cup of instant coffee, and was headed back to the bedroom when I stopped her.

"Please," I said. "We need to talk about Roberto."

"Give the next nurse the information," she said gruffly. "I gotta bring this to him."

"No." I said more sternly. "You have to hear this. Bring him the coffee and come right back or I'll come in there and talk to you both."

"Don't you come in there," she warned, narrowing her eyes. "He don't like nobody in the morning."

"Okay, then if you want to avoid that scene, you deliver the coffee and come back."

I waited five minutes, then started toward the bedroom. The mother met me at the door, and in a strange sort of dance, we more or less herded each other back to the kitchen alcove.

I told her what I had suctioned from her child's lungs, showing her the specimen cup.

She winced and covered her mouth. It was the first appropriate *human* reaction I'd seen from any of the adults.

"I'm not making judgments here," I lied. "And I don't want to offend you. But your baby cannot stay in this environment. They must have told you at the hospital that this kind of thing could kill him."

I became aware of how rigid and controlled I was. But I knew that if I loosened the stays, I would lose it and horrible things would come out of my mouth. In my mind's ear, I could hear myself screaming, *My God, you live like animals! Worse than animals!*

I waited until I was relatively sure the information had sunk in. The impassive expression which seemed to plague the entire family had again settled over the mother's features. She shrugged but said nothing.

As if to challenge the woman's apathy, I added that I had notified the pediatrician, and glanced at my watch.

"Dr. Flores is going to call here to speak with you around seven-thirty. She's going to tell you why Roberto has to go back to the hospital."

I don't know what reaction I expected, or perhaps hoped for. Anything—tears, rage, remorse—would have been a whole lot less frustrating than the big fat nothing I did get. Again the woman shrugged, and without another word, went back into the bedroom.

Never once had she even looked at her son.

I waited by the window until I saw the day shift nurse heading up the walkway. From the window, I shouted for her to stay where she was and that I would give report outside.

Feeling like Mary Poppins with a nursing degree, I kissed Roberto's furrowed brow and wished him the best of luck. He was not the first child I had wanted to take home with me. I didn't usually dwell on those feelings, but today the picture of how this baby in particular would thrive on the love and affection I could give played over in my head until the pain choked me. One more kiss and I left, feeling all the separation anxiety of a new mother.

On the sidewalk, I gave report, glad that the nurse had been fore-warned by the agency as to the recent developments. She asked to see the specimen I was dropping off at Dr. Flores's office.

It was with a puzzling reluctance that I allowed her to examine the thing. Glancing around furtively, I was engulfed by an overwhelming sense of shame.

I hurried past my car, down the block to the corner.

The bus stop was deserted, which suited me perfectly. I sat down on the bench and dumped out the contents of my purse and my kit.

I had once heard a story about a nurse who had done a shift in the same sort of home and accidentally brought a stowaway roach to her car. Within a month, the car was completely colonized. It had cost her over three hundred dollars to get them out of the dash.

Not wanting to repeat the same mistake, I went through my belongings with a fine-tooth comb. I checked linings and pockets, opened lipstick tubes and ballpoint pens. Every piece of paper was scrutinized. In the end, only things like my checkbook, credit cards, and whatever was completely sealed went back into my purse or kit. The rest, I threw in the trash can.

I brushed my hair vigorously, shook out and examined the sweatshirt I had used to camouflage my purse. Assured I was unobserved, I quickly took off my uniform, socks, and shoes. My slip, bra, socks, and panties, I checked and shook out as best I could without removing them. The uniform was added to the other trash. The shoes, I took apart, checking under the inner soles and the tongue.

As I slipped into my husband's sweatshirt, I noticed five dead roaches and a couple of roach eggs lying under the bench. As I stared at them, I again felt the odd, dismaying sense of shame. I could only guess it partly stemmed from the revulsion and fear of that which symbolized poverty. Mostly, I realized, it was due to the apathy which man often exhibited toward his less fortunate neighbor. It was the same feeling I'd had each time I'd ever turned my eyes away from the limbless man begging in the street and claimed no responsibility. It was a shame for the human condition in the raw.

Thus half dressed, I ran to my car, grateful that the only person who saw me was an elderly man in a Dodge station wagon of similar vintage. Laughing as he passed, he'd honked and pointed.

In the VW I threw on a wrinkled but clean spare uniform and set my bare feet back inside my shoes. Taking a last look at the orange door, I pulled away from the curb feeling guilty that I could not "save" Roberto and his siblings, or any of the hundreds of children I had and would care for who did not get the love due them.

For the first twenty minutes of my drive home, I kept thinking, *I can't do this anymore. I can't . . . I just can't.* I felt like I'd failed somehow—after all, aren't nurses supposed to give and give? I work inside a home health care system that has the potential for being the best—the most ideal—nursing care available. Yet sometimes the system, the agency, or the recipients themselves just won't allow it to be that way.

When I got tired of the negative thoughts, I replaced them with one positive one: I had done my best, and perhaps whatever love or comfort the infant received from me would, in some positive way, make a difference.

It was all I could hope for.

James F.

This is a short one from James F., an ICU nurse from New Orleans. The visuals were just too good to pass up.

Clara was in her mid-nineties and living in a rest home. Clara had been one of those huge buxom blondes from the forties and fifties, who fade overnight like a burst balloon. She'd worked on presidential campaigns and been in the *Who's Who of Women*, so you know that this was one dynamic babe who still had a mind of her own.

One day, Clara decided she was tired of life and didn't want to go on anymore, so she took matters in her own hands. She hoarded all of her sleeping medications and all the drugs she was supposed to have taken on a daily basis for about two weeks. With a bottle of scotch she'd bribed from one of the nurse's aides, she downed 147 pills.

They brought her into the ICU after they'd found her. Unfortunately—to Clara's way of thinking anyway—she woke up in the ICU. Once she was able to speak, this was how the dialogue went word for word:

"I'm dead?"

"No, Clara, I'm afraid you aren't."

"Yes I am!"

"No, Clara, you may wish you were dead, but someone intervened and you are in fact alive and well and in the ICU in New Orleans, in the United States of America."

"No! That's a damned, bold-faced lie. I'm dead, and I'm in heaven!"

At this point, there were a few of us that were laughing about her insistence, and we were coming up with all these ideas of how to make her believe she wasn't dead.

Well, the head nurse of our ICU was the biggest, fattest, ugliest drag queen of a guy you would ever want to set your peepers on, so I tell Billy to come on over to the bed and I said, "Now Clara, I want you to take a good look at this person."

Clara blinks and squints, and I put on her glasses for her and she makes an awful face at the sight of this big, ugly bruiser with his buck teeth, Coke bottle glasses, and hints of lipstick and eyeshadow.

She drew as far back from Billy as she could.

And then I said, "Okay, so I ask you, Clara, could there be any angel this ugly in God's heaven?"

Clara put her hands over her mouth and looked at us totally horrified. "Dear God," she whispered. "I've gone to hell."

Then she shook her head. "Damn it!" she said with real vehemence. "I knew this would happen if I worked on the Nixon campaign!"

Thomas R.

I know, I know—this is supposed to be a book of nurses and their stories, but I just had to include one story from the nurse's right-hand army—those incredible men and women who do the initial work out there in the field: the paramedics.

It is 9:30 A.M. Sitting across the table in this quaint New England café, the six-foot-three fireman-paramedic drinks his orange juice without seeming to taste it. The polished brass name pinned to the dark blue uniform jacket reads "Thomas R."

Thirty-nine-year-old Paramedic R. has just gotten off twenty-four-hour duty. Despite his handsome face, he looks haggard and exhausted. When I mention this to him, he is quick to assure me that it is not the usual state he's in when he gets off work. He sadly—almost apologetically—explains that he has just returned from a 6:00 A.M. call that was "one of the ones that take the wind out of everybody's sails."

Nobody likes calls like this, so the whole crew was pretty down. At about 5:50, we get a call for a six-year-old hanging from a rope.

So we get there and this little guy is hanging from a tree in the backyard. He must have been a pretty smart little fella, 'cause he tied the rope to a dog's choker chain and then threaded the other end through it so he could tighten it up real good. He put the chain end around his neck and jumped off a kitchen chair.

He was only six, so maybe he weighed about fifty pounds. He was about three feet eleven inches tall. What in God's name could have compelled the little guy to do that? Shit, I don't know. I've been to that house two, maybe three times on domestic violence calls. The boyfriend of the mother is a convicted felon who's done time on some rather heinous things. I don't even want to think about it.

So, by the time we got there, the mother's boyfriend said he'd done CPR like he'd seen on the TV. I don't have any idea what the fuck that was supposed to mean, so I kind of pushed him out of the way and did my assessment.

The kid was breathing but unconscious, fortunately. We did everything we were supposed to—spinal precautions, IV, vitals. The BP was about 90. I put oxygen on him, but both pupils were blown wide open and fixed.

The house is out in the boonies, so we put him on a board and called Lifeflight. In the end he was diagnosed with hypoxemic encephalopathy [damage to the brain due to lack of oxygen]. They'll probably pronounce him that way too.

It was weird, though, 'cause he had a negative Babinski, and he did come around a little at the end, but his pupils stayed blown throughout. An hour later, we called the hospital and were told the prognosis was guarded but good and that his pupillary response was improving, so we were all really upbeat over that news. That lasted about ten minutes, when the nurse from ICU called to say the kid took a straight dive down the tubes and was having seizures and all that other brain stem shit. So that's the end of that, huh?

Man, life's so fucking unpredictable—everything can change or be over in one minute. *Boom!* Gone! Six years old? A hundred and two? A bum? A fuckin' beauty queen? It doesn't matter who or what you are, not one motherfucking bit.

The guys I usually work with? One's about twenty-five and a Jesus freak, although he definitely has some interesting un-Christian attitudes about certain races. Another is about my age, got a kid, and works at a fruit farm. He's got a good, level head on his shoulders—a responsible guy, so I guess I identify more with him. My lieutenant is about forty. He's been at this about seventeen years, so he can take it—in one ear and out the other. My partner is a woman, and she's the best in the field that I've ever seen. She was my mentor when I first got out of paramedic school, so I'm real lucky to be paired with her.

I got into this not for any compelling need I had to help people, like some other wonderful persons who get into this. I just needed an extra job. I used to run a dive business and I'd see these young guys come in with brand-new cars and diving equipment sometimes on a Tuesday morning, or a Thursday afternoon, and I finally asked what kinda job they had. I thought they were dope dealers or pimps or something.

But they said they were firemen-paramedics and they worked one day on and two days off. It sounded too good to be true. So I took my state tests to be a fireman and then got my EMT certification. Not being a guy who likes being pushed around and told when to wipe my ass, I decided I wanted the autonomy of being a paramedic. That meant paramedic school for another year.

That was the easy part. Getting the job was a bitch. For every job there's a line of people applying. Then there's the internship, where you have to complete five hundred hours of riding on the rig as the junior medic.

The stressful part of my job is making the decisions in the field without a doctor's order. After ten years in this job, I can justify most all my decisions. I read and study a lot too, though. I spend a good deal of my time reviewing protocols and pharmacology, and how I would handle general situations.

Every morning I go over my equipment, because when the poopoo hits the fan, believe me when I tell you the equipment is *not* where you can be slack.

At work I'm serious as a heart attack. When a call comes in, we have to be there within eight minutes or we get written up for not responding appropriately. I mean, you could do a whole lot worse if you call and it's my crew who responds. You know how they say the first hour after the response to a call is considered the "golden hour"? Well, in my book it's the "golden twenty minutes." The faster you can stabilize them and get them into an ER, the better.

I maintain that level of professionalism so that I don't have any of the post-traumatic stress shit going on. Not to say you don't feel it sometimes anyway. I mean, I can watch a movie sometimes and because of certain calls that I've had, I'll let go and end up crying like a baby. But at the scene, I put those emotions to work. I get the most value out of the fear and the horrific stuff by putting that energy into doing the best job that can be done.

Where the company is located, we get a good cross section of ages. Geriatric calls on the people over seventy-five that don't turn out good don't usually bother me, because there's usually some preexisting conditions and they've had a full life. I do the best I can no matter what age they are, but I won't think as hard about a ninety-two-year-old that craps out in the rig as I will about a seventy-year-old.

The ones that bother me most are the old people who are terminal and they'll sometimes reach up with the last bit of strength and grab my hands while I'm trying to intubate them. I hate it that their last dying moment is spent looking up into my big hairy fucking nose and feeling like they don't have the right to die the way they want. You don't have to be a brain surgeon to realize that this person should be allowed to just die. But unfortunately, some Jello-O brain relative at the last minute gets scared and guilty and calls anyway and screams, "SAVE THEM!"

Other difficult trauma calls obviously are for the young people that no matter what you do, they still die. Even worse are the young ones with spinal cord injuries . . . the future quads and paras of America. I've seen my share of those heartbreakers, I'll tell you.

Kids calls can be rough, but as long as you can justify your actions, and you're trained well, and you have a good crew, it makes it a little easier to handle.

I guess if I had to pick one call that got to me, it was a kid who was about twelve who was out with his buddies roaming the strip malls, just fooling around. Apparently they discovered that if they jumped on a soda machine all at the same time and rocked it back and forth, they could get a couple of free sodas and maybe some change.

According to the young man who had the sense to make the 911 call, they'd found a big machine—and let me tell you, that damned sucker was twenty-five hundred pounds—and they were doing their thing, but the machine got away from them.

This one kid who's in front gets his sneaker stuck in the slot where the cans come out, and as the machine goes over, he can't pull it out, and he doesn't have time to maneuver himself, so the machine lands flat on top of him. That's twenty-five hundred pounds of steel on top of a one-hundred-pound boy.

As soon as we got there and I saw him, I determined that had that kid lived—and I'm sure you're going to think, *Who the fuck are you? God?*—he would've been a vegetable of the lowest form.

The fucking machine had almost severed his neck, and he wasn't breathing and hadn't been for a long time. There weren't any reflexes. I'm glad that kid didn't survive. I don't think I could deal with knowing that because of my efforts, someone was doomed to live another fifty years as a carrot.

Another thing that I have to get out is that people don't realize how hard it can be to stabilize someone in the field. The paramedics don't have the support of medical teams with pharmacists, doctors, surgeons, lab techs, and nurses. We don't have the high-tech equipment. We're working in the dark. We've got two people. You can't do airway, IV, administration of drugs, and EKG within thirty seconds with just two people. The mental presence one has to have to work this job comes through experience—you don't get it overnight.

So much has to be taken into consideration at the scene, not to mention prequalifying safety and protection in regard to communicable diseases. You'd be surprised how many emergency personnel are injured or killed each year because they don't park the rescue rigs correctly. The whole thing is a mind-set of prioritizing.

One: Get parked out of the way. That's five seconds.

Two: Gloves and eye protection. That's another three seconds.

Three: What am I going to need there? A spine board? An airway? That's another few seconds.

Get in there and determine within a few seconds if you need an air transport. Secure airway and C spine precautions, call for assistance if needed.

On the highway? Shit, I can't tell you how many hazardous materials are being transported on the common roads you and I travel every day. There's everything out there from moderately radioactive materials to caustics, propane, alkaloids, and acids. When these huge semis get hit and they're carrying this stuff, that has to be taken care of before you can initiate patient care.

Sometimes you have to stand there and watch someone die because you can't go in there. It's a save-yourself-first situation sometimes. We just had three firemen—all under thirty years old—die of a nasty cancer that they each got when they responded to an overturned truck that was carrying some carcinogenic crap. The shit got on their coats and equipment, and later, when they took off the coats and were cleaning the equipment, they got it on their skin. [He snaps his fingers.] Just like that! One year later they're all dead just from touching this shit.

And this shit's being carried on the same road that your kid's school bus travels every day? Scary. If people only knew the truth about what corporations are shipping on our roads, they'd shit, man.

Anyway, no matter how you train for it, you can't always avoid the dangers. You can respond to a call, and have some asshole open the door and you get your head blown off by somebody who's just plain pissed off. There's a lot of anger out there. Most of our trauma comes from vehicular traffic, true, but there's a lot of shootings and stabbings too.

To me a good call is where even if the person dies you did the best you could do, airway went in easy, IVs went in, meds were well documented, and the doctor looks at you and says, "Yeah, you did good."

The things about the job that get to me? Well, like the other day, we responded to a suicide attempt of a young man with AIDS. It still amazes me and pisses me off to see people in the field who have a distinct aversion to dealing with AIDS and no empathy whatsoever.

I get real annoyed with the EMTs who are lackadaisical about their jobs. I think those guys are dangerous. Face it—this isn't exactly the kind of job where you can have a bad day. I mean, you can't come in and say, "Well, shit, I think I'll just fuck off today." You are on every freaking minute of every freaking day. With this job you can get an 80 percent success rate with a 150 percent effort, so you've got to have your mind set right. That's real difficult sometimes.

The twenty-four-hour day is hard. Try rousing yourself out of a sound sleep, roaring out to a scene, and managing a cardiac arrest.

The worst is seeing the reactions of the loved ones. Grief is grief and you'd have to be pretty inhuman not to recognize when people are profoundly affected by the loss of a loved one.

Oh yeah, another difficult kind of call are the burn calls. I've been really fortunate in the worst I've ever had to deal with was a forty percent second and third degree. People go into shock right away. A lot of times if you have to wait for the helicopter more than fifteen minutes, the patients [he laughs] start to hit you. It takes a while to reassure them. I just had a nine-year-old boy with some bad burns over thirty percent of his body, including the genitals—that was a tough one.

The humor in the job? Well, I've had people tell me jokes as they were dying, and I've sure heard some wild stories in the back of the rig.

Once I had to help a little old lady pull her britches down so she could pee, and she kept telling me she hadn't had a man take off her panties in over forty years. [He laughs.] Said she kinda liked it now that she'd remembered. That gave me the grins for the rest of the day.

Oh, then there are always the guys who are sticking their tally-whackers into strange places and we have to go out and get them unstuck.

I guess I don't think in terms of this job having much humor. Maybe that means something too. I guess it takes a pretty weird fucker to choose a job where you're constantly exposed to people who are sick and dying or just in dire need. And when you consider the rush you get from working on an arrest or a trauma call, it seems perverse.

There's got to be a repercussive stress that'll get to each of us eventually. I mean, you've got to be a fucking robot not to be affected by this kind of job, right?

Nancy D.

Nancy D. looks a good fifteen years younger than her fifty-three years. Her impeccable dress and grooming make me think that if I met her on the street, I would guess she'd had a career in modeling.

As she speaks, her smile is always present and her hands are never at rest. Easy laughter punctuates many of her sentences. Unlike many of the nurses I have interviewed, there is an obvious lack of the signs of stress that tend to linger on nurses' faces. What is the same, however, is the knowing behind the eyes.

I graduated from nurse's training in 1965—at the age of twenty-one—and I didn't leave nursing until last year, so you can see I've been a nurse for a long time. As I look back, I never thought I would be anything else but a nurse. My aunt was a nurse, and she was my favorite person when I was growing up. Also, I was told by a high school counselor that I could do anything I wanted to in the sciences, and since I was a female, that meant, of course, I would become a nurse.

Psych nursing was my special interest, but on the day that I interviewed for my first job as a psych nurse, some man dove through the plate glass window right next to where I was sitting, and that was the end of that. I never applied for another psych position.

After I received my RN, I took a job in pediatrics for about six months, until one night when I had a very traumatic experience. They'd staffed the unit with only one RN—me—and two nurse's aides. About 3:00 A.M., an infant came in directly to me from ER. The pediatrician was nowhere to be seen, I had no orders, no diagnosis—nothing.

The child—I think he was less than one month old—was very dehydrated and extremely critical. I did everything I could do for that baby, but he died in my arms within thirty minutes after arrival. I was completely and utterly devastated.

That baby's death was a deep trauma for me. It made me realize the vulnerability of the little ones and how narrow their ranges of life were during certain periods of illness. I didn't have the heart or the courage for that at that time, and so I left.

Next I worked in ICU and then I went into coronary care. The last twenty-two years I've spent working in postanesthesia care [recovery room] and then in surgical day care.

While I was in CCU, I went back to school for my bachelor's degree in public health nursing. I also worked part-time in home health care, and at the Women's Health Center. Around 1983, I became a volunteer for La Familia, traveled to north Guatemala, Chile, and Peru working with Doctors without Borders in plastic surgery, obstetrics, and general surgery.

The longer I've been a healer, the more I've gotten into the holistic type of healing. I feel like a liaison between the Eastern and Western concepts—I like to call them complementary concepts of healthcare.

I've seen so many changes over the years. As women's roles became stronger and more defined, my role as a nurse became more defined. Although there is still enormous progress to be made, nurses have gone from the assistive, abused handmaiden role to the independent, professional performer, but now . . .

I've seen hospital nursing change a great deal. It's become less oriented to high-level service and more to financial considerations of how much can be done by whom and how fast. That's extremely difficult for me as a nurse because it's hard for all nurses and it's potentially very harmful for nursing as a profession.

Because I began nursing at such a young age, I think I grew in many ways long before my time. I saw a lot of death and pain and talked to many people who freely offered their wisdom on such things. I was grounded in the realities of life—pain, death, celebration—in my twenties.

I never burned out. Yes, I did leave nursing a year ago to travel around the world with my husband, but it wasn't because I was burned out.

This whole business of burnout is very interesting to me because at the same time I realize I don't want to go back to nursing, I know that if I hadn't left to travel, I would have been perfectly content and happy to continue on as a nurse.

One of the reasons I didn't burn out, I think, was that I had been working only a three-to-four-day work week for the last twenty years. I am lucky in that I live simply. I never had the need to work full-time, and I never had children—a conscious choice on my part. I knew there were a lot of things I wanted to do, and I needed that freedom.

Another reason I didn't burn out was because postanesthesia care and surgical day care had the luxury of having more than adequate staffing with very wonderful and giving people. I think I kind of lived in la-la land that way, because we were so well staffed we didn't really go through some of the awful stresses that the other units have.

A major reason—and you might find this strange—I didn't burn out was that when I was head nurse of the CCU at the age of thirty, I suddenly realized that I had seen huge numbers of young men—men in their forties and fifties—die. Many of them had said to me: "You know, I have all this stuff—money, power, material wealth, a wife and kids— *but* . . . I'm dying and my life is despair. My wife and kids don't know who I am, and I've never done anything I wanted to do."

I took that very seriously. After about eight years of hearing that same story over and over again, I decided to go part-time and live a simple life.

There was another thing too that helped me decide to change my path in life and in nursing at that time: an experience I'd had in 1968 that was one of the most profound things I ever saw.

I know this is going to sound a little woowoo, but bear with me.

It took place one autumn afternoon in 1968. At the time, the hospital was only one floor with about a hundred beds, and I was assistant head nurse in an eleven-bed combo ICU/CCU.

Coronary care units were really a new concept at that time, and we were doing a lot of pioneer work. [She laughs.] Gee whiz, we were giving three and four hundred milligrams of Xylocaine IV push [about four to six times the normal dose], so you can imagine how exciting it was.

I remember coming to work one day, when I got an extremely panicky call from the head nurse down the hall saying: "Open the doors stat! We found Mr. James dead in his bed and we're rolling him in to you!"

Mr. James was a really fine, lovely gentleman who was in his mid-eighties. Prior to this phone call, he'd been in our CCU for about two weeks with an extensive heart attack and congestive heart failure, but he'd been transferred down the hall a few days before because he was doing much better, and was actually getting ready to go home.

Well, this man was sharp and very interesting, so we talked a lot, and over the weeks had formed a really sweet friendship.

Once he confided to me that he'd had a full life, and he was ready to die, but that he didn't want to leave his wife, with whom he'd had a wonderful, loving marriage for over sixty years.

So as soon as I put the phone down, the door flings open and in comes Mr. James. And sure enough, he was pretty dead.

The nurses were doing CPR; his pupils were dilated. We threw the bed into room 4 and connected him to the monitor. He was in ventricular fibrillation, and he was looking very bad. There wasn't a doctor in the house at that time, so I ran the code.

I defibrillated him so many times I was afraid I'd fry his heart. We gave the drugs and intubated him and got him on the old bird [an outdated ventilator].

For the rest of the shift, he went in and out of V fib, so we continued to shock him and bolus him with whatever drug we had. I don't recall that his pupils ever did come down. By the time I left that shift, the doctor said he didn't have a chance in hell to survive for more than a few hours. It was a very traumatic day for me because I'd really loved that man and I knew how much he wanted to live.

Please realize that at this time in my life I was very young and clearly had no religious or spiritual awareness about anything. At the time, I was more interested in bridge games and waterskiing, and decorating my house with fancy things to impress my neighbors and friends. That's where I was.

Well, the next day, I walked into the unit and there was Mr. James sitting up in bed, chatting with the day shift nurse, drinking a cup of tea.

I was so happy I ran into his room to hug him, but when I approached the bed, he warned me to get away from him. He wouldn't talk to me. He was so angry with me that he couldn't even be civil.

I was just devastated over his behavior, so I pleaded with him to at least tell me what I'd done, when he finally said, "I know what you did to me."

When I asked him to explain what he meant, he said, "Yesterday, I had this terrible pain in my chest and I died. All the pain was gone, and I didn't feel old anymore. I felt blissful and at peace. I was surrounded by this wonderfully warm, white light."

Now remember, this was 1968. Accounts of white light stories were unheard of at that time. Certainly I'd never heard of anything like it in my life. So, because I'm sitting on the edge of his bed just speechless, he says: "There were a lot of people in the room, but you kept on doing something to my chest with a machine. I was sitting on the curtains up there, and whenever you did that thing, I would get jerked back down into my body and I would have that terrible pain again. I wanted you to stop, but you wouldn't. You were being mean."

Mr. James had no idea I was on duty that day. He didn't know anything about medicine or defibrillators or that there were a lot of people in the room. He was brought to us unconscious; there was no way he could have known that.

I was in shock and totally mystified by his story, but finally, I told him that from what he had told me about not wanting to leave his wife, and by his very presence in the hospital, we'd had sort of a contract for me to do my best to keep him alive.

With that approach, he told me I was right and he was just angry because the white light was so wonderful and he wanted to stay there.

Well, I didn't know what to do with his story, it was so bizarre and disturbing. I certainly didn't tell anyone about it. Then, in the mid-seventies, I heard Kübler-Ross talk about life after death, and of course, people have written and talked a lot about this white light phenomenon since then.

Mr. James's experience taught me to allow death to come even in the most tragic situations in a way that left dignity to the patient. It also left me with less fear of death. Death was no longer the enemy and I accepted it as a natural part of life.

So, at the age of thirty, I was also propelled into seeking out nature, which is a very authentic spiritual thing for me. It certainly wasn't a religious experience I sought. I was very alienated from church and religion, having been raised in a strictly religious atmosphere. But there has been this slow, steady progression toward a connection with earth and spirituality. And if I didn't say this, I might as well be blowing smoke, but the fact is, I love nursing. The rewards have been tremendous. Personal growth, understanding my body, being there for others who need knowledge and support, giving advice, helping people die with love and dignity, taking away pain. Yeah, on the technical stuff I did a pretty decent job too, but my greatest reward was with the interaction with the patients and the families.

I also think nursing paid very well. I made a good living, and the perks were excellent. It also gave me a clear identity in this world. I am, have been, and always will be a nurse. It was something I respected doing. I never could figure out why other people in nursing didn't respect what they were doing. I thought it was an opportunity of a lifetime to be present for people in their pain and fear.

Another thing that helped maintain me as a whole human being was that I started taking classes at the local college. I think I took every course that the humanities, arts, and literature departments offered. To depend strictly on one's job for personal growth is limiting. For me, to know more about the world and who I was made a big difference for me as a nurse.

I made sure my world was larger than nursing. I've done a lot of things. I taught backpacking and rock climbing for years. I teach environmental education to grade school kids, I'm a docent at a bird sanctuary, and I also run a business where I lead vision quests into the mountains.

If there was one thing about being a nurse that I hated, I'd have to say it was my interaction with the doctors. I'm not one who gets sucked into the negative flimflam stuff going around in nursing these days, but I must say I never found my relationship with doctors to be consistently pleasant. I disagreed with who they were and what they stood for most of the time. I really disagreed with how they see themselves in the overall healthcare-provider chain. I didn't and still don't like most of them as human beings.

I've been married many times, which has allowed me to experience a number of lifestyles. However, I have been married to the same man for going on six years now. This is really a wonderful time in my life and a very generative period for me.

I don't feel I need as much nurturing and I can really return a lot of gifts to other people and the world. I miss family and patient contact, but I'm finding I can have that same sort of nurturing relationship outside of nursing.

Olivia P.

Forty-one-year-old Montana nurse Olivia P. was laughing so hard when she told me this story that I started to laugh, and then we both got to wheezing so bad I had to finally shut off the tape.

In our ER we had one of those really superuptight arrogant doctors. You know the type. Every ER has one—or if you're really unlucky, two.

Well, this guy also suffered from LMS—Little Man Syndrome—because he was only about five foot one inch tall. In his case, the nurses also called it the Chihuahua syndrome, because he liked to bark orders and commands. In short—oops, no pun intended—he was an insufferable human being who was generally shunned by all.

One day a code came into the ER, and he did his usual arrogant-doctor stuff and was shouting out orders and having temper tantrums and throwing things at people. Basically, he was having himself a grand old time.

Well, he decides for some unknown reason that he doesn't like the way the nurse is doing CPR, so he orders a step stool to be placed next to the gurney, and he climbs up there and starts doing CPR like there's no tomorrow—which there wasn't for the patient, because he was dead and there wasn't any bringing him back.

So he's up there and he's hyper as the devil on wheels. And he starts screaming that he wants the results of the last blood gas—and when someone didn't give it to him in less than half a second, he started jumping up and down on the stool, screaming and turning purple.

Well now, I suspect that it was during this jumping-up-and-down part of the tantrum that his lab coat got caught on the IV pole.

When he tried to step down, the stool fell over, and he ended up dangling from the pole like a puppet from a string, or a man being hanged by a rope. Yep, there the little guy was, flapping and flailing in the breeze, his feet not touching the floor.

He started yelling for us to unhook him, but the whole staff decided to leave him there until he calmed down. Meanwhile, our head nurse was out in the hall trying to get as many hospital staff as possible to come in and take a gander at this guy.

The clerk took a photo.

By the time someone let him off the hook—sorry!—at least fifty staff members had gotten a good laugh.

Danglin' Doc—as he came to be known—has long since left, but his picture still hangs in our glass case as a warning to all new docs.

Richard Y.

"Whenever you see a patient coming into the psych unit carrying a teddy bear, it's a bad sign." —Richard Y., forty-seven-year-old psychiatric nurse, Los Angeles, California, formerly a civil engineer, fireman, commercial pilot, and EMT

After I graduated in 1983, I worked in ICU and CCU before I burned out and moved on to chemical dependency. [He laughs.] Not me—the department.

The main reason I burned out in critical care was making the discovery that we were keeping patients alive way longer and more often than we should have. I'm not touting mercy killing, but we take it too far . . . the whole bit with prolonging life. We're here to alleviate suffering, not prolong it.

I remember one lady, she was ninety-eight years old, weighed eighty pounds, had three types of inoperable cancer, and had been contractured in the fetal position for over twenty years. The family rarely ever came to see her, but they were Catholics, so by God, they wouldn't let this poor woman die. The family still wanted us to do everything we could. When she finally went, we did as little as we could get away with legally.

I recall another situation with an eighty-five-year-old man who'd had a heart attack. He and his wife lived in a mobile home on their retirement savings. He only had Medicare, which didn't pay for anything.

Well, about the third day we knew this guy wasn't going to make it, but we kept on going, giving him more and more stuff to bring him back to life, because the doctors weren't thinking . . . or didn't care. He lived for two weeks more. Of course, the wife had to sell the mobile home and use up all their life savings to pay the medical bills. In the end some relatives took her in as a welfare case.

When that happens over and over, you have to ask yourself whether or not you're doing the right thing. I knew I had the skill to save lives and keep them alive, but there were too many times that I was saving lives that aren't meant to be saved. After a while, I decided I couldn't continue in critical care.

From there I went to work for the registry for a while, but the problem with registry is that you get the worst patients. The regular nurses think they can dump on you because you don't know.

Well, we *do* know. Plus, you can never get help when you're a registry nurse. The staff nurses just don't care.

I've been through burnout a couple of times for various reasons. Nursing hasn't really changed, it's me who has changed because of what I've seen. I got into nursing because I wanted to make a difference and improve the quality of people's lives. From what I've seen, people really don't want to make the changes they need to in order to make their lives work right.

There was a study done that showed that eighty percent of people who are discharged from the hospital on lifesaving medications will stop taking those medications within one week of discharge. It's similar in chemical dependency—you can try and try to help them help themselves, and only about one in ten will get out and stay clean.

After I'd bounced back and forth between ICU, ER, and chemical dependency, I came to where I am now—night shift supervisor in an adult psychiatric unit.

One thing I've learned being a psych nurse is that nobody else in medicine wants to deal with psych patients. They get rubber-stamped through medical and sent back to us right away. Sometimes these patients are really sick and we'll have to send them back out to critical care, and quick as a switch, they'll come right back within a few hours. We had a couple of patients with potentially fatal blood alcohols that ERs have medically cleared and sent to us.

Even departments like housekeeping don't like coming into the unit. We take in all the geriatric psych patients, and one of their favorite things to do is to be incontinent and then wipe it all over themselves and the walls and furniture. We have had more than one housekeeping employee literally quit on the spot in our unit.

We have a lot of great things to use in psych nursing, like guided imagery or hypnosis. They're techniques that have been around for a couple hundred years and they're really effective, but they aren't *cost-effective* as far as the hospital is concerned.

I developed this simple program in psych in order to cut down on the number of meds we had to give out. The first night they'd come down and demand their sleeping pills, we'd tell them they had to listen to the relaxation tape first. They'd go nuts, screaming and yelling—then come back and slam the thing down and get their pill.

Second night, they'd grumble, but take the tape. About forty percent wouldn't come back because they'd fall asleep with it on.

The third night, about eighty percent wouldn't come back for the pill. But little by little, the headsets disappeared, and then the tapes, and pretty soon the hospital stopped replacing them, and so we went back to giving pills.

When patients come into the psych hospital, they get evaluated for intake and assessment. They'll show up with as many as six suitcases full of their worldly possessions, because the family just drops them off and they think they're going to stay for the rest of their lives.

Some of the patients have what's called borderline personality disorder. They're the worst because they live to cause trouble. They thrive on attention and will do anything—including deliberately initiating conflicts—to get it.

We had one borderline woman who sat in front of the nurses' station one night and told this story about how her mother had tortured her with a steak knife when she was five. As the story went, the family dog had had a litter of puppies and the mother ordered her to kill them one by one. Every time she refused, the mother would slice her with the knife.

At this point in her story, she would show off the scars that covered her belly and her arms. Her audience—mostly male—started to get more and more upset, and the next thing that's happening is they're demanding she get her medications and then the therapist be called in, and the staff is upset and divided over how to deal with the situation, and eventually, the patient has all this wonderful attention from both the staff and the other patients, and she's allowed to get an extra dose of her medications and she goes to her room and sleeps. The other patients were upset for days over this.

About two weeks later, the same woman is admitted, and lo and behold, she starts telling this exact same story—the same voice inflec-tions, the same pauses, the same timing of the sobs. This time, however, her audience is mostly female, so the puppies are now kittens.

It was a beautiful performance, but needless to say, I nipped it in the bud before she could so much as wring one helpless baby kitten's neck.

A month later, I came into work one night and found that she'd been admitted again. When I came out of report, I noticed she was on the phone. Well, we all go on about our business, and eventually she hangs up and goes to her room.

About ten minutes later, two policemen come to the door and ask to speak to me. Apparently this woman has reported that I had made death threats against her.

Now I'm in a bad situation, because I can't reveal anything about the patient because it's all confidential, and the nurses' notes are all confidential. This is stressed even more so in a psych hospital because of the stigma that's still attached to the psych patients.

I explain to the officer what a borderline patient is, and that I've not had any contact with the patient at all during this admission. Well, this policeman talks to her, and he's convinced that nothing like she re-ported had happened, so he lectured her about how using 911 to report a false emergency is a crime, and that was the end of that.

Except there are two hours' worth of paperwork that needs to be filled out—incident reports and notification notes. I also have to call the doctor involved, who wants her put into seclusion.

So we put her into locked seclusion, which is more paperwork to log that in, and of course she won't go until there's a crowd of other patients around, all of whom end up getting upset, and then they all have to be medicated and calmed down, which is more paperwork and time.

Manipulation is part of the game here. One of the funniest things that we've noticed is, here you have all these psychotic patients who are stumbling around, being crazy, talking crazy—*until* there's an earthquake.

I'm telling you that when there is an earthquake, you have never seen so many people get so normal so fast. Their speech is no longer slurred, they stop shuffling, they make complete sense. They come to the nurses' station in an orderly manner and want to know, one, what's going on, two, where should they go, and three, what do they need to do?

It's funny to watch—it's instant cooperation and organization. It lets us know who's playing games.

Even though I only work four nights a week, I don't know if I'll stay in psych nursing. Every day I deal with people who aren't psychologically wired right, so I'm seeing people at their worst. If you're in this environment long enough, it sneaks up on you and you begin to get depressed. You don't notice the depression until life loses its qualities and you realize all you're doing is sleeping, getting ready to go to work, and dealing with psychiatric patients.

After a while you find that you become suspicious of other people's motives. It's difficult to socialize when you're always wondering what kind of psychological profile people have. Too, I think psych nurses get used to keeping their emotions in check. It's not easy or healthy. After a while you don't take as good care of yourself as you should.

Appreciation is another problem. The one time I did get a note of thanks was from a nurse. She was going through some hard times—her marriage was breaking up, and then a boyfriend killed himself after that, then another relationship broke up. It got to the point where she was considering suicide. I spent a couple of all-nighters talking to her and finally got her to a therapist so she could get the help she needed. I got a Christmas card from her that said: "Thank you for saving my life." I still have that card. I read it every Christmas. It lets me know that I have made some kind of difference in at least one person's life.

Echo Heron

I wanted to share this story for two reasons. One is a lesson I learned about never underestimating human will. The second is that even when you think you've seen it all, there's always something lurking around the corner, just waiting to take your breath away.

I was whistling when I showed up at work. It was one of those days that I was happy as Larry to be alive and healthy and not in need of any of the services I was about to give in the Coronary Care Unit.

Then I looked at the assignment board. The whistling stopped abruptly. I'd been floated to ICU.

For some of the CCU nurses, myself included, ICU was scary territory—filled with unfamiliar procedures, obscure diagnoses, and strange equipment. It was one of the most unpopular places to be floated to, not only because it was scary, but also because the floated-in nurses always got the train wreck patients the regular staff didn't want.

Sure, I dealt with a lot of the same problems whenever I worked in ER—gunshot and stab wounds, massive head injuries, exotic diseases— but emergency medicine was a different kind of nursing. ER nurses stabilized the patients and got them out as quickly as possible—we didn't take care of the aftermath.

The ICU staff—made up of tough-as-nails nurses who knew their stuff inside and out—was pretty scary too. I generally tried to stay as far out of their way as possible, hiding in my patients' rooms or moving at such speed through the unit that I was an unrecognizable blur. I was always afraid one of them might ask me a question like: "Hey, what's Mr. Jones's ICP reading?" and I'd think: *Mr. Jones has an ICP line? So that's what that thing is coming out of his head!*

I received report from the day shift nurses. I was to care for two non-English-speaking Mexican brothers who were STS (sicker than shit), but after ten days, no one had been able to figure out why. I had a two-day postop laminectomy patient whose fever could not be brought down below 104. He was somnolent and each time he was moved, he'd vomit from the headache pain. He was on every-thirty-minutes vital-sign and neuro checks.

My fourth patient was Emma Swenson.

I knew about Emma because I'd been the one who received her in the emergency room two weeks before. Then, the following day, I'd had her as a patient in CCU. Now I was going to have her again—kind of like leftovers that would not die.

The story, as revealed by the chart history, the daughter, and eventually the hairdresser herself, went like this:

Mrs. Swenson had had a standing appointment with Nancy, the hairdresser, for a wash, tint, and set every Tuesday morning for the last six years. She'd never missed an appointment.

On this particular Tuesday, the six-foot Swede had driven herself to the beauty salon and stumbled into the chair, barely making sense. Nancy noticed Emma was perspiring and pale gray—Emma, not her hair.

Nancy also couldn't help but notice the unpleasant odor the woman gave off. Still, Emma insisted she felt fine and would Nancy please get a move on because she had a book club meeting in an hour?

As the beautician laid her client back in the chair, she noticed that the lower half of Emma's dress was soaked with something which, judging from the smell, she thought was a broken colostomy bag. Being too polite to say anything, she continued to wash while Emma continued to get more gray and sweaty until, halfway through the shampoo, she had a seizure and 911 was called.

By the time we got Emma in emergency, she was in shock. Emma's daughter told us her mother was a diabetic who was on steroids. She had complained of an abdominal "upset" from time to time over the week, but refused to go to the doctor even though she had a fever and no appetite.

What we found when we took off her dress was a necrotic hole through the upper right quadrant of her abdomen. Amazingly, she had infarcted her bowel in the recent past and the bowel, the abdominal wall, and the skin had been necrosed by gram-negative bacteria.

How in God's name she had managed to function through the pain and the sepsis was beyond all of us. Then again, what would we have expected from a person who had a hole through her belly but only complained of an upset stomach?

Perhaps if she'd been smaller she would not have had the resiliency, but at six feet and 186 pounds, she was working with a lot of reserve.

Then, on top of that, she was in atrial fibrillation, which had to be controlled before she could go to surgery. Thus I took care of her the following day in CCU.

I don't know what happened the night she was admitted, but when I came in to work CCU the next afternoon, I could hear her screams from the first floor. CCU was on the third floor.

By the time I got report and went to her bedside, she'd been converted out of her fibrillation, and preop routines had been initiated. No amount of pain medication could control the woman's agony.

Her daughter was present. So was the priest. Last sacraments were administered, and the surgeon told the daughter to say goodbye—her mother's chances of surviving the surgery were one in a thousand.

I signed over Emma's chart to the surgical tech and told him the situation was "grave"—no pun intended. Halfway through surgery, the surgical ward secretary called to inform us that Mrs. Swenson's heart had stopped twice, and they were having a big problem keeping her blood pressure up, no matter how many vasopressors they poured into her. She also mentioned that so much of the woman's bowel had necrosed that the surgeon was considering stuffing it all back in, closing her up, and letting her go.

So sure was I that the woman would not survive, I shipped her belongings to registration, which was where the daughter would be sent after her mother was pronounced. I had her room cleaned and gave it away to another patient before I left my shift.

To say I was incredulous when I discovered that the Emma Swenson in the bed in front of me was the same Emma Swenson who was at death's door two weeks before is an understatement. I was rendered speechless—an extremely difficult thing to do in my case.

Peter, the nurse who'd taken care of Emma on day shift, started report by asking how many other patients I had. When I told him, his eyebrows shot up to meet his hairline.

"She's my only patient," he said, "and I haven't been to lunch yet. Didn't they explain about her dressing change?"

I shook my head. I wasn't sure who "they" were. If he meant the charge nurse, she'd hidden when I came into the unit.

Peter gave me a glance that an executioner might give before pulling the trapdoor. (It was the *God help you, you poor bitch* look.) "Well,"
he began with a deep sigh, "she's on reverse isolation, and her dressing
change has to be done twice during your shift."

"Uhn-huh." What was the punch line?

"It's a wet-to-dry dressing."

"Yeah?" I was tapping my finger on my knee. Waiting.

"And it takes about an hour and a half . . . maybe two if you count
gathering your equipment first."

"Two hours? You mean, like one hundred and twenty minutes for
each dressing change?" I thought he was kidding.

He nodded. "Yeah, maybe give or take a few minutes either way."

I'm terrible at math. I mean, I carry a twenty percent tip chart when
I eat at restaurants, and I still use my fingers for subtraction and addition. But I do know that two and two makes four.

"Four hours? I have three other patients—what are they supposed
to do while I'm spending four of my eight hours in here?"

Peter shrugged. "Maybe somebody can help you."

"Oh please. I wasn't born yesterday, Peter." I was furious. "She's on
every IV antibiotic and every treatment known to modern medicine.
There's no way I can—"

I stopped ranting. The aphorism that I had learned to live by over
the fifteen years I'd been in that particular hospital came to mind and I
relaxed: *I'll do what I can with the one brain and the two hands and legs I
have. Other than that, it's out of my control.*

"Now, tell me about this famous two-hour dressing change."

Honestly, I didn't believe him. Even after he went over it step by step.

I wrote down the list of what I'd need: eight boxes of these, six
packages of those, a bushel of them, four bottles of that. I made an overall estimation of the procedure: pull out the old dressings, pack in the
new—saline-soaked ones first, then damp, then dry.

Okay, no problem.

In my mind, Peter's credibility went to hell when he described
the surgical wound. "Cavernous" was the main word he used. As a
writer, one learns early on in the game that the more one embel-
lishes, the more spellbinding the story. But—I still worried over it.
Even though Peter was a fiery-tempered Italian, he was not an
embellisher.

He also told me to medicate Emma with ten milligrams of IV morphine an hour before beginning the dressing change, because although she claimed not to feel pain, she had a tendency to get anxious and move around a lot if she wasn't completely under, and, he said, "She really needs to be under, Ec. Like, waaaaay under."

Okay. So I'd medicate her—way under—and tend to my other patients. I was sure that what had taken Peter two hours was going to take me about twenty minutes tops.

I mean, a dressing change is a dressing change is a dressing change. It wasn't like I was going to do a spot of brain surgery here.

I'd preordered the list of dressings, gathered every conceivable supply I might need, and gowned up for isolation.

Emma was pleasantly snockered and snoring by the time I was ready to change her dressing. Her vital signs and general assessment were fine, all within normal limits. I hung new IVs and hyperalimentation lines, tidied her room, and set up saline bowls and an elaborate sterile field for my dressings.

What an exaggeration, I thought as I unpinned the scultetus binder—a sort of jumbo cummerbund which held the dressings in place. Why would Peter purposely mislead me?

Using a pair of hemostats, I pulled back the flaps of the binder and removed the top layer of dressing, which consisted of five thick pads that were maybe twelve inches by nine inches by one inch thick.

As soon as they were all off, my mind went into hyperscramble, and my jaw unhinged of its own accord.

My first take was that some jokester of a surgeon had painted a huge mouth on the woman's belly—for just under the rib cage, a red strip of raw flesh about thirteen inches long was peeled back, resembling the upper lip. Then there were the "teeth"—a ten-inch-wide gap that was filled with white gauze dressings. The red "lower lip" of flesh was situated just above her pubis.

The corners of this mouth turned up into a smile which ended at her hips.

Okay. Now, I've had people hand me limbs, ears, fingers, toes, once a nose, twice scalps with the hair still on them. I could do the job, I said to myself. No problem.

Uhn-huh. I was feeling uncomfortably warm and slightly nauseated.

I checked the clock and began picking out the gauze pads, one at a time, layer after layer. They were all saturated with fluid ranging in color from clear to yellow to light green to light pink. The smells ranged from medicinal to bad.

About three inches down into the hole, I began to feel dizzy. I kept looking at the way the edges of her flesh were all curled back. I had instant recall of my anatomy class with Dr. Ryno and Fred, the twenty-semester-old cadaver. Fred was like working with a big, man-shaped piece of beef jerky.

Emma was like beef in the process of being dried for jerky.

I wanted to get my face out of there. I wanted to look at something else, but had to pay attention to what I was doing.

The wastebasket was overflowing, yet I could not bring myself to crush down the contents with my foot. I didn't want that mess on the bottoms of my shoes. With the side of my foot I pushed a clean waste-basket across the room.

Peter had said to make sure all the stuffing was out before I began restuffing. He'd said to lift up the flaps (lips?) and look up inside for stray gauze pads. Use a flashlight, he said.

I was sweating by the time I changed my gloves. I'd been instructed not to change into a new pair of sterile gloves until I was ready to soak and repack, but I was too far inside the abdominal cavity to be comfort-able with that.

I picked up a flap of something—no idea what structure it might have been—and found a wad of stray gauze. A kind of dull whooshing sound started inside my head, and the overhead fluorescent light sud-denly seemed unbearably bright.

Following Peter's advice, I found a flashlight and set it down on one of Emma's ample thighs, aiming the light into the cavity.

I regloved and reached under the upper lip . . . er, I mean flap, lift-ing it up. I looked into the hole—it was like looking inside a two-hundred-pound turkey ready for stuffing. Pat dry, then lightly sprinkle with salt and pepper.

I swear on my cat's ninth life that I could see the apex of her heart beating. My hands grew unsteady, and I had to use my shoulder to wipe the sweat beading on my forehead. My mask was saturated and starting to slip down my face. The noise roaring through my head rendered me deaf.

Then I saw it. Far up—at the very top of the cavity—was another wad of gauze. I leaned over the cavern, snatched the wad, and stepped back to get some air and check my stuffing mix.

Then I looked back at Emma. I was far enough away to be able to take her in as a whole. It wasn't such a good idea, because she looked exactly like a woman who'd been sheared in half. Her upper body was large and stately. She had a lot of white hair, a big face with strong features, and very broad shoulders and chest. Then there was raw carnage, and then a sudden rising of huge hips and legs.

Blue and white spots swam past the periphery of my vision, a warning sign that I was going to pass out. All I could think of was what would happen if I fell into that hole. Would I die? Would Emma die? How long would it be before they found us? What if my waist-length braid escaped my hair cover and got snagged on something in there—would they have to cut my braid off? What if I got some of that green stuff in my mouth—would I have to be hospitalized or would I end up in the psych unit as a stark raving lunatic?

The blue and white spots were taking over my vision as quickly as the roaring train in my ears got louder.

One of the more interesting features of most ICUs is that there is absolutely no privacy. ICUs are usually either one big room where the beds are separated only by curtains, or rooms with windows for walls. This was the glass wall type of ICU.

A passing housekeeper's attention was drawn to the overflowing wastebasket. When she looked up and saw the pale gray of my face, she had the presence of mind to call a nurse's attention to the person swaying over the patient.

Not stopping long enough to don isolation garb, the nurse ran in and caught me as I fell. She (and about ten other people as well) told me when I regained consciousness that I was aimed—face first—right for the dark cave.

I still had to finish the dressing change, although the nurse in charge made me sit down to do it. She ran a strap around my chest and attached it to the back of the chair so that if I passed out again, I wouldn't go far.

When I was finished, I checked the time. The whole procedure, including my brief attempt at escaping reality, took just two hours and five minutes.

The one thing I took from that experience—other than a recurring nightmare about being sucked into a giant turkey cavity—was the conviction that Emma would not live.

I would have wagered everything I owned (all previously owned by Goodwill Industries) that this woman who seemed to be cut in two, her insides open and begging to host any opportunistic bacteria floating around, would be dead inside of seven days. I had been only inches from her innards. I mean, Christ on a bike, I'd practically breathed on her liver.

But no—Emma walked out of the hospital a couple of months later and immediately went to get her hair done.

I was happy for Emma. I believe in miracles, and Emma was a walking miracle.

Then, just about a week ago, I was talking to Emma's gastroenterologist, who said she complains from time to time of a fleeting sharp pain in her gut that comes on with a sudden position change. She says it's not anything she can't live with.

How nice for Emma. I'm the one who can't live with it—to the point where I've been losing sleep.

See, it wasn't until the next day, when I could bear to look in a mirror, that I realized I was missing one of my earrings.

Of this I am sure—somewhere in Mrs. Swenson's cavernous belly there swims a small, twenty-four-karat dolphin which belongs to me.

Colby B.

"There's no easy way to say this, but I guess if you're the patient and you're mangled and barely hanging on to life, and are being kept alive with all this technology, then you see me as the angel of mercy.

The family members probably see me more as the angel of death.

Whatever it is, I'm dedicated to assist these people and their families and the physicians in letting go."

Colby B. has been an R.N. in the ICU of a large Massachusetts hospital. The eighth of ten children born to Italian Catholic parents, he grew up in a small mining town in Minnesota. Immediately after high school, when the Vietnam War was at its peak, he joined the military as a corpsman.

Following the military, he went to work at a small hospital and began college as a premed major. After being rejected by fifteen physician's assistant programs ("I was a white male with a low GPA—a perfect affirmative action specimen," he laughs), he was sidetracked into the environmental sciences. He graduated with a degree in marine biology and went to work for the National Marine Fisheries Service.

"But the intensity of the whole hospital scene was in my blood. After three years of researching the effects of pollutants on striped bass, I said hey, these are fish, not people. I need to feel like I'm doing something worthwhile.

"I immediately quit and went to a hospital where I was hired as a phlebotomist. I knew the first day I walked in that this was where my whole being needed to be. That environment was for me."

Colby went to nursing school and has worked in the intensive care unit ever since his graduation eleven years ago. Presently, he is working toward his master's degree in healthcare administration, although as he comes closer to graduation he says, "I'm beginning to wonder what the hell I'm doing this for. I'm having a lot of feelings about not wanting to leave bedside nursing, because, you know—I really do love it."

My role as a nurse has developed over time. When I started I was basically a gung ho technical guy who loved all high-tech stuff and the trauma, and I went at it full force. Now, I see that my real expertise has come down to helping people die.

My first significant experience with terminating care on an individual took place in a seven-bed, dark and windowless ICU which was tucked into a far-off corner of the hospital. I had been assigned to a gentleman in his mid-sixties—a dentist. This guy had a long history of depression with many suicide attempts and had been under the care of psychiatrists for quite some time.

One morning he'd been walking along the road in front of the hospital and decided to put a shotgun to himself and blew the front of his face off. At that moment, one of our more illustrious plastic surgeons happened to be driving into the hospital parking lot and actually witnessed the whole thing—fortunately for the guy's face.

The first three days were just a god-awful mess. Even though the plastic surgeon had done a great job, the guy's face was still pretty grody. We had him on a respirator and scads of IV drugs. Then, about day three, the doctors and the shrinks all got together and decided to let this man go.

I remember being galled by the decision. But being a very young nurse, and not really knowing how to handle the situation, I went into the gentleman's room, roused him a little, then told him that the decision had been made to let him go.

Well, at that point he became agitated and began to cry.

This unglued me no end. Here I was going to extubate this guy who would surely die as soon as I did, and he was seemingly not happy with that decision even though his life had been a wretched mess up to that point.

As I was breaking down and losing it and not knowing how to handle myself, this psychiatrist—an elderly woman—saw I was having trouble, put an arm around me and pulled me aside. She then proceeded to tell me that this was what he really wanted.

I extubated him an hour later. I was upset for days, but I also realized that this guy had taken extreme measures to kill himself a number of times.

The experience was significant for me, too, because it was really the first time I realized the extreme fragility of life and what power physicians and nurses have over controlling life and assisting death.

Much of my experience with handling the dying comes from the neurologic patient. A short time after the dentist, I took care of a woman in her late forties. One of her three kids was getting married and they were out shopping for a wedding dress. As she was getting into the car she turned to her daughter and said, "I've got the worst headache I've ever had in my life." Those were the last words she ever spoke.

She passed out in the parking lot. She had a cerebral aneurysm and a major bleed and we kept her alive for about a week. On the third or fourth day she showed signs of brain death. Of course, the family was just devastated.

The husband reminded me a lot of my father. He was one of those men full of pent-up emotions who couldn't express any of them and was just dying inside over what had happened. The kids weren't much better. I knew what the husband must have been going through, so I managed to get him to open up to me, and as a result we got pretty close.

Dr. M., an internist specializing in respiratory problems, was on that case. As my primary mentor, his kindness and compassionate way of handling situations have taught me how to be gentle, how to be open, and how to be honest. When someone's time has come, it's come, and a lot of the artificial means we have of keeping these people alive is ridiculous.

We did decide to let this lady go. I brought in the whole family and Dr. M. shut off the respirator. I made sure I stood close to the husband.

Of course it only took her about six minutes to die, and everyone, including myself and Dr. M., broke into tears. I wrapped my arms around the husband. He bawled and thanked us for all our care and . . . it was . . . very ah . . . tough time . . . It . . . [Colby stops the tape.]

I went home at the end of one of those days knowing that I had really contributed to the universe. Letting someone die and assisting families and coping with the stresses of a dying parent or spouse is a lot of work. It takes a lot out of you. But the satisfaction that I derived from helping these people whose universe has been ripped right out from underneath them is amazing.

They look at you with those pleading faces. *How did this happen? What is going on? Oh my wife, my mother, my son . . . How can this be?*

And you, as the nurse, have the strength to help these people through to the other side.

A good example of someone who could not deal with the stress was Maurice. He and Susan had been married for only a year, when Maurice woke up to find Susan unconscious. She too had had a cerebral aneurysm, and was not brain-dead, but the damage to the brain was so severe that she would never return to any conscious state.

We had her during her acute phase after the initial surgery for about six weeks. Once she was stabilized, she left ICU and went to rehab—not so much for her, but to teach Maurice how to care for her body.

Susan returned to ICU about four or five times with either pneumonia or fever of unknown origin, and each time, Maurice would be at the bedside, and each time he'd be more and more emaciated and wasted and torn emotionally. He could not let go.

Every time he'd come in, I got a little closer to him. Ultimately he began to hear what I said. To most of the staff, Susan and Maurice were a travesty. We could not understand how anyone could force someone they loved to live on like that—without dignity as the body deteriorates and contracts.

It was much easier for him to talk to another man, and I think he was grateful to have me there. Ultimately Maurice decided to let her go, and of course the sad thing was, when we pulled the tubes out, she didn't die.

There is a real fine point with a neuro patient where you've got to make a decision relatively quickly. Making the decision quickly in a patient who's had a brain hemorrhage is a very difficult thing to do.

Think about it. Here you have an individual who has just sustained a major injury. The likelihood that this person is going to come out of a comatose state and not remain vegetative is very slim. On the other hand, it is also very likely that the body—the physical self—will survive this injury given time. If we put a patient on life support and keep him going for two or three days, and the swelling goes down, many parts of the brain will remain intact and this person will stay in the vegetative state indefinitely.

Once we decide that this person does or doesn't have a chance, then we need to give this information to the family as fast as possible so they can make their decisions. That's where my role comes in, and it is one I play strongly. I gather all the information I can from all the sources, and all the physicians; then I can work with the family about their loved one.

I feel them out first by asking simple things such as, "Are you aware of what the prognosis is? Do you know that if your loved one survives, they will never be able to communicate with you in any way? Do you know the best he will ever be able to do is blink?"

For the families, this is almost unimaginable. After all, just two hours ago that son, or that daughter, or that lover was a vibrant human being doing what they did in life and then . . . *wham!* Now they're comatose in bed, and some stranger who they have never seen before is suggesting that their loved one isn't going to return to them as the person they were.

It isn't something that the average person can even comprehend, let alone make a decision in twenty-four to forty-eight hours about turning off life support.

When presenting bad news to the family, I find that it's best to be frank and open and slightly to the harsh side. You have to be as honest as you can—none of this "Well, there's a slight chance . . ." shit.

You must learn to say, "It looks like your daughter isn't going to come back anything like you remember her. The chance that she'll recover anything short of a vegetative state is almost nil. The best thing we can do is withdraw life support. Think about what her life will be like. Make this decision now before it's too late . . . before you have a vegetative individual."

And you know, we don't always make right decisions either. I remember a young gentleman, seventeen years old, who was in a motor vehicle accident and he presented with all the bad signs, with decerebrate posturing, blown pupils—everything that said this guy ain't gonna recover.

He went to surgery and part of his frontal lobe was removed because there was so much swelling. With all that information and the neurosurgeon extraordinaire's experience, and my experience, we were all consistent in our belief that this kid had no chance of recovery.

We attempted to convey this to the boy's family. It was a divorce family. Mom and Dad didn't talk. They had two separate camps—Mom's and Dad's. The mother was in concurrence with us and could grasp this concept of letting him go.

Dad was another matter altogether. There was no way in hell his son was going to remain vegetative and not come out of this. He didn't care what we told him and there was no way he would allow us to stop anything; he was going to see to it that we did everything that could be done.

We of course had to do what he wanted, but we thought it was a great injustice to this young man, and that we were right and the father was wrong.

A month later we sent this kid off to rehab. One month after that, the young man came into the unit walking, talking, and making jokes.

When you're wrong it can work against you too. There was another case that was publicized nationally. A young kid was visiting his mother for the summer here from the East Coast, and decided to get a job and stick around. Well, one night he's walking home from work, and he steps off the curb, and *wham!* he gets smacked by a bus.

Well, it was the full-court press: surgery, intracranial pressure monitoring, ventilator, pressor support—looked really bad. The ICPs kept falling out, ventriculostomy tubes [a shunt to drain fluid from around the brain] had fallen out and been reinserted, there were high ICPs with very little perfusion to his brain. God, it was pathetic.

I believe it was the third ventriculostomy tube that had fallen out when the mother put her foot down and said, "That's it. No more. I don't want you people to do anything more to him. Take everything out. Enough is enough. Leave him alone."

So we extubated the young man, pulled all his lines out, said our goodbyes, and I'll be damned if the kid didn't wake up the next morning.

The reason stories like these two work against you is that the next time you talk to another family member with another comatose patient, they say, "Yeah, but I read about this kid that got hit by a bus and woke up. . . ."

Then we have to explain that eighty-eight to ninety percent of the time, they don't wake up. These kids' story is rare. If we can't convince the family to turn things off, then they are left with this vegetative body for however many god-awful years it takes for the person to die.

I've made my share of mistakes, believe me. It's a part of my life that I never learn anything well until I blow it. Then I go, *Ah gee, I guess I really fucked that one up! Time to do it another way, Colby.*

A good case in point here was a thirty-two-year-old gentleman who had some arterial-venous malformations in the past and had had several surgeries to try and correct the problem, without much success.

His right arm had some partial paralysis, but he worked like a son of a gun to overcome it and was apparently a guitar player. According to his parents, he was also "full of life."

Well, this guy just lived to play his guitar, which, I was told by several people, he did quite well. Anyway, when we got him, he'd had another bleed from an AV malformation, and it didn't look good.

There were signs of brain stem function, but no higher signs of life. The family was having problems with letting him go, although the physicians were suggesting he needed to be taken off life support.

Well, feeling like the miniexpert that I feel like sometimes, the family came into the room to visit and I thought that I would try to impress upon them the fact that he really was gone, so I decided to demonstrate to them some of the clinical signs of brain stem damage.

First I took his right arm—at this point I didn't know that he was partially paralyzed and that this was the arm he loved to play the guitar with—and I squeezed his nail bed very hard to show them that he didn't withdraw from pain.

Well, they're all looking at me with this look of absolute, abject terror.

So then I said, "Here, let me show you something called doll's eyes—another sign of brain stem damage." So I took his head and sharply turned it side to side, and of course his eyeballs basically stayed fixed, staring straight ahead.

Well, again I got this look of absolute horror, and all of a sudden the father says, "That's enough. We have to leave now." About fifteen minutes later the sister comes in and tells me her father wants to talk to me.

So I go out to the waiting room and the father lit into me with all the force of a hurricane. He said, "Who in the hell are *you*? How do you get off doing these horrible things to *my* child? That was the most despicable, disgusting display I've ever seen in my life . . . You have no respect for human life."

Then the mother cut in: "You caused him pain in his bad arm. How can you live with yourself?" Then the sister proceeded to rip me to shreds for fifteen or twenty minutes.

Well, I was in tears. I could not believe I had fucked up this bad. I was trying to demonstrate to them what the story was, and never stopped to think that this was not something you showed the parents of a dying son. This was not compassion, this was not caring. So, I never did that again. I found another way.

A recent experience I had that I'm still trying to work through was with a thirty-two-year-old gal—just a beautiful woman named Melanie. Melanie was single, physically gorgeous, a VP of an accounting firm, very bright.

She'd been at a party on a yacht. She met a man and they decided to go to dinner at one of the restaurants on land. Even though she'd had a few drinks, and he hadn't, she insisted on driving her car. For some reason he agreed to this, and they went to her car. The road that went out of the parking lot and to the highway had a pier that angled off of it. She took the pier instead and went right off into the bay.

When the divers found them, all the windows were up and they were both in the back seat. It looked like they'd tried to get out but . . . It was a very traumatic scene. They were both submerged underwater for a minimum of fifteen to twenty minutes.

The man did not survive, and she arrived to us asystolic and looking pretty anoxic. She was converted back into a sinus rhythm, put on a ventilator, and had an ICP inserted.

What got me initially was that this girl had so many friends and parents who loved her very much. There was such a lot of outpouring of emotion, and ah . . . [He begins to cry. The tape is stopped.]

I took care of her all three days she was with us. Her friends— hordes of them—came on an hourly basis and would tell me stories about her.

I'm still working out why I did, but I think . . . Well, actually my wife brought this out . . . I think that . . . [a long pause here] It bothers me to even say this, but ah, I think I loved that girl. She was like every girl I'd ever dated: she was gorgeous, vibrant, and smart. I can't explain it. I wanted more than anything to take care of her. I wanted her to get well. I wanted to do everything I could to save this precious woman. And yet it was evident there was nothing left to save. She'd been without oxygen for too long. But still, I did everything I could. I went the extra ten miles for her so that if by some miracle she could recover, she would.

But it was all for naught and I knew it. So, at day two I began my usual speech to the family and the friends. "We have to come to some decision here. It looks bad. All the information says Melanie will never be the same. . . ."

The third day it was more and more evident that Melanie was beginning to go downhill. She got edematous and began to look dead.

There is a point when a patient takes on the look of death and you know that their soul has left their body and that they are nothing but so much flesh lying on a mattress hooked up to so much artificial stuff.

I'm sorry but I've got to stop for now. I can't talk right. . . . [The tape is stopped.]

I think the really sad thing about Melanie's case was that on her driver's license she had indicated that she wanted to donate her organs. It was evident that she wasn't going to survive, but it was also evident that she wasn't brain-dead.

Often in people who have a cardiac arrest and have an anoxic injury, they have an intact brain stem, and to be clinically brain-dead, you have to show signs of brain death. You can't breathe on your own, your blink reflex has to be gone, and no gag reflexes, your pupils don't work. Melanie did have working pupils and she did take a few breaths on her own.

So, despite all the tragedy here and her desire and her family's desire to donate her organs, it was going to be impossible because she was not brain-dead, and there isn't any way to make someone be brain-dead.

When they disconnected her from life support, I had to leave. I couldn't deal with it. I was fried. She died about seven hours after the disconnect.

I went home an absolute zombie. I couldn't talk to anyone. At the time, my wife didn't know what was going on.

The next day I got on-line and wrote E-mail to all my brothers and sisters and told them everything about Melanie's case. It proved to be a real catharsis for me, because I got out how horrible I was feeling, how tragic it was, how fragile life is, and how instances like this slap you upside the head and show you that your life is all you've got, buddy, and it can be over in a flat instant.

I'm married and have two kids, a boy and a girl—five and three—

and I love them all to death. I wouldn't be able to do the things I do without being able to go home to them and be with them.

Appreciate what you've got. Hug your wife and your kids, because you could be dead tomorrow. I call it "stopping the world." Melanie stopped the world for me.

Lesa B.

Lesa is a twenty-four-year-old nurse whose mother and grandmother were nurses. ("It's a genetic thing.") Now a divorced mother of two, she has worked in long-term care facilities, Alzheimer's facilities, dialysis units, and detox wards. She also works as a paramedic on her off days.

When I asked her how she felt about nursing as a career, her answer was instantaneous and direct: "It's not a career—it's a lifestyle. It is your whole life. We are the ones who really see and take care of the patient. You have to be open-minded and compassionate and never lose your perspective . . . keep your head no matter what is going on around you and take care of it. In other words, you have to be one hundred percent nurse."

I did many of these interviews over the phone, and usually the nurses had one or two stories in mind that they wanted to talk about. Not Lesa. She rattled off a list of stories, one after the other, giving each about a thirty-second spot. She barely took a breath in between.

I went over the tape four or five times, trying to figure out which stories to present and what style to use, when it hit me that I'd just list them exactly as she did.

Well, there was one time on the ambulance when we got a call from the sister of a woman who had a bad infection in her leg, and she was telling us that her sister was delirious she was so sick.

So we go to this house where these two eighty-year-old spinster sisters live. It's the middle of July and it's about 100 degrees and we walk in, and they've got the heat cranked up to 90. The whole living room was wall-to-wall garbage bags, and the stink was horrific. When we asked them why they had the garbage stacked in their living room, they said they just couldn't bring themselves to part with it.

After we get in there, these two sisters are fighting because the one called 911 on the other. She really didn't want to go, but we went ahead and took the one to the hospital anyway, because even though she wasn't delirious, she did have a bad open sore on her ankle and had been wearing the same sock over it for three months.

In the ER she was screaming obscenities and throwing things at the nurses. Nobody could touch her, so we had to bring her back to the house. Well, the second time we drive up to the house, the driver noticed that every garbage can in the whole neighborhood was painted bright, neon colors but each one was completely smashed and dented. When we asked one of the policemen about it, he said that these two women still had their licenses and they always drove with the Club still partially attached to the steering wheel.

Every time that location comes up as a call on the scanner, everybody freezes.

Then there's our Scottish Alzheimer patient. Every time someone takes her to the shower, you have to sing Scottish ballads with her or she'll try to get you with the shower hose or throw the soap at you or something.

One day, the nurse taking care of her stopped singing . . . you know that song, "You take the high road, I'll take the low road . . ."? Well, this old lady turned on the shower hose full force and wouldn't let anybody near her. One of us finally surrendered and went in there and sort of wrestled it away from her.

I had another Alzheimer's lady who was really mean when she first came in. She'd bite and scratch and yell obscenities, but for some reason, I was the only person this lady liked. Except she started calling me Dorky, and I remember saying to her, "Hey, what kind of talk is that? That's not very nice to be calling me a dork, you know."

That went on for a few weeks until her daughter came in and I found out that her best friend's name was Dorkus.

One night we've got a patient in the back of the ambulance and we roll up to the hospital, but it has a gate that requires the entry of a code. So I go up to the door of the ER and I pound on the door and this nurse comes up to the window and says, "Yes, may I help you?"—she sounds just like Lily Tomlin doing Ernestine.

I told her I needed the numeric code to get in the gate, because we had a patient for them. Then she says that she can't give me that information.

Now I ask you, there I am in my uniform with an ambulance behind me, we've already radioed ahead to tell them we're coming in, and this bingo brain says she can't give me the code?

So we're arguing back and forth when a janitor walks by and takes it all in and gives the nurse a dirty look and me the code.

Sometimes the ER nurses really don't seem to like us when we bring in patients. Like last week we were bringing in a couple of stab wounds and as soon as we walked in, the nurses started yelling at us to go away. I don't blame them. They were treating a walk-in gunshot wound, a triple electrocution—somebody touched a live wire, and then somebody grabbed him, and then somebody grabbed that guy . . . sort of like a chain electrocution? There was a mother-and-child spinal meningitis case, three victims of an earlier MVA, and another stabbing, which had happened right outside the hospital in the parking lot.

My favorite story is about this Alzheimer's patient who twenty years before had quit smoking. Well, one day she told us that she needed a cigarette.

We told her she didn't smoke, but that didn't cut it with her, so she ended up screaming all night that she wanted a cigarette. Finally, one of the nurse's aides cut a straw to the length of a cigarette, painted one end red and the other end light brown like a filter. Well, for weeks, this woman was completely happy with her plastic cigarette. We even made her a pack of cigarettes and gave her an ashtray.

She'd ask for a light, then just sit there and smoke it for a while, then put it out. We'd find ashtrays full of her "cigarettes."

The best part was when she finally started to complain that her cigarettes didn't have much flavor.

Sometimes, working in an Alzheimer's unit, you've got to get a little nutty. I remember this one forty-eight-year-old man who'd had a stroke and had come down with MRSA pneumonia and was on a vent in our subacute unit. Well, you'd walk in there and you just knew that somebody was home behind those eyes. I felt we had to keep him going somehow, so whenever we'd go in, we'd tell him jokes—even dirty ones. He loved those. You could tell he was laughing, because he'd start bucking the vent.

With MRSA we all had to be masked all the time. So we'd paint teeth and lips on the outsides of the masks with big smiles . . . or just goofy things like that.

One day he was really depressed—you could just tell by the look in his eyes. Well, I went out and got a couple of the aides and we took a

bunch of face masks . . . the kind with the ties? And we tied them together and made ourselves these sort of string bikinis which we painted
with nipples and other anatomical details and then put them on over
our uniforms . . . We walked in and his face just brightened up so much.

We also have an Alzheimer's lockdown unit, and usually their dinners all come up at the same time. One night they all got strawberry
shortcake for dessert. So, as was my habit, I went from room to room
making sure they were eating and that everything was okay.

Every one of those patients had put their peas on top of their strawberry shortcakes. By the time I got to the last room, my curiosity was
killing me, so I finally asked this one lady why they were all putting
their peas on top of their strawberry shortcake—was it a secret code,
like a secret handshake or something?

She said: "It's good, girlie, so don't knock it until you try it."

We had a retired R.N. with Alzheimer's who went around taking
care of the patients; she'd wake them up and give them bed baths and
take their pulses, and try to feed them things. We also had a patient
who was a retired police officer who had worked the night shift for
thirty years. Well, every night at eleven o'clock, he'd get up and walk
the beat, which was the halls. He'd look in each room just to make sure
everything was okay and there wasn't any criminal behavior going on.
Every once in a while we'd give him a flashlight and let him check the
rooms. That always made him happy.

He'd go to bed at 7:00 A.M. and sleep until late afternoon. It had
been his schedule his whole life and we weren't about to change it.

Oh, and then there was the time we got a bomb scare, and the time
a patient's bra was hooked up wrong and the daughter reported us to the
police. And there was the patient we had who . . .

Oklahoma City Bombing

I remember hearing the news come over the radio on April 19, 1995, that a bomb had exploded in Oklahoma City. My first thought was if there would be enough medical personnel to cover the event. Silently, I blessed the nurses and docs in my own agnostic way and wished them all the best. Little did I know that almost two years later, I would be talking to five of those nurses, hearing their stories firsthand.

This was not an easy chapter for me to write. I taped all five nurses during live phone interviews. After the first interview, with Courtney Nield, I had nightmares about wandering around blown-up buildings. By the time I finished my last interview with Jan Williams, I realized I hadn't been able to get through any of the tape transcriptions without weeping.

In the weeks and months following the bombing, we all read and heard about the many acts of bravery and dedication. No American who saw the now famous photo of fireman Chris Fields holding the lifeless body of one-year-old Baylee Almon went untouched by the horror of this American tragedy. On our television screens we watched firemen and police going into the rubble to pull out the victims both living and dead. What we did not see were the countless scores of nurses and physicians who worked in the chaos behind the scenes to save those who could be saved.

The following story is about a handful of those unsung, behind-the-scenes heroes who went beyond the call of duty in Oklahoma City.

WEDNESDAY, APRIL 19, 1995

5:15 A.M.

Dana Scholl, twenty-five-year-old staff nurse at Presbyterian Hospital ER, didn't particularly want to be a nurse. In high school, she saw nurses in the same distorted light as most others did—the pill-pushing, bedpan people. After working as a registration clerk in Presbyterian ER, she decided there was a lot more to the profession.

One of "Presby's" youngest ER nurses, she has been an R.N. for exactly one year as she begins this day in her usual leisurely way. Dressed in her scrubs, she eats cold cereal, catching snippets of TV news.

5:30 A.M.

Jan Williams, forty-one, has practiced nursing for twenty years in Oklahoma City emergency rooms. Fascinated by anatomy and physiology, and considering that "God has done such a wonderful job in creating the human body," she decided in high school that she wanted to know how it worked and how to fix it when it broke down. An LPN for eighteen years, she has been an R.N. and Presbyterian Hospital ER's assistant head nurse for two.

On this morning, Jan is fighting a stomach virus. Getting ready for work is slow going due to intestinal cramps which keep her running to the bathroom every few minutes.

In lieu of breakfast, she sucks on ice chips while driving the twenty-one miles to work.

6:00 A.M.

Georgia White, R.N., thirty-eight-year-old director of Presbyterian Hospital ER, begins this mild spring day with the usual chores involved in running the small farm where she lives with her husband and son.

A nurse for twenty years, she has worked in oncology, ICU, nursing homes, chemical dependency, and health education. It is, she says, the flexibility of the profession which has allowed her to change her life.

During the thirty-minute drive to work, she thinks about the first order of business on her schedule—an 8:30 A.M. supervisory enhancement meeting in which she will learn about the latest hospital policies and how best to put them into place with her staff.

6:45 A.M.

There is nothing unusual about Dana's eleven-mile drive to work. When she pulls her Camaro into Presby parking lot, she makes a mental note that it is going to be another sunny spring day.

Inside the department, she greets Jan Williams, who is treating a patient left over from the night shift—a diabetic nurse from another unit suffering from low blood sugar.

Dana turns the radio on and commences the routine beginning-of-shift activities of restocking equipment carts, general cleanup, counting drugs and narcotics, and taking report from the shift going off duty.

APPROXIMATELY 8:50 A.M.

Jan tends to a seven-year-old boy with conjunctivitis.

Dana thinks it might be a slow day for the ER.

9:00 A.M.

For no particular reason, Courtney Nield, R.N., EMT, wakes suddenly from a sound sleep and jumps out of bed. Still tired from being up late the night before, the twenty-seven-year-old gets back into bed thinking she'll get a few more minutes' sleep before she begins her day.

Following in her grandmother's footsteps, she has wanted to be a nurse for as long as she can remember. She has worked in Presby ER for almost two years.

9:02 A.M.

Three miles from the Alfred P. Murrah Federal Building, thirty-three-year-old Katharine Cranwell, R.N., EMT, paramedic, is sound asleep when a loud explosion violently rattles the windows of her house and knocks her onto the floor. She realizes almost at once that there has been an explosion and expects that if she looks out the window she will see her neighbor's house blown to bits.

But next door the house is intact—along with the rest of the normally peaceful neighborhood. Her neighbors are streaming from their homes to look around. In the background, sirens begin to wail.

She goes back into her house and turns on the TV. There are no reports of any explosions, but when she picks up the phone, the line is dead. In the next room, a news broadcast breaks into the regular programming with the announcement that there has been an explosion in downtown Oklahoma City.

Presbyterian Hospital ER, where she has worked on the 3:00 P.M. to 3:00 A.M. shift for a year and a half, is less than two miles from the explosion site. Knowing she will be needed, Kathy automatically gets into her scrubs and prepares to head to the hospital.

At the supervisory enhancement meeting, Georgia is sitting at the back of Presby's auditorium. She recalls: "I was bored. I had my knees up against the back of the chair in front of me, and my head was back. All of a sudden I was jarred out of my chair by a loud explosion which rattled the windows."

Looking around, Georgia sees the three elevators just outside the auditorium. She is convinced that one of them has snapped its cables and crashed.

While people are getting to their feet, asking each other what has happened, the five-foot-nine nurse is up and running toward the walkway which leads to the third level of the parking garage. Long-legged and moving fast, she gets there before most other people. When she looks out over the city, she sees a perfect brownish gray mushroom cloud rising into the sky over downtown. She thinks a gas main has blown.

All around her, people are gathering and confusion is mounting. People are still asking each other what has happened. Suddenly focused, Georgia has one thought: to get to the emergency room stat. Running across the garage, she passes the hospital's vice president. "I've got to get to ER," she yells to him. "I've got a feeling a lot of people are going to be coming in."

In the ER, Jan has had another attack of cramps and has just come out of the bathroom, when she feels the floor move under her feet. Immediately she thinks of earthquakes, then thinks to herself, *Wait a minute. We don't have earthquakes in Oklahoma.*

Convinced that the disturbance has come from the construction going on at the end of the block, she thinks, *No big deal,* and begins typing out discharge instructions for the conjunctivitis patient.

9:07 A.M.

Dana, sitting Indian style on a chair at the nurses' desk, has not felt the explosion.

Georgia bursts through the back doors of the department, hanging on to the door. "There's been an explosion at a building downtown," she announces loudly.

It does not register with Dana exactly what she means.

Jan walks over to the nurses' desk and says that she felt the ground shake, although she is convinced that Georgia is overreacting. She wants to tell her to calm down and relax, and that it's probably no big deal—only construction going on.

Dana initially interprets the disruption in a similar way: "I was thinking: *Wow, this is kind of cool. I want to go out and see if I can see any smoke.* I was heading out for the parking garage to see what I could see, when Georgia put herself in front of me so I could see her face. She said, 'Dana, this is a disaster. There was an explosion and there's going to be a lot of injured people coming in here.'

"And it was like, BOOM! All of a sudden I saw the panic in her face and I couldn't swallow. My stomach went into knots. I realized suddenly that I had never seen Georgia flustered before."

Dana runs to the parking garage and looks toward the downtown area, where a huge cloud of black smoke is billowing into the sky. The reality of the situation clicks into place and she switches into high-gear adrenaline output.

Okay, she thinks, running back to the ER. *This is it. This is a real disaster. We've got to get ready stat!*

She stops at the outpatient eye surgery department behind the ER, and tells them she needs their beds. No one there is aware there has been an explosion. As she pulls out the extra beds she knows will be needed, she tells them a building has collapsed.

Georgia recalls that the television was on in the ER: "There were a couple of regular ER patients who'd come in for treatment who were now glued to the screen of the TV. As soon as they understood what had happened, they just said, 'Hey! We're outta here. See ya later,' and were gone."

9:08 A.M.

Courtney is awakened by a policeman friend, who has called to ask if she has been mobilized. In the background, she can hear sirens. When she asks what he's talking about, he tells her, "There's been a gas explosion downtown and a lot of people are walking around cut."

She turns on the television and flips through the channels trying to find some news. Stills of news reporters are on the screen with voice-overs saying, "We are on our way downtown in response to reports of a major explosion . . ."

She throws on a scrub top and tries to call Presbyterian, but because all cell phone and land-line capabilities have been lost, she cannot get through.

Within minutes, Courtney is speeding to the Broadway Extension and drives fifteen miles south to Presbyterian. From the highway, she sees a large plume of black smoke rising into the sky.

9:10 A.M.

Kathy leaves her house. On the drive to the hospital, she is extremely aware of what she will describe as "a weird atmosphere." Despite the police cars racing past her, the air is very still. The same eerie stillness is noticed by many others on this day.

9:15 A.M.

At Presby the decision to call a disaster has just been made. Unable to get through to outside ER personnel, Georgia manages to reach the hospital operator and tells her to page the triage officer to the ER.

Georgia has turned to Dana, Jan, the ER doctor, a fourth-year resident, and the tech to give directions on how to set up the rooms and how they will oversee the flow of patients, when multitudes of hospital staff and onlookers pour into the ER. Georgia remembers: "All at once at least two hundred people poured into my ER."

A woman who has been in an auto accident unrelated to the blast comes into the department at that time. Jan does a quick assessment and hands her over to a surgeon who has responded to the disaster call. He does one of the fastest treatments she has ever seen in her twenty years of ER nursing: "He looked at the patient and said, 'Chest contusions. Admit her,' all within fifteen seconds."

When Jan goes out into the main room, it is like the entire hospital has descended on the ER, causing more chaos than she feels is necessary. "I walked around saying, 'Get all these people out of here! I don't want them in my ER.' But nobody seemed to pay any attention to me."

No one, she notices, leaves.

9:17 A.M.

Georgia, Dana, and Jan begin distributing the medical talent, placing several doctors in each trauma room. Each of the twelve treatment rooms and the two trauma rooms have at least one ER nurse. Three physicians are sent to do triage in the parking lot.

Georgia's best friend, Margie, an R.N. in the cath lab situated directly above the ER, walks into ER with five of the cath lab staff. At one time or another all six nurses have worked in Presby ER.

Margie hugs Georgia and says, "Here we are, babe. Where do you want us?"

For Georgia, the appearance of the troupe is like a gift from God.

9:18 A.M.

Dana runs past the two-way emergency-systems radio where Debby Kumm, the ER tech, is taking calls from EMSA (Emergency Medical Services Authority) ambulances that are on their way into the hospital. It seems to Dana that the tech is almost in shock. The calls are constant, one coming in immediately after the other has disconnected. Debby repeats, "Yes, we accept. Clear. Yes, we accept. Clear," over and over without a pause. Dana estimates that the ambulances that have managed to get through on the radio are only half of what is actually on the way.

Out in the parking lot, nurses, doctors, residents, triage officers, transport, and even the hospital engineers are lined up ready to do what they can.

Dana recalls an engineer approaching EMSA personnel and saying, "We don't have medical training, but what can we do? Please, we need to help."

He is told more back boards will be needed. By the time the need does in fact arise, the engineers will have made enough back boards to replace those used.

9:21 A.M.

When Courtney pulls into Presby parking lot, there are cars everywhere. In front of the ER, several neat rows of empty stretchers run all the way into the street, and boxes of medical supplies sit in piles all over the lot. A triage area has been set up to one side of the lot. One of the regular ER doctors is there, waiting to sort out the wounded as they come in. The walking wounded will be given a card and told to go to one place; the more severely hurt will be sent inside.

When she goes inside the ER, a person she does not recognize asks her name and then checks it off a list of employees. Courtney asks for details of what has happened and is told that a building has blown up and that the first wave of victims will soon arrive.

She doesn't recognize any of the people who are milling around her department. There are nurses and doctors she has never seen set foot in the ER before. A crowd has gathered around the TV in the ER lobby. It is the first time Courtney sees the nine-story Murrah building after the bombing. She believes someone at the TV station has gotten mixed up and is showing pictures of Beirut instead of Oklahoma City. It does not sink in immediately that the catastrophe she is looking at is just two miles from where she is standing.

Stunned, she walks to the receiving dock of the ER, where a car full of wounded pulls up to the curb. "Suddenly," she will recall later, "time just sped up."

9:22 A.M.

The first patients arrive in the back of an El Camino. The doors open and five bleeding people emerge. These five people were across the street on the south side of the building—the side opposite the bomb crater.

The majority of the north side of the building was made up of windows. With the explosion, all nine stories of glass became deadly flying projectiles. The first injured are suffering from typical blast injuries—ruptured eardrums and lacerations from flying glass, wallboard, and concrete. There are—and will continue to be—a high number of eye injuries and lacerations.

Immediately, more private cars, trucks, and minivans pull up and more wounded pour out.

Dana takes one look at the people being filtered through triage and runs back into trauma room 1. She orders the nursing students to begin spiking IV bags.

The first patient Jan sees is a man whose eye is bandaged. The EMT tells her it is hanging out of its socket and needs to be treated ASAP.

9:23 A.M.

Kathy pulls into the ER parking lot and stares at the scene taking place.

"There were injured people everywhere. I was full of emotion and thinking: *This is the real thing. I am an emergency room nurse and this is really happening right now.*"

She runs into the ER, where nurses, doctors, and medical supplies are packed into every available hallway and corner. Outpatient eye surgery personnel are suturing lacerations. Floor nurses are starting IVs and bandaging. A few of the regular ER nurses are having to act as gofers because they are the only ones who know where the supplies are.

All around her, patients are being transferred quickly to different areas depending on their acuity and the extent of their injuries. Right away, Kathy notices that none of the patients have IDs or charts. She finds this factor particularly distressing.

"I was so afraid that patients would fall through the cracks during the confusion and be lost. The inborn nature of an ER nurse is to document every detail about a trauma patient. We didn't even know any of these patients' names."

Outside, Kathy sees Courtney and Georgia standing on the ER receiving dock and heads in their direction.

9:31 A.M.

A paramedic opens the back of his rig and pulls out a large stretcher with a small child lying in the middle of it. The bundle is covered with concrete, ash, plasterboard, and blood.

Georgia looks at the face caked with blood and debris and thinks, *Oh my God, this kid is dead.* Courtney is not even sure what the form on the stretcher is. Kathy remembers seeing a small child without a face.

The EMT tells them it is a critical pediatric patient who needs an airway stat.

Kathy yells out that an airway is needed as Courtney and Georgia run with the carrier to trauma room 2. Pulling off concrete and dirt, Courtney discovers a child's face and determines his age at about three. As she wipes the caked-on blood away from the child's nose and mouth, he moans. He is barely breathing.

What is left of his clothing is in shreds. She finds that a bandage has been hastily wrapped around his head, and when she pulls off the dirty wrapping, what she believes are pieces of brain matter come with it.

Georgia turns away from the stretcher as a swarm of pediatric-neonatal intensivists—nurses and doctors alike—enter the room and surround the child.

At this moment, Jan enters the room to make sure the supplies are in order. As soon as she sees the serious laceration over one of the child's eyes, and the hole in his skull, she is convinced he will not live and wonders why the staff is working on him.

For a brief moment, she feels as though she is being watched. Her eyes automatically go to the ceiling. "There was such an eerie feel to that room," Jan recalls now. "When they told me later that the child didn't die, I said to myself, *That was his angel with him. That's who was watching.*"

No one knows the child's name is Brandon Denny and that he is one of only six survivors out of the twenty-four children who were at the America's Kids Day Care Center in the federal building that day.

9:32 A.M.

Jan calls out that an anesthesiologist is needed for a pediatric emergency in trauma room 2. She recalls being frustrated by the "fifteen thousand residents milling around the ER, doing what they wanted." Later, she will say, "It really wasn't fifteen thousand, exactly, but they were in my way, so it sure seemed like it!"

Kathy "latches onto" a terrified patient lying on a back board. Alert, he keeps asking what has happened. Wanting him to feel safe, she brings him into an empty treatment room and takes over his care. As she untapes him from the back board, she sees that strapped down with him are chunks of plaster and concrete. At that moment, the magnitude of the explosion becomes clear to her.

She splints his broken leg and gives him a tetanus shot. He is immediately taken to surgery. Kathy will not see him again. Later in the day, she realizes she never knew his name or what happened to him.

Dana treats a woman with bilateral fractures of her lower legs and a compound fracture of her right arm. The patient keeps trying to use her arms, but the staff holds them down. Days later they will discover that the patient is deaf and trying to use sign language.

"The weirdest thing about this period of time," Dana says, "is that I don't remember the patients' faces exactly. I only remember their injuries and the looks in their eyes. Scared. Shocked. Hollow. I also remember their clothes hanging in burned shreds from their bodies."

Jan also notices a common expression. It is, she says, "not so much the look of pain as disbelief . . . like they are in a dream. The unnatural silence and stillness of the air added to the dreamlike quality of the day. It was very disturbing."

Georgia recalls vividly: "Everyone needed to help. I can't tell you how strong that feeling was that day. We had transport techs, and high school students and the engineers all begging to help. There was a need for everyone to be a part of it—it was amazing. Every one of those people would have done anything to help out."

9:45 A.M.

Outside, chaos reigns. Ambulances arrive one after the other; the area of the driveway that has been set aside for triage is filled with people. The once neatly lined up stretchers are now scattered helter-skelter all around the parking lot. Many of them are occupied by bleeding patients.

An African-American woman, possibly in her twenties or thirties, is pulled from the back of an ambulance. As far as Courtney can see, her clothes do not exist. The woman's skin is covered in glass and dirt. One side of her scalp is completely torn away from the skull. Her screams echo through the emergency department.

Courtney takes hold of the woman's right arm to begin an IV, and her fingers find nothing but mush. Someone behind Courtney yells that the ambulances are calling for help at the site of the explosion.

9:47 A.M.

Georgia is directing the traffic inside the ER, when she sees a woman go by on a carrier with what looks like half her face torn off. She notices an ear is missing and the muscles to her neck and shoulder are exposed.

Georgia's most vivid memory, besides Brandon Denny's face, will be the amount of blood draining off of carriers, carts, and people. It is more blood than she has ever seen in her life.

It will be noted later in the new disaster plans that the need to clean bloody, grossly contaminated wheelchairs and stretchers was unanticipated but adequately dealt with. In an area outdoors, ancillary help—outfitted with protective gear—use garden hoses to rinse blood, glass, and concrete off the equipment, then wipe them down with disinfectant.

9:50 A.M.

Dana is treating a primary blast injury patient who has a variety of fractures, lacerations, and a large chunk of flesh and tissue missing from her neck. The patient is awake and alert, although she is intubated and cannot speak. Dana starts an IV and splints her fractures. Almost immediately the injured woman is sent upstairs to surgery. On the patient ID card, Dana writes: *Blond hair. Blue eyes. Splint left leg.* There is no time to write anything else.

Dana uses bottle after bottle of saline trying to wash dirt and concrete out of wounds. Runners who know the ER are constantly in motion, fetching supplies for the doctors and nurses.

Dana's next patient is a man with a bad laceration whom she will not forget because he is so happy to be alive. In shock he repeats the same question that is on most of the victims' lips—"What happened?"

A few seconds after tagging the happy laceration man, Dana runs past trauma room 2 and notices there is a great deal of hustle and bustle. People are running around trying to find an intraosseous needle (a needle which goes into bone—used only on young pediatric patients). She asks why they need it, and is told they are trying to start an IV on a child and cannot find any other access site.

Moving to the right side of the gurney, she sees a large jagged piece of ceiling tile covered in blood. One of the nurses turns to her and says, "He was in the day care center. We pulled this out of his head."

"He was surrounded by doctors and nurses so I couldn't see the baby," Dana says, "except for his little feet lying on the gurney. That and the piece of ceiling tile was all."

As she leaves the room several of the nurses say, "We're gonna lose this kid." In reply, the doctor says, "No. No, we're not."

Dana thinks: *This is a baby. This is just a baby. Why has this happened?* She allows herself to think about the small feet for only a few seconds more. She knows she has to keep moving.

Patients are walking in every door. Georgia is circulating to make sure everything is going smoothly. "I couldn't get involved with patient care. I needed to be able to see the whole picture in order to turn chaos into order."

Kathy is assigned as the tetanus shot nurse. Since most people don't know their tetanus status, an ER doctor tells her to give one to every person who comes in.

APPROXIMATELY 9:55 A.M.

"I remember around ten o'clock I started wondering about how long the rush of patients was going to last," Georgia says. "I knew my people weren't going to last forever and still maintain that level of energy. I knew I needed to start looking ahead."

Dana is heading back to trauma room 1 when she hears her name repeated over and over again in a bloodcurdling scream. Heading toward the source of the screams, she finds a young African-American woman lying on a gurney. From her right ear to the back of her head, the scalp is flapped over on itself. The nurses and doctors are trying to clean the area with saline.

Dana does not recognize the woman, and realizes the name probably belongs to a family member. But each time her name is screamed, her nerves go into a crunch.

Outside, near the lounge TV, there is complete silence among those who have gathered to watch. Dana dares to look at the screen, which has film coverage of the north side of the federal building.

"I absolutely could not believe my eyes. The air around the building was still filled with smoke, and I could see the rescue workers, but no one was coming out of the building. The sight of it was too much. I could not process what I was seeing."

Dana turns her eyes away and back to the bedlam at hand.

Jan tries to comfort the confused, screaming woman, who asks over and over what has happened and where is her sister, Daina?

10:05 A.M.

Georgia sees two African-American boys about three or four years of age sitting silent on a stretcher—two more of the six children to survive the blast.

"They watched the doctors and nurses running around, with those big, brown eyes open wide. In the middle of all that chaos, the sight made me smile."

APPROXIMATELY 10:30 A.M.

Sixty miles north of Oklahoma City, as Timothy McVeigh is being pulled over on I-35 for not having license tags, Courtney walks out of the room where Felysha Bradley is yelling for her sister. She is told by Mary Jack, another Presby ER nurse, that EMSA has called again, asking for nurses to come to the site.

Georgia knows that Courtney and Mary Jack are EMTs and have paramedic training. Feeling like a strict parent, she wants to say, "Don't go down there. Go back to your rooms and don't come out again," but she realizes that there are too many people in the department and that things are beginning to slow down. Soon she will have to begin sending people home.

With excavation of the federal building just beginning, the experts have said it will be a while before the second wave of victims hits the ER.

What no one realizes at the time is that with a bomb blast of such magnitude, there is no second wave of survivors.

APPROXIMATELY 10:40 A.M.

Courtney and Mary hop into a police car and are dropped off three blocks from the Murrah building. Courtney walks for a while and finds herself at the southwest corner of the building. Everywhere she looks, she sees broken glass.

There are ambulances and triage sites and hundreds of medical personnel standing around, but there are no patients. She notices people entering a hole on the south side of the building where there used to be doors. She expects to see victims being brought out, but no one is coming back out.

People are passing equipment and medical supplies into the building, although there seem to be more lines passing pieces of the building out.

Someone shouts that a worker has fainted. Courtney grabs an IV set and goes over to the fallen worker. She is waiting to see if he needs an IV, when to her right she notices a small playground.

On the ground lie body bags. Small body bags. And they are filled with children. Sticking out from under one of the bags she sees a foot wearing a tiny tennis shoe.

She is overwhelmed, unable to take her eyes off the shoe.

APPROXIMATELY 10:45 A.M.

At Presbyterian ER, most of the first-wave victims have been transferred to other departments for treatment and care.

Dana receives a page from her boyfriend, who is a paramedic. He is across the street from the site, he says, in a lawyer's office. His voice, which is normally deep and calm, is higher and speeded up as though, Dana recalls, "he had a thousand things to say and only thirty seconds to say it in."

He tells her that initially people were pouring out of the building. If they could walk, he told them to just keep walking to St. Anthony's Hospital, eight blocks away.

In the Water Resources Building, which stands across the street from the blast, he found a pregnant woman under a desk. Deeply embedded in the ceiling directly above her were large shards of glass and debris. He tells Dana that he intubated the woman and made sure she was transported out, even though he knew she was already dead.

Dana hangs up and springs into action with a team of students restocking and spiking more IV bags.

Kathy remembers overhearing the medical director say, "Now that the adrenaline rush is over, it's just going to be hard work." His words don't sit well with her. *We are nurses and doctors,* she thinks. *This is our work.*

They continue to wait for the second wave.

11:00 A.M.

In the administrative suites, Georgia attends a conference called by the CEO. It is a sort of regrouping effort—an examination by management of what mistakes have been made on the first wave and how they will improve on the second.

11:20 A.M.

Kathy and the rest of the ER staff are still waiting for the second wave of survivors which has not yet come. A woman from central supply tugs at Kathy's sleeve and hands her a yellow plastic gown and goggles, with the explanation: "Miss? I think you need to change or put this on."

Kathy looks down and sees blood covering her left pants leg. She has no idea where the blood came from.

Dana remembers it was hot and smoky inside the ER, the air smelling of plaster. She is still pumped up with adrenaline, ready to go. She walks around thinking, *Come on, let's go! We're ready. This is what we're trained for . . . this is why we are here. Please bring us more survivors. Let us do our job!*

12:00 NOON

The sister of one of the ER night shift nurses brings in platters of sandwiches, Cokes, and lemonade. Kathy goes to the break room to have a snack and catch some of the news.

A nurse she does not recognize is crying. Kathy puts her arms around the woman and asks if she's okay. In response, the woman shakes her head and tells Kathy that her daughter was in the day care center.

Shocked, Kathy asks what she's doing at the hospital and tells her to go find her daughter.

The nurse replies, "I could go home and drive myself crazy crying, or I could go downtown and add to the confusion, or I can stay here and care for patients. I just hope and pray that another nurse here in the city is giving my baby the same kind of care."

Kathy holds the woman tightly for a moment and lets her go. She will never see the nurse again, nor does she know what happened to the woman's child.

12:15 P.M.

Kathy picks up a call from the EMSA director requesting help. He wants to know if there are any nurses who can come to the site. Doubly trained as a paramedic, Kathy goes to Georgia for permission to leave.

Kathy feels her first priority is her emergency room, but since the ER is overstaffed and she is paramedic-trained, she thinks she may be needed more at the site.

Accompanied by several coronary-care-unit nurses, Kathy climbs into the back of a senior citizens' van, normally used to transport seniors to and from their nursing facilities. As the van wends its way through the city, she is amazed at the extent of the damage. Five blocks away from the site she sees broken windows and cars twisted into metal balls.

As the north side of the building comes into view, Kathy will remark, "I was horrified. Never having seen destruction like that before, the sight of it literally took my breath away. There was yellow police tape all around the front of the building. Hundreds of people were standing around in total disbelief.

"I remember someone on a loudspeaker saying they had more rescue workers than they needed and people should go back to their facilities."

Kathy does not heed the directive, but instead weaves her way through the crowds until she finds a paramedic crew she knows.

APPROXIMATELY **12:30 P.M.**

Mary Jack returns from the site and goes directly to the ER with the news that there will be no second wave. The realization descends on the staff in numbing silence: Those still left in the building are all dead.

Hope gone, the staff take on glazed expressions, staring at one another in disheartened silence. The personnel go on doing what they have to do to get cleaned up.

Mary goes next to the conference in the administrative suites and informs the managers of what she has been told.

Dana looks around the ER. There are two hundred IV bags spiked and ready, there are still multitudes of doctors and nurses . . . all ready to go.

When Georgia returns to her department, she also makes note of the spiked IV bags and all the supplies. The same two hundred people who were in her department when she left are still there.

Except there are no patients.

"It was eerie," Georgia says, "because it was so quiet. There wasn't any joking and hardly any talking going on. Some people were just staring, trying to take in what had happened."

APPROXIMATELY 1:00 P.M.

Kathy is on the south side of the building talking with the paramedic crew, who have requested her help in transporting a patient out of the building. As she walks closer to the building, she looks over to the lawn and sees what has become the temporary, makeshift morgue.

"That was the point at which I began to lose it," she recollects. "I just don't remember much of what was going on around me after that. I remember the sounds of crunching broken glass under my feet with every step I took, and seeing chunks of concrete all over the ground. I remember carrying a survivor out of the building, but I can't remember her face or her injuries. I only remember it was a female with dark hair who was conscious and talking. I can't remember anything she was saying."

A man approaches Kathy and tells her: "There's a young woman down there with her leg trapped. I need you to find a surgeon and send them down around to the back of the building."

Kathy climbs on top of a pile of rocks and starts to yell that she needs a surgeon.

A few moments later, Dr. David Tuggle approaches her. Kathy explains the situation and he disappears around to the south side of the building.

APPROXIMATELY 1:15 P.M.

Courtney has lost track of time. In her haste to leave her apartment, she has left her watch at home. She guesses it is sometime around one o'clock or after by the position of the sun in the sky.

Chris, Courtney's best friend and an intermediate paramedic, finds her in the crowds and tells her that there is a young girl trapped alive inside the building whom they have been with most of the morning.

Courtney's first thought is that she wants—needs—to help in some way. She is in the middle of this thought when a nurse appears and asks how good she is at starting IVs.

"I told her I'd done my fair share, so she handed me a hard hat and told me to follow her."

Courtney finds herself part of a group of two physicians and two nurses who enter the building through the hole which has been created in the south side.

"We all went down a ladder and then a partial staircase. I couldn't recognize anything as a building—only pieces of building. Bare wires were hanging down and blocks of concrete were lying haphazardly around. There was water everywhere and water pumps were running. Somewhere, it sounded as though jackhammers were in use.

"For about five seconds, I thought I really shouldn't be there inside that building, but then I saw a small group of people all standing around a young woman who they were calling Daina."

Daina is trapped on the ground floor by several large pieces of the building, her right leg crushed under a large concrete block. The block has stopped only a few inches short of crushing her entire body. The space in which she is imprisoned is dark and small—coffin shaped. Only one person at a time can be near her.

Courtney is told they are waiting for the engineers to come and tell them where and if they can cut the concrete block pinning Daina's leg.

When Courtney crawls inside the space and kneels down next to the girl, Daina looks at her and asks, "Are you going to try too?"

"I told her yes, I was going to try to get an IV line in, but when I picked up her arm it was icy cold and covered with dirt. The light was very bad, and I couldn't see or palpate any veins. I saw where others had tried and failed to get in, and I realized there wasn't any way anyone could have gotten a line in on her.

"I wondered if someone could do a cut-down, but it was just too dark and small a space to try. I could tell she was hypothermic. I didn't understand at first why her body was so cold, but then one of the nurses explained that when Daina was found, she was almost completely submerged under water pouring in from the broken water mains. They had to pump the water out."

Courtney is handed a bucket of medications by a doctor who was called to assist another trapped victim just around the corner.

Inside the bucket Courtney finds a lot of Demerol and a few syringes of Versed, a sedative. Dr. David Tuggle looks into the bucket and says, "You know, we may end up having to use all of that on her."

Courtney looks at him and at once understands what he is saying: If they cannot free the young woman, they at least plan to make her comfortable.

While they wait for what seems like forever for the engineer, twenty-year-old Daina continues to ask about her family, who had accompanied her to the Social Security office that morning where she was applying for a card for her four-month-old son, Gabreon. She asks if her three-year-old daughter, Peachlyn, her twenty-three-year-old sister, Felysha, and her forty-four-year-old mother, Cheryl, have been found. None of those present know that Daina's children and her mother have all died in the blast.

While she waits, Courtney studies her surroundings as they etch themselves in her memory forever. Blood is literally oozing out of the walls and dripping onto people's hard hats. She can hear moaning in the rubble, and to her left, she sees a human hand in a pile of debris.

Courtney is not entirely sure this is reality. She thinks she might still be in bed asleep and having a horrible nightmare.

APPROXIMATELY 1:30 P.M.

Outside the building, Kathy and over a hundred other medical personnel are standing around waiting for clearance to enter the building for more rescues. She is speaking to a paramedic when a Red Cross worker comes by with a box of Taco Bell beef burritos. Several of the paramedics grab a couple, while Kathy, a vegetarian, declines.

Suddenly someone yells, "Run! They've found a bomb!" All around her, police officers and firefighters begin running for their lives. A man runs past her full speed; on the back of his shirt is written "FBI BOMB SQUAD." The Red Cross worker drops the box of burritos and runs.

A passing firefighter scoops up the box on his way to safety.

In the most terrifying moment of her life, Kathy finds she cannot move. A paramedic pulls her into a nearby ambulance, where five other people are huddled together. The paramedic tells her the ambulance is the safest place to be because the vehicles are built to withstand explosions.

In the back of the ambulance Kathy is scared—not just for her life, but for Oklahoma and the United States. The other paramedics attempt to lighten the tension. Kathy remembers a few random comments: "So, Kathy—I'll bet this is your greatest fantasy—you with five good-looking men in the back of an ambulance?" and "Hey, anybody got a burrito?" and "Gee, I wish I had a Coke."

2:00 P.M.

At Presbyterian, the air is beginning to cool off, but it is still smoky and smelling of plaster. Everyone continues to stand by and wait for the second wave. Dana has realized that if victims are not out by now, they probably will not be coming out. No one knows for sure how many people were in the building at the time of the blast, but they do know the number has to be greater than five hundred.

APPROXIMATELY 2:15 P.M.

After what seems like hours to Courtney, the engineers give their consent to cut the concrete beam under which Daina Bradley is pinned.

Cutting through the piece of beam will free up an area of Daina's leg that Dr. Andy Sullivan, the smallest doctor on the scene, wants to get to to amputate. The beam cannot be completely removed because it is holding up a significant amount of debris. It is later found that the block of cement which has pinned Daina is holding up the center portion of the building.

After explaining to Daina what he is about to do, Dr. Sullivan crawls back out.

He asks who has the medications. When Courtney steps forward with the bucket, he jokes with her and Dr. Tuggle about how much Versed she thinks he ought to give.

Without an IV line, and considering that Daina is hypothermic, hypotensive, and having respiratory problems, Dr. Tuggle crawls in and gives Daina five milligrams of Versed intramuscularly.

Dr. Sullivan then enters the space again and lies on top of Daina, his face toward her legs. A few seconds later, Courtney remembers, Dr. Sullivan says, "Okay, we're starting now. Here we go. Here we go."

"And then," says Courtney, "the screams began. To this day, I still hear Daina Bradley's screams in my sleep."

Over Daina's screams, Dr. Sullivan asks for another knife. In the next ten minutes, he will go through several amputation kits because the saws and knives he uses keep dulling from hitting concrete.

"Dr. Sullivan asked for an instrument that none of us had," Courtney recalls. "I saw him take something out of his pocket but didn't realize that it was his own pocket knife until he told Dr. Tuggle that he'd used it to finish the procedure."

"Okay. I've got it," he says finally. "Let's go."

Courtney helps pull out the woman, whose right leg has been amputated through the knee.

With Daina on a spine board, the group heads out of the dark building, stepping over blocks of concrete and plaster. Chris steps into a hole and her leg is flayed open on a piece of rebar. Courtney steps into the same hole and aggravates a previous muscle injury in her leg, which will require three surgeries to repair. Behind her, a fireman curses as he injures his knee in the same hole.

Weeks later, Courtney will take comfort from the information that Daina remembers nothing of the incident.

2:30 P.M.

Georgia and one of the neonatal intensive care nurses take a break and drive around the block. As they drive, Georgia's husband pulls up next to them in his truck. Through the window he hands his wife a "survival kit"—a six-pack of Coke and some candy bars. He kisses her through the window and tells her he'll see her when she gets home—whenever that might be.

3:00 P.M.

Jan tends to a man who has walked into the ER complaining of chest pain. Calmly, he explains that he was on the fourth floor of the Murrah building working, when suddenly his computer and desk fell forward, taking him with them. He says that had he fallen backward he would be dead, because when he looked, there was nothing there. No floor, no building—just empty space.

It is the look on this man's face which finally makes Jan comprehend the full significance of what has happened.

When she finishes treating him, she goes to the lounge and looks at the TV. "It was the first time I saw it," she recalls. "I just sat down and cried."

APPROXIMATELY 3:30 P.M.

Jim and Claudia Denny walk into Presby ER asking if anyone knows the whereabouts of their three-year-old son. They have been informed that a Baby Doe with reddish blond hair is in surgery at Presbyterian Hospital. They believe it is their son, Brandon.

Jan notices that Claudia Denny is very quiet. Her husband seems scared. They tell the staff that after searching at the site and several other hospitals, they have located their two-year-old-daughter, Rebecca, at another hospital. Rebecca has a fractured elbow requiring surgery, and her skin has been peeled off the left side of her body by concrete and glass. A chunk of one-inch blue plastic, thought to be from the barrel encasing the bomb, has narrowly missed her jugular vein, drilled through her cheek and tongue, and lodged in her mouth. Although her injuries look worse than her brother's, Rebecca Denny will fare much better.

In ICU, Brandon is unrecognizable under his bandages. Jim Denny identifies his son by the birthmark on his upper left thigh. Only fifty feet from ground zero, both of the Dennys' children are miraculously alive.

3:45 P.M.

It begins to rain.

Transported to an ambulance staging area some four blocks from the building site, Kathy realizes she is wasting her time and heads back to Presby, where her regular 3 P.M. to 3 A.M. shift began forty-five minutes before.

In the Presby ER lobby Georgia sees a film clip of the bombed-out shell of the Murrah building and thinks it is Tel Aviv.

The chief of medicine comes to the ER and informs the staff that an employee of Presby had gone to the federal building on her break that morning. A widow of just seven weeks, she was going to apply for SSI benefits. No one has seen her since she left.

3:50 P.M.

Dana receives one of the last survivors—a young woman who was trapped under a desk. She started out on the fourth floor, but as the building shifted, she'd slid down inside the building.

"I don't know where I finally ended up, but I knew that water was rising around me," she tells Dana, giggling.

Dana is astonished that the woman laughs as she tells her horror story, but then realizes she is simply happy as a lark just to be alive.

"I was underneath the desk and EMSA was there to get me out," the woman relates, "when all of a sudden they said they had to leave because they'd been ordered out due to another bomb scare. I begged them not to leave me. When they came back I was just so happy."

Amazingly, she has sustained only scratches and bruises.

3:55 P.M.

Courtney helps Chris find her supervisor so that she can go to an ER and have her leg sewn up. As they walk around the north side of the building, Courtney sees the blast site for the first time.

She is so stunned by the view that Chris has to shake her "to snap her out of it."

4:15 P.M.

Courtney does not recall how she ended up back at Presbyterian ER, but when she walks in, she asks the first person she sees about the little boy who was treated in trauma room 2. Someone tells her he is dead. For her it is the last straw in a day of horror and destruction.

Jan is at the nurses' desk talking with her husband, a lieutenant with the OKC Police Department, when she sees Courtney walk in still wearing a hard hat. In a trembling voice, Courtney verifies that there will be no more survivors and that the blast was caused by a deliberately planted bomb.

Until now, it has never entered Jan's mind that the disaster was the result of an intentional act. Her world was shattered, Jan says. "I couldn't believe that someone could be filled with so much evil and have that much hatred for God and their fellowman.

"I was raised in a town of two hundred where you left your keys in your car and your house unlocked and open. People love. They don't hate."

As Courtney relates her experience of that day, Jan can see she isn't handling things well. She thinks that the young nurse will have problems later on dealing with the disaster because of the horrors she has seen that day down at the site.

Dana is shocked by the hollow look in Courtney's and Kathy's eyes. "It was as if I could look right through them and see the terror, disbelief, and helplessness. It's a look I still sometimes see on their faces almost two years later."

4:30 P.M.

"I don't remember the drive home at all," says Courtney. "I do remember taking off my scrub top and seeing that it was soaked with blood and dirt. I was so exhausted. God, I was exhausted, so I thought if I could just lie down to sleep . . ."

5:00 P.M.

Among the calls pouring in from neighboring cities from nurses and doctors offering their services, Kathy's sister calls her from Seattle to make sure she's okay.

Kathy is momentarily confused—her sister has never called her at work before. When she asks her sister what she means, her sister tells her that the Oklahoma City bombing is worldwide news. Her sister explains that there has been nothing else on the television all day.

6:00 P.M.

Kathy and other ER staff stay on the phones trying to identify John and Jane Does. They begin networking with other hospitals in an effort to connect unidentified patients with the people who have been coming in all day with photographs of their missing loved ones.

Several groups of staff have begun informal debriefings among themselves. Kathy refuses to talk about what she has seen that day.

Some of the staff are crying. Kathy is not one of them. Her attitude at this time is: *I'm strong and I can deal with this. It was a bad day and bad things happened. We did our best, we don't need to dwell on it. Let's just move on.*

Jan recalls: "We all talked about how intense the day had been, and how none of us ever wanted to go through that again. But did we sit down and talk about our *emotions*? No! We went over what we did for the patients—never how we felt inside."

7:00 P.M.

Dana is talking with some of the other staff when Rita Cink, the triage nurse, comes back in tears. She tells them there is a female patient who has come in with a broken jaw. She was in the building at the time of the blast, having just dropped off her eighteen-month-old son, Blake, at day care.

Despite her injuries, the woman refused to leave the site all day, telling rescue workers again and again that if she just found her baby, then everything would be all right. She has been to all the hospitals searching for her child without success.

She has found one of her baby's shoes in the rubble of the building, and will not let it be taken out of her hand.

Dr. Jerry Childs, a Presby ER doctor who has four children of his own, goes into the treatment room where the woman is sitting with her husband. When he emerges some time later, he is weeping in earnest.

With that, Dana, Jan, and Georgia leave for home.

APPROXIMATELY 7:20 P.M.

A woman comes in looking for her husband. Happily, she tells Kathy that someone from the Red Cross has called and told her he is at Presby waiting for her.

As Kathy calls around to the units, and then to the other hospitals, she watches the woman's face slowly change; the hope which lighted her face dissolves into a dark pain.

Kathy cannot believe the cruelty of the incident, after it is discovered the woman's husband was killed in the initial blast.

7:30 P.M.

When Jan drives into her driveway, her twelve-year-old son opens the garage door, wanting to know if she is okay. He tells her he felt the blast at his school, which is twenty-three miles away from the site. Part of his day, he says, was spent with two classmates whose father had been killed in the building.

Mentally and emotionally drained, Jan lies down and begins to watch TV. As soon as she sees the film footage, she understands why there will be no more survivors.

8:00 P.M.

Kathy receives another call from her sister in Seattle, who tells her her four-year-old niece, Jacquie, has seen the news and asked many questions in an attempt to understand what happened.

When Jacquie was told that her Aunt Kathy was there helping the hurt children, Jacquie ran to the phone and said, "We have to call Aunt Kathy because she is very sad."

Fifteen hundred miles away, Kathy's sister and her four-year-old niece sing the children's song "Sara Sponda" to her over the phone to make her feel better.

At home, Georgia talks out with her husband what has taken place that day. It is when he tells her that her mother has called from Pennsylvania to see if she is okay that she realizes the incident is national news.

10:00 P.M.

Dana debriefs herself at home by calling her mother and telling her what has happened. She also talks at length to her roommate, whose grandmother has been injured in the blast.

Shortly after, she falls into an exhausted sleep.

10:30 P.M.

Trapped by debris for over thirteen hours, Brandy Ligons, fifteen, is the last survivor to be pulled from the building.

Seventy-seven people have been treated at Presbyterian Hospital since 9:22 P.M. Twenty-three of those were admitted within the first four hours. All twenty-three will survive.

The reports on the final tally will vary, but it is estimated that there were approximately seven hundred to a thousand people present in the Murrah building at the time of the blast. The grim toll is 168 dead, and approximately 675 injured. Of the dead, almost all must be identified by fingerprints and dental records. Three of the deceased children are identifiable only by DNA testing.

10:35 P.M.

Unable to sleep, tortured by sights and sounds of the day, Courtney dresses and heads back to Presby just to be around other people who have also experienced the horror of the day.

11:00 P.M.

Georgia and Jan find themselves glued to their TV sets, also unable to sleep. As they watch the film clips and begin to comprehend the numbers of innocent people and children killed, they both feel angry and violated.

Jan, feeling for the rescuers who are finding the remains of victims, will call Presby ER five times during the night wanting to know if they need her to come back in.

11:30 P.M.

Courtney returns home emotionally and physically drained. She feels as though she has experienced in one day what most nurses see over an entire career.

Falling into bed, she tosses and turns all night, only dozing intermittently.

12:00 MIDNIGHT

A young African-American couple come in searching for their aunt. Kathy looks for her name on the lists of Jane Does and does not find it there. Finally she calls ICU and tells them she is looking for a forty-year-old black woman.

The ICU nurse tells her they have an unidentified woman but there is no way she could possibly tell her age due to the extent of her injuries. Kathy decides to bring the couple to ICU, explaining to them on the way what they might see, so they will not be shocked.

As they walk closer to the unidentified woman's bed, the young woman stops in her tracks and shakes her head. "No," she says emphatically. "No way. My aunt would *never* paint her toenails red."

While Kathy lingers in the ICU, one of the nurses tells her that the child "Brandon" has made it through surgery. She looks through the doorway of his room and sees a heavily bandaged child on a ventilator. She remembers him from earlier in the day as the little boy without a face.

THURSDAY, APRIL 20, 1995

Courtney returns to the site because of a driving need to be doing something helpful. She gives first-aid tetanus shots to the workers, many of whom are exhausted and suffering from lacerations and exposure.

Courtney makes note that many of the rescue people are still hoping to find survivors.

Dana gets up early and turns on the television. For the rest of the day she will not move from the house—she cannot stop crying long enough.

How could anyone do this to people? she asks herself in despair. *Especially here in Oklahoma City.*

Jan cannot bring herself to turn off the TV, positive that the building is going to collapse and injure the workers. She is thinking that the nightmare that was yesterday will be lived all over again. She continues to call Presby ER several times over the day to make sure they do not need her.

After an exhausted sleep, Kathy checks the news from time to time, but goes on with her daily life. That night she has a first date with a man who also works at Presbyterian. During the course of the evening, neither of them mentions what has happened the day before.

Georgia returns to work as usual, aiding in the cleanup, reorganizing, and debriefing which goes on all day. She recognizes that some of her staff are beginning to decompensate emotionally. She notes that staff who "wear their emotions on their sleeves" fare the best.

Presbyterian ER patient traffic is slower than usual—very few patients are seen.

FRIDAY, APRIL 21, 1995

AT 4:00 A.M.

Georgia volunteers to give tetanus shots to the workers for four hours.

She recalls seeing the building for the first time: "It was standing in the pitch-dark with all these floodlights pointed up lighting up the building and the rubble . . . It was a very powerful moment for me, one I will remember forever."

Later that morning, Courtney returns to the site for four hours. The triage tents have been closed down, but a sort of "quick shop" tent is open and dispensing snacks, beverages, and analgesics to the workers.

The body of Presbyterian Hospital employee Pam Argo, thirty-six, will be found and counted among the dead. Two of Dana's high school classmates will also be found.

Another nurse, Teresa Alexander, thirty-three, present in the Social Security office at the time of the blast, is pulled from the rubble, and her body identified.

SATURDAY, APRIL 22, 1995

The rescue dogs are growing more depressed because they aren't finding what they are sent into the building to find. The police send people in to hide just so the dogs can find them. It helps lessen their depression.

Jan returns to work day shift in ER. She notices that things are quieter than usual and business is slow. She later recalls that business did not pick up again until after the building was demolished—as if it were the ultimate signal saying, *Okay, now let's move on.*

Jan feels particularly bad for the medical examiners: "We were the ones blessed. We got the patients who were alive—not a perfect body, but at least repairable. The medical examiners received sometimes just a leg or a part of a face . . . I've heard the stories."

She packages up candy and sends it to them with a letter telling them how much they are appreciated.

That evening, Courtney returns to Presby for her usual shift. During the course of the night, she mentions to Kathy that she is particularly depressed over the death of the little boy she helped bring into trauma room 2. Kathy informs her that the child is in fact alive and in ICU.

Courtney runs to the unit and looks at the boy's face to make sure it is the same child. Until this moment, she has not even known his name. "I had gone through Thursday, Friday, and most of Saturday thinking that nothing had gotten accomplished. As soon as I saw this three-year-old alive, it made everything better."

SUNDAY, APRIL 23, 1995

Kathy is at church when her pastor says to the congregation: "I want all of my police officers and firemen to stand up and take our thanks for all your help."

Feeling like she's been slapped, Kathy stands up too.

After the service is over, a friend comes up to her and says, "I was thinking about you on Wednesday and I hoped you were doing okay." As he hugs her, she breaks down and cries—something she has never done in public.

At first she is surprised at herself. "The way I was raised," she explains, "you could not show that you were upset or that things were bothering you, so I coped by suppressing emotions."

Then she thinks, *Everyone here knows I'm an ER nurse, and if I'm not that perfect strong person I always try to be, who cares?* It was, she says two years later, "a freeing experience."

On this day, nurse Rebecca Anderson, the 168th victim, dies of injuries sustained when a piece of concrete fell on her as she went into the building to help pull out survivors.

MONDAY, APRIL 24, 1995

Dana is touched by the fact that drivers—including many out-of-state cars and trucks—are driving with their headlights on day and night as a way to pay their respects to Oklahoma City.

Kathy makes note of the fact that stores and movie theater marquees have replaced their usual billings with other messages: "God Bless Oklahoma," "Pray for the Victims, Survivors, and Rescue Workers," "Oklahoma City United."

TUESDAY, APRIL 25, 1995

Dana volunteers to go to the site and gives tetanus shots to the workers. The smell which hangs in the air, she recognizes immediately as that of rotting flesh.

"People who didn't know better, would walk by saying, 'Euew, what's that smell?' The medical people knew what it was, but did not say."

For the next ten days, the odor can be smelled all the way to Presbyterian Hospital.

WEDNESDAY, APRIL 26, 1995

Exactly one week after the explosion, at 9:02 A.M., the state of Oklahoma stops for a minute of observance. The workers at the site bow their heads; all traffic in Oklahoma City comes to a complete halt. In small towns all over the heartland, church bells ring.

"Oklahoma," says Jan, "showed how great it is. We might be down, but we are not out!"

SATURDAY, APRIL 29, 1995

Kathy goes to the site. The block is surrounded by a chain-link fence with police stationed at the entrances. A makeshift memorial has been started outside the northwest corner of the fence, where people have placed flowers, teddy bears, cards, letters, photographs, and even money.

Kathy passes a twisted wreck of a car on her way to the first-aid station. She recalls thinking: *A week and a half later, and this car is still here. Who did it belong to? Was it someone killed in the blast? Someone recovering in the hospital?*

"I looked around at the surrounding buildings and thought about how the bombing had destroyed more than human lives and property. It had destroyed the security I have always known living in the United States."

TWO WEEKS LATER

Dana discovers one of the infrequently used linen closets stuffed with cookies, candy, pizzas, and Cokes—obviously placed there as an emergency stash on the day of the bombing. Dana still laughs when she thinks about it.

The two African-American boys who sat so quietly on the gurney on the day of the blast have come back in with their grandfather to get the stitches removed from their heads and faces. As the ER doctor is removing sutures, Kathy feels a lump about the size of a quarter under the child's scalp. When she points it out to the doctor, he laughs and says: "I can't imagine how many pieces of that building are hiding inside people."

Jan is sitting in the emergency room reading a story in the *Daily Oklahoman* about how a worker found a flag in the rubble which was torn and had blood and body tissue on it. Without warning, she begins to cry. For two hours she cannot stop, and finally goes to talk to the chaplain.

TWO AND A HALF WEEKS LATER

Courtney does not go to the debriefings despite the notices posted around the department. "I didn't want to talk about it. I couldn't talk about it. I had so much stress in my life at the time. I was dealing with the loss of a close relationship, plus a divorce. The bombing was the final straw.

"I was averaging about four hours of sleep a night because I kept waking up hearing Daina and Felysha Bradley's screams. I woke up in a pool of sweat seeing the building and things blowing up around me."

Losing all coping mechanisms, Courtney makes what she calls an unconscious "M&M" attempt to take her own life by "snacking" on pills to help her sleep. "I just wanted to be able to sleep without waking up in sweats and seeing everything I saw, and hearing those screams over and over again."

Admitted to the hospital with a diagnosis of post-traumatic stress disorder, Courtney cries for four days straight. "I couldn't . . . I kept seeing all . . . All I could see was what happened down at the site. I just couldn't get my life in order. It was like I couldn't think about my life and not think about the bombing."

Finally her counselor tells her to concentrate on the good things that have come out of the disaster.

She concentrates on Brandon, who is doing well.

Dana is just getting a handle on dealing with the typical nonemergent patients who come into ER. Since the bombing, both her own and Courtney's feelings about the patients coming in for treatment have been: My God, how can you possibly come in here for something like that after what we've just been through? You don't know what sick is.

Georgia recalls the strange sensation that everything was moving in slow motion for a long time after the bombing. "It was similar," she says, "to standing outside watching a movie run at an incredibly slow pace. No one was up to par, as though all of a sudden there were other things in the world more important than oneself.

"Nothing got back to normal for a long, long time."

NINE MONTHS LATER

Kathy and Courtney begin to talk about the day of the bombing. Kathy realizes that her life feels unsettled and she is becoming increasingly irritable. She is frustrated and discontent. Recognizing the symptoms of PTSD, she contacts Project Heartland, a counseling service offered to anyone affected by the bombing.

By mistake she is sent to a victims' support group instead of a rescue workers' group.

"It was pure hell," she says in an edgy voice. "I stayed as long as I could to be polite, playing Elton John songs over and over in my head to keep from hearing them talk."

Later, she explains to her counselor that she feels like she didn't do enough, that she had the skills and wasn't needed. She wants to know— *Could I have done more?*

ONE YEAR LATER

Courtney and Kathy decide to go to the first-anniversary memorial service, but have a hard time finagling tickets. They are both bitter about the fact that the ER nurses who worked that day are not offered tickets, although they are being given away to firefighters and policemen coming in from New Mexico, Washington, and California. Kathy notes that although EMSA has been invited, not enough tickets have been made available for everyone to attend.

Kathy has discovered that the general attitude of the public seems to be: "Well, it's all just part of a nurse's job—whether you do it in a hospital, a blown-up building, or a doctor's office. Quit complaining about recognition. It's your job."

"No one looked at the nurses or paramedics as heroes," she says.

Jan stewed about going to the memorial service. "I wanted to go and I didn't want to go. It was really more for the families than for the rescuers. It was a time for them to make closure. I knew I would cry if I went—for the families, not me. My heart hurt for them, not me."

MAY 23, 1995

AT 7:01 A.M.

What remains of the Alfred P. Murrah building is imploded in eight seconds, with 150 pounds of explosives.

TWO YEARS LATER

COURTNEY NIELD:

It is still very rough for me to talk about everything I saw that day. It was frustrating because I didn't think that I did enough. I felt like my skills weren't used to the fullest.

It's been almost two years and I'm still trying to get back into the flow of things. I'm feeling pretty angry too. So many people got recognition—deservedly so—but the people who got ignored were the medical people. There were hundreds of medical personnel down there, and it's like we were forgotten.

The main things I took away from that day? Besides the image of Brandon Denny's face, I realized how fragile life is, and it made me look at how I deal with people and handle stress.

The most important thing, though, is that I am a survivor, and I am a nurse. That's what I wanted to be all my life, and it's what I will be for the rest of my life. I help people, and I was there on April 19 and I did everything I was able to do.

And, you know, I would do it again.

DANA SCHOLL:

Nobody is immune to disaster like this. I think I feel more vulnerable now—like, this can happen anywhere, anytime.

The good thing which came out of this for me was how people pulled together. In a time of crisis we're all pretty strong, you know. We didn't buckle. Oklahoma City has a lot of good people in it.

There are times, though, when I wonder why this happened. Those kids were so young and innocent. They had their whole lives taken away because . . . Well, we still don't know why.

I question if I did my best. Maybe I should have gone down to the site. Maybe I could have pulled someone out. I don't know, you just have to question yourself sometimes.

The nurses didn't get a lot of recognition for the part they played.

The firemen got most of that. I think the only nurse who was ever really recognized was Rebecca Anderson, who died. But see, the media was all down at the site where the firemen and the police were . . . so those were the people who got the coverage. The people behind the scenes were forgotten about.

We did get recognition from other nurses from all over the country, though. They sent banners and letters, cards, and food too. A whole class wrote us letters saying how proud they were of us and that they all wanted to be nurses or paramedics, and asking, "How are you doing?" and, "Are the babies okay?"

I never go down to the site. Never. I want to remember it the way it was before. The way the site has been commercialized and all the media? It's like it's supposed to be Oklahoma City's claim to fame. It isn't right. That's not what it was all about.

The one thing I will never forget through all of it was seeing Brandon's little feet on that gurney and the bloody ceiling tile. I will eventually replace that memory with the child I saw only two days ago—a bright-eyed, giggling Brandon, holding his father's hand, and half walking, half running to keep pace. Behind them, happily holding her mother's hand, was his sister, Rebecca.

GEORGIA WHITE:

As far as I'm concerned, just knowing what I and the other personnel did that day is enough recognition in and of itself.

That I could survive something like that and be capable of running an ER through mass chaos gave me confidence in my professional knowledge. Plus, just think about this: Most people will never be a part of anything like what happened here. We rewrote the disaster policy in our hospital. The information I got, I got firsthand. I didn't need to read somebody else's stuff—I lived it.

Like Dana and Courtney, the one image I can never forget is Brandon Denny's face.

If I could change one thing about that day, it would have been that there was a second wave and all those people weren't dead.

I just wish I could have done more.

KATHY CRANWELL:

The best thing is that I'm a more free person now. I mean, I cry—I don't have to hide my emotions. I'm not afraid of what people will think of me. If I'm hurting, people will know. I don't have to pretend I'm strong.

The one visual that I cannot shake is the face of the woman who came in looking for her husband after someone called to say he was alive—and then watching her growing frustration and fear as we searched for him.

Yes, I'm grateful too for all those people who came in from the outside, but I was there too, and I still live here. I live with this on a day-to-day basis.

JAN WILLIAMS:

The best thing was the coming together of all the people of Oklahoma City. It was like the whole city just stopped for a couple of days. There was no crime, and the gangs quit fighting for a while.

Even though I did not meet them, I feel close to the rescue people. They are a part of Oklahoma history forever.

I am a Christian woman, but when they arrested Timothy McVeigh, I never felt like I could hurt someone except for that day. I really thought someone would shoot him, like they had Oswald. I expected it. I wanted it. It was something that should have happened, and I was upset that it didn't.

The image that sticks with me is the expressions on the victims' faces . . . not your common accident victim in pain, not hysterical pain. They were all so calm and quiet. Maybe their calmness kept us calm.

I don't worry about who gets the praise and glory. God didn't put me here to be in the spotlight. My reward was knowing we did our jobs well. My rewards come from a patient's smile, a hug, or an "I love you" for just the smallest kindness. It makes my heart smile.

I never saw the bombed building in person. It was a conscious choice on my part not to go down there. I just didn't think I could deal with it.

Yesterday, I drove past the site. Ohhh, I just break out in chill bumps now just talking about it. . . . Where the building stood they've planted grass in there and they have a chain-link fence all around it that people have decorated with banners and little mementos to the memory of those who died.

I hope someday everyone can find peace with what they did, whether it was finding the bodies, counseling, taking equipment to the site, or just giving a needed hug.

"There was a large parking lot across the street, where all the cars blew up. Somewhere in that parking lot there's a tree that's still standing. It was completely burned, but now I believe it's sprouting again. They call it the survivors' tree."

—COURTNEY NIELD, R.N., OKLAHOMA CITY

Calista H.

Forty-nine-year-old Calista H. was born in St. Louis, Missouri.

When he returned from Vietnam after the war, he was sent to the Soviet Union as an embassy Marine. From there, he decided on a profession in healthcare, although he could not make up his mind between premed and nursing. The deciding factors came during a short stint of hospital volunteer work. There, he realized that while doctors had the final authority and led the team, they spent little time with the patients. Nurses did all the work, had the time to care for people, and saw the results of their work.

Having graduated from college in the meantime with a B.A. in biology and chemistry, he entered the "whiplash school of nursing" in 1978 and graduated with his bachelor of science in nursing in 1979.

He started as a labor and delivery nurse—his first love. "It was challenging and tough, and if things went wrong, it's really bad, so you've got to know what to do. Initially wary, the moms liked me. I'd walk into a lady's room and I'd say, 'Hi I'm Cal, your nurse. I've got a beard on my face, and a tattoo on my arm, and I'm going to help you through your labor.' "

Moving farther out west, he continued to hone his critical care skills in a variety of units until he found a full-time job working as an emergency department nurse manager.

Eight years later, the warden of the state penitentiary asked him to take the job as nurse in charge of the institution. "It really was," Calista says dryly, "quite a different kind of nursing."

Presently, he works as the director of an emergency department in the Pacific Northwest. His wife is a deputy court clerk. They have a son and two daughters.

Even though M. was only in his late thirties, he'd been on death row for many years when I met him. Originally, he'd been incarcerated in a county jail for drugs. Drugs were how M.'s fortune had been made—that, and smart investments in property and various stocks.

While M. was still in the county jail, he got into some kind of hassle with the county attorney, who would not allow several of his properties to have water or access rights. Somehow, he arranged to have the attorney's house blown up. It killed the attorney, his wife, and one of his two children.

They found the people who did the job, who turned state's evidence for a minimal sentence. The prisoner was tried and got life imprisonment.

M. decided—while in the penitentiary—to seek revenge against the person who'd turned him in. He arranged another murder.

When the man who had turned state's evidence was released from jail, he was abducted, taken to a roadside rest station, tortured, and killed. During the course of the investigation, the prisoner was again found out and tried for the death penalty. The case was controversial, to say the least. Trying a man for a capital offense that he did not actually commit but had only arranged and paid for while he was already in prison was a twist.

However, on the case was a very famous and clever prosecutor who did his job well. M. was found guilty and condemned to death.

As the date of execution came closer, the warden in charge of the penitentiary relied on me as the nurse to help him arrange it. There hadn't been an execution in the state for over twenty-five years, and the previous one had been in the old penitentiary in the gas chamber. Since then, the statutes had been changed and executions were now to be done using the lethal injection system.

I'd never been involved in anything like it before, never heard about it, never read about it, so I did a lot of studying. Some prison system people from Texas helped us out, since they have a lot of executions down there by lethal injection. I discovered that I was the one who had to order the drugs, and someone had to be chosen to start the IV. At first the warden even thought he might start the line, but we decided that wouldn't be very successful—I couldn't imagine some man strapped to the table and having an unskilled amateur sticking him ten times or more trying to start the IV on him that is going to end his life.

I talked to the state board of nursing to find out what my limitations were as a registered nurse to be involved in such a thing—I mean, it certainly wasn't something that could be considered nursing care.

The board said that as a nurse I would be able to start the IV, but could not inject the drugs. As it was, state law called for a citizen to be selected and paid by the warden as the person to push in the drugs.

So, as we got closer to the day, and it didn't look like there would be any more stays of execution, I ordered the drugs from a pharmacy. It was a standard recipe: sodium Pentothal: 2,000 mg [2 grams—five times the normal dosage], to be given IV push, followed by 100 mg of pancuronium bromide, followed with 100 mEQs [millequivalents] of potassium chloride. Usually they stop breathing with the sodium Pentothal. You give the Pavulon—the pancuronium bromide—to paralyze the respiratory muscles so they definitely stop breathing if they haven't already. The potassium chloride causes the heart to stop pumping.

It was spooky, doing something like that in cold blood. I didn't have a lot of previous contact with the prisoner—he was a pretty healthy guy who hadn't needed much healthcare. He had kept himself in good shape on the exercise machines provided on death row, and he didn't really have any contact with other prisoners.

I talked to M. a few days before and told him exactly what was going to happen. The warden and the guards and the counselor all said he was a personable man, intelligent and warm. I had to agree with them. He was a home-grown boy, not from some big East or West Coast city. He'd never been disagreeable, but M. was stubborn as hell—wouldn't give in to anything if he didn't have to. When he appealed his case, he did so as best he could, but never with anger.

I asked him if he wanted to donate his organs. I'd already checked with the organ procurers. It was a different kind of situation than they were used to dealing with, but they thought it would be okay since technically there wouldn't be anything wrong with the organs; the medications weren't poisonous or damaging to them. Initially, M. was a little surprised, and then amused by my question, but he didn't want to give anything away.

A few days before the execution, I practiced with the guards about how they would bring him out and strap him down. I set up the IVs, and taught the citizen how the injection would work.

The mood of the prison was not terribly antiexecution, believe it or not. The prisoners are a fairly practical bunch; most of them realize they're in prison because they screwed up—even if they don't admit it. They knew this particular person wasn't someone they would want to be involved with, but at the same time, it made people unsettled and nervous.

The execution was scheduled for midnight. There were demonstrations outside the penitentiary with news crews and reporters and the whole circus. I'd picked up the citizen at a private location, and then drove him to another location, where he was picked up again and driven inside in an unmarked vehicle. We arrived early to avoid all of that mess and waited in a quiet spot inside the penitentiary.

Just after midnight, the guards came in and strapped the prisoner down to the table, which was in a grilled cage outside of two isolation cells. There were curtains over the entry windows and the vehicle bay windows, so that no one could see me or the citizen.

Outside one of the entry windows was a room where witnesses could view the execution. We entered the compound wearing surgical outfits—gowns, masks, gloves, hats. I hooked M. to a cardiac monitor and then proceeded out of the room to get a few things I needed to start the IV with. An IV bag of normal saline was already hung and the tubing had been primed.

As I prepped M.'s arm, I didn't talk much—just a few words here and there about what I was doing. He didn't say anything at all. I started the two required IVs and taped them down.

At the very end of this task, M. asked: "How soon?"

I answered: "Five minutes."

I have to say that it is a rather remarkable thing to be so accurate when telling someone when they're going to die.

I went back behind the screen and the warden and I brought in the citizen—someone known only to the two of us. The warden went out and read the final order and instructions to the prisoner and asked him if he had anything to say.

At that time, M. changed his mind about having witnesses watch him go through the execution. He decided not to because he didn't want anyone to see him die. He didn't say anything about his guilt or his innocence. He said that the act of executing him made the warden and everyone involved in the room killers just like him.

The warden raised his hand to his tie, which was the signal that the injection was supposed to start. I hooked the syringe to the IV port and told the citizen to go ahead and start injecting the way I had taught him. The sodium Pentothal went in first.

The only thing we heard was the inmate start to say, "Yeah, I can feel . . ." and that was it. He went right out.

We went through the drugs one after the other. On the monitor, the prisoner's heart went from a regular beat to a slow bradycardia and then to nothing.

We waited for three minutes, which was a very long three minutes. Two physicians who had been just outside came in, listened to his heart, checked his pulse, and pronounced him dead. That was it.

We had the coroner vehicle nearby and the guards helped remove the body. The coroner took him and delivered him to the funeral home. The people outside left. I took the citizen with me and drove him away from the penitentiary.

Now this citizen was someone who was strong and definitely a complete believer in capital punishment. He broke down and cried for quite a little while. I consoled him as best I could. There wasn't much to say except "I understand" and "That's okay." After a while he stopped crying, and by the time he got home, he was relaxed.

It didn't hit me for a while, I think because I regarded the inmates, the warden, the guards, and the rest of my staff as being my responsibility. They needed support and someone to do the job right. I had to make sure they were all okay with what had happened. We talked about it, and had critical-stress debriefing for the guards who were more intimately involved.

I don't think there's been another execution there since that one.

It wasn't until weeks later that I broke down and cried. It wasn't that I had any regrets—it just all seemed very sad that people did those things and then deserved to die like that.

Sophie E.

Set nurses—the best-kept secret in nursing. This branch of nursing is con-trolled by a privileged few who protect their prize jobs like rabid pit bulls.

For the number of hoops I had to jump through while doing research for this chapter, one might have thought I was attempting to steal top-secret mili-tary information from the government. After a month of trying to find some-one in the union who would agree to talk to me about the details of the job, I was finally warned away by one of the union office's nurse-secretaries: "Don't you dare tell anyone about this branch of nursing," she cautioned. "The few of us who do get the good feature films have had to work our way up through commercials, sitcoms, and shorts. We don't want a bunch of out-of-work R.N.s trying to muzzle in. There're barely enough films to go around as it is."

Sophie E., forty-seven, was an out-of-work nurse who knew someone high up in "the industry." From there, she managed to step over the heads of the pit bulls and into the dream job—or, as Sophie said, "It's actually more like stepping into a scene from A Nightmare on Elm Street.*"*

The producers decide to begin shooting the low-budget ($19 million—pffft, chicken feed) film in July. It is so hot and muggy, and the air pollu-tion is so bad, everyone—men, women, and children—uses inhalers. Everyone complains of sore throats and runny eyes and noses . . . they keep saying it's just hay fever. I know better. It's Los Angeles—Pollution City, U.S.A.

It is the first day of the shoot, and my first day as set nurse. The daily call sheet indicates that I am supposed to be the first on the set and the last to leave—a very scary thought when I think of the sections of L.A. we'll be shooting in. I've seen grown men turn pale at the very mention of some of these locations.

I have been on the freeways in and around L.A. trying to find the

213

location. I don't like driving, and I especially don't like driving in a city where, in the slow lane, the slowest you can go without being run off the road—or shot at—is seventy-five miles an hour. I foolishly assumed that at 4:00 A.M., the freeways and highways would be empty. Not. In L.A., the highways are busy twenty-four hours a day. I want to stick my head out the window during one of the frequent long-distance crawls at 3:25 A.M. and ask those who pass me where the hell they're going at that hour.

Our first location is at a boys' school in Pasadena. The scenes we are going to shoot today feature all five of the film's stars and 150 children. I am responsible for the health and well-being of every single one of them, plus the crew. Considering that I left my apartment in the heart of L.A. at 3:45 A.M., I'm already tired.

The man who is setting up the honey wagons—the trailers that house the toilets—directs me to the production trailer parked at the end of a long row of identical trailers. Timidly I stick my head inside and announce that I am the nurse. The assistant director (cigar already in hand) and a production assistant glare at me much in the same way I would expect to be glared at by a roomful of surgeons. The PA says: "So what?"—also much in the way a surgeon might say the same.

I tell her I've been instructed to pick up a radio and a headset so that I might be "in the loop"—privy to everything that goes on on set between the director, assistant director, the PAs, and the main crew members.

Once I have the bulky black box clipped to my belt, I find myself adopting a sort of swagger. Only the key players in the making of a film are in the loop. I hold my head, with the headset conspicuously placed, a bit higher. Little do I know that before five days of this four-month ordeal pass, the intercom radio—that thing which invades your privacy every second of the day—will become the bane of my existence.

The cast and the rest of the crew begin arriving around nine o'clock. I have staked out a sunny corner of the playground and have been trying to keep myself warm with hot cocoa and decaf coffee generously dispensed from the craft service truck. I read the newspaper, pace, and do exercises. I see other people talking away on their radios, but I don't hear anything on my radio.

I devote a few moments to paranoia. Maybe I'm not so important, I think dejectedly. Everyone except me is on a special channel . . . I'm not really in the "in crowd" at all.

I brighten with the thought that my radio might be broken. I begin fiddling with dials, when a PA screams "MEDIC!" at the top of her lungs and waves me over to the other side of the playground. I notice several other people around her have also begun screaming "MEDIC! MEDIC!" over and over. Two of them are jumping up and down, waving their arms.

I have worked emergency room for most of my career; when someone uses this particular tone of voice, it means something is very wrong—the death of a child, or imminent death of the hospital administrator or a surgeon. Heart racing, I take off running at breakneck speed. When I reach the screaming, jumping parties, I ask where the victim is and if CPR is in progress.

"Ms. A. [the main star] wants a vitamin C and some hot echinacea tea," answers the PA, looking down her nose.

Automatically, my hands go to my hips. "You called me over for a vitamin C and some herbal tea?" I say through clenched teeth. I'm about ready to recite the don't-cry-wolf fable when the second assistant director rapidly approaches. Her face is a snarl of rage. The veins in her forehead and neck are distended.

"Goddamn it!" she screams. "Why haven't you been answering your radio?"

I stare at her blankly. "I haven't heard a thing," I answer.

She reaches over and unhooks the radio from my belt, then yanks the headset off my head, taking several strands of my hair.

"It's not even turned on!" She scowls as she flicks an obscure button. "J. wants to talk to you now!"

"J.?" I ask.

She looks at me, filled with disgust. It fairly drips from her pores. "Your first assistant director," she answers as she marches across the playground.

"You're dead meat," she says over her shoulder, sounding very much like some nurse-managers I've known. "One of the crew needed an aspirin an hour ago."

"Nobody showed me how to use the radio," I plead weakly. "I didn't know it wasn't turned on."

"I hope you didn't quit your day job" is her comment on that.

I am paraded through the set of lights and cameras and make-up artists to the side of a good looking man who is about six foot five inches tall. The second AD shoves me forward like a prisoner. The first AD takes his cigar from his mouth and blows the stinking blue smoke over my head—except he misjudges and it ends up in my eyes.

"Who the hell are you?" he roars, so loud I instinctively cover my ears. The man standing next to him—one I recognize from the covers of movie magazines as the dark-eyed Adonis of Hollywood—smiles and gives me an up-and-down look like you see in the movies.

Looking up, I tell J., "I'm the set nurse and no one showed me how to use my radio and this is my first time on a movie set and see, I'm really used to working in the ER, so when someone uses that tone I think someone is dying, but don't worry about anything because nobody really needs anything except some vitamins and herbal tea, big deal."

J. blinks a few times. The Hollywood god laughs and tells J. that after he's done firing me, he needs a nurse in his trailer.

"This your first time as a set nurse?" J. bellows finally.

I nod.

He slaps his forehead and rolls his eyes, then brays, "Oh Christ! Just what we need. A civilian traipsing around, gawking at the actors, tripping over wires and walking into scenes. What goddamned moron hired you?"

I name the name of my friend, the big muck-a-muck. J. immediately goes silent. "Oh," he says—quietly. Then, in a low voice, he asks, "Why would he do something so stupid?"

"Because I need the money and because I have twenty years of emergency room experience and because he thought you, especially, might need a good nurse." I eye his cigar and the extra tire around his waist.

J. personally shows me how to work the radio.

No sooner is the headset in place than another hysterical call "MEDIC!" comes through. This time, I ask what the situation is, and exactly where the patient is located. The response chills me—a child has been badly injured in the playground. It is, someone in the loop howls, either a broken neck or internal hemorrhaging.

I move at the speed of light, pulling my stethoscope out of my fanny pack as I go. The "badly injured" child is one six-year-old who has fallen and received a bloody nose. He is sucking on a Popsicle and giggling when I arrive. The anxious mother hovers, on the edge of hysteria. "His face!" she screams, wringing her hands. "His career is ruined!"

I look long and hard at the ruined child and see that his lips are stained slightly orange from the Popsicle, but other than that, there is nothing there but a normal kid's face. With freckles.

I look back at the mother, who is being comforted by a circle of the other mothers. Most of them are cooing the names of plastic surgeons who might be able to help the "poor child" and his disfigurement.

Suddenly I realize I am in the presence of those Hollywood Mothers I've heard so much about. My focus of care shifts from the child to the mother, who is working herself into a dramatic hysteria worthy of an Oscar. I give her two aspirin and tell her to go to one of the honey wagons and lie down. Wiping Precious Petey's nose, I send him off to play on the same nasty jungle gym that threw him down and ruined his career.

The mother is led away by one of the lower echelons of PAs as I receive another panicky "MEDIC!" call. This time it's for a bucket of Sea Breeze, aspirin, and Advil.

"MEDIC!" One of the female stars tells me she feels depressed, and since I'm a "real" R.N., do I carry uppers or maybe a line or two of cocaine?

"MEDIC!" The other female star wants some downers because she's nervous.

"MEDIC!" A splinter in the pinky finger of a grip. He asks me if I will send him home on disability.

"MEDIC!" The head of transport has a cut on his elbow that he refuses to show me. He assures me it's only a scratch. After fifteen minutes of begging, I convince him to let me see his scratch. It is a deep laceration that will keep a good surgeon busy for an hour.

"MEDIC!" This time, I am ordered to Mr. Hollywood Adonis's trailer to dress his toes.

Yes. Dress his toes.

I bring my med cart with me—a converted 1950s TV cart with three plastic boxes held down on it by bungee cords. Outfitted with everything except prescription drugs, the boxes are in fact a mini ER. I knock on the trailer door. There is some shuffling around and then the door flies open and out stumbles the location supervisor. As she trips lightly down the stairs, I notice her bra hanging by its hooks from the back of her skirt.

Adonis is lounging on the bed as though it is his natural habitat. He pulls off his socks, explaining as he does so that he's just had his ingrown toenails removed and needs his feet soaked, massaged, kissed, dried off with my hair, and dressed. With a straight face he tells me his feet are his second–most sensitive erogenous zone. He reaches around me and locks the trailer door.

I am being backed against the wall when I accidentally step on his toe. While he is howling, I run some warm water into a dishpan which I just happen to have on my cart and pour in a box of Epsom salts. When he has both feet immersed, I begin to explain how the tissue heals and what the signs of infection are. I'm about three sentences into the standard home-instruction speech, when his hand slips from my arm and lands—still groping—on my crotch.

I push his arm away, and put a little pressure on the surgical site with my thumb . . . to check for capillary return.

Mr. Adonis decides, at that moment, he doesn't have time to waste. Without so much as causing waves with his feet, he stands, picks me up, throws me onto the bed, and is on top of me, pawing at my breasts. His tongue is halfway down my throat.

I've always worked in the relatively secure environment of critical care. Most of my male patients either have been badly injured or are dying, so I've never really had to deal with anything even remotely like this. I mean, the last thing on a man's mind while he's having a heart attack or bleeding to death is sex. But here, in this trailer, there isn't a call bell I can pull out of the wall, and who would come to my aid if I screamed, anyway?

I fight him off, taking advantage of his soaking toes. He cannot believe it. Affronted, he rolls off and stares at me, his mouth agape.

"How can you turn me down?" he asks. "Nobody ever turns me down!"

"There are a lot of cretins out there," I say, then add, "I'm a nurse, Mr. Adonis, not a whore, nor a fan. I'm here to care for your feet, not your sexual needs."

He thinks I'm being coy, and begins to lick my neck.

"Stop," I say, and slip to my knees, where I remove his feet from the Epsom soak and wrap them tightly in a bath towel. I do a quick-look scan of the healing tissue and scowl just as his hand gropes my breast.

"Oh jeez," I murmur.

He stops dead in his groping tracks, seeing my worried frown. "What is it?"

I shake my head and purse my lips. I point to a perfectly healthy portion of his toe. "See this here? It looks just a touch ecchymotic to me."

Mr. Adonis backs off, an expression of nervous concern filling his face. "Oh my God!" he whispers. "What's ecchymotic?"

I shake my head, the look of concern settling into a grave, defeated expression. "It's quite serious and excruciatingly painful." I look into his face. "Just how much do you use your feet, Mr. Adonis?" I ask, trying to sound deeply troubled.

The question jolts him into a standing position, except his ankles are still bound together with the towel and he falls back down.

"Your fly is unzipped," I point out, and then run a Q-tip loaded with antibiotic cream along the surgical site of his toes. "See this reddened area here?" I ask. Mr. Adonis is examining his toes with the expression of someone who will never see that part of his body again. He's gone pale and sweaty. For a minute, I'm afraid I've pushed him over the edge and try to remember where I put the ammonia poppers.

"I should probably inject those toes with some antinecrosis medication," I say, pulling out a 50cc irrigation syringe and waving it in front of his face.

Mr. Adonis jumps up, kicks the towel off of his ankles, and bolts out the door, yelling for the PA.

Biting my tongue to keep from laughing outright, I clean up my equipment and head for the honey wagon to check on my hysterical Hollywood mother, when I hear a scream, "MEDIC!"

I keep the floodgates of adrenaline locked and continue to walk to the honey wagon. "Medic here," I respond, opening a stick of gum. It was probably a call for an Advil or some tofu compresses.

"It's burning! He's in there . . . the . . . Oh my God, medic, help."

I stop chewing. There's no fake hysteria in this voice. I ask where the problem is located. I'm directed to a trailer that is at the other end of the set—a quarter of a mile away. I wave down a transport truck and have the driver lift my cart into the back. As soon as we pull out of the playground and onto the street, I can see the smoke.

Less than twenty-five seconds later, I am at the burning trailer where a crew member is lamenting piteously over his new Calvin Klein jeans, which are in charred, smoking shreds. In a quick once-over, I see that he has first degree burns on his legs, arms, and face. His right hand hangs at his side, bleeding. On examination, I find that his hand has sustained a combination of second and third degree burns. Wishing I had some morphine or Demerol to give him, I rinse off the seared flesh and wrap it with a sterile dressing soaked with sterile water.

As I turn to the transpo man to tell him to take the patient to the nearest ER, I see one of the grips leaning against the water truck, the canvas hose at his feet. He is holding his hand—or what is left of it—looking like he's going to go out. I grab a box of dressings and run to him just as he slumps to the ground.

I look into his eyes for explanation.

"Got it caught in the hose reel," he says, and vomits.

Recognizing shock, I lay him on the ground and call for a blanket and the transpo man while I look at his hand. The thumb and the entire base of his thumb is severed from the rest of his hand and is hanging by a thread of skin.

With sterile saline, I rinse the wound and set that part of his hand back to where it belongs, wrap it with sterile dressing, elevate and immobilize it, and ask the transpo man how fast he can drive without killing them all. He says he drove an ambulance for ten years. He promises me he can have both patients at the ER within five minutes. I believe him and make a judgment call. The patients loaded, I wave them off like a flagman at a speedway.

From the headphones comes J.'s booming voice. "LUNCH!" The word triggers a stampede you might see in a cartoon. Approximately sixty crew members charge toward the caterer's truck, and for a moment, I am afraid the children who are still in the playground will be trampled.

Lunch is an incredible affair under a lovely white tent. There are five different salads, baskets of homemade fresh breads, any choice of entrées—including filet mignon and chicken cordon bleu—fresh steamed vegetable of one's choice, and desserts to die for. I am one bite into my lightly steamed broccoli, when there comes a hysterical "MEDIC!"

Tampons for the set decorator and the script writer.

One bite into my veggie burger and another call—

Sunblock for the other male lead, and a tube of Blistex for his precious, wonderful lips.

A first bite of salad—

An antihistamine for the director, who is simultaneously eating a hamburger, reading *Variety*, and having his hair braided into haphazard sections by one of the male hairdressers. The end effect looks like a spider with wobbling legs.

Back at the tent, I dip a spoon into my frozen yogurt—

Calamine lotion and more antihistamines for one of the prop guys who has gotten into poison ivy.

After lunch, it is a constant dribble of antihistamines, minor cuts and bruises, minor therapy sessions, several calls for illegal drugs, and sunburns. At four o'clock, I am ordered by the producer to be close by the set because a violent scene is being filmed—without stunt doubles.

The lead female star has to attack one of the minor actors. It involves lots of kicking and screeching. Surely, I mistakenly think to myself, the actress won't really hurt the guy. An hour later, I am cleaning out a deep bite wound on the arm of the lesser actor.

"You couldn't fake the bite?" I ask Ms. A.

"I had to make the scene believable," she sniffs. "I live my art."

I insist that the actor go to the hospital for a tetanus shot.

"Do you think it will scar?" he asks anxiously.

I look at the depth of the bite and nod. "I'm afraid so. She really took a chunk out of you, buddy."

Beaming, the actor gets into the transport van, starry-eyed. "Good," he breathes in relief. "I can tell everyone I was bitten by A. in a violent fit of passion."

In between being summoned for vitamins, sunblock, and antihistamines, I manage to read the entire script—which is, to my dismay, one of those extremely violent action films. All four adult stars and the one child star insist on doing their own stunts. Currently it is considered "extremely cool" for an actor to do his or her own stunts.

The script contains three complex fistfights, two scratch-and-bite fights, someone having his head swung at with a golf club, a strangulation, a two-story fall, a stabbing, an attack by a live crow, a person burning, someone's eye being poked out, a child being chased through woods alive with poison oak and dangerous creatures, and a child walking down the middle of a freeway at night.

By 6:00 P.M. the 150 children are getting tired and cranky. Despite my warnings, sugary treats and soda pop are handed out freely. Chaos escalates, and I am constantly running from one bloody nose to the next bruise.

As the light fades, we send the kiddies home with their call sheets for the next day and switch to shooting some of the indoor scenes. The notation on my call sheet says "Closed Set." This means that only the director, a skeleton crew, the producers, and the medic are allowed in on the scene.

In all of my movie business ignorance, I think that the reason for the skimpy crew is because of the small space in which the scene is shot—a closet inside one of the schoolrooms.

Imagine my surprise when Mr. Adonis and Ms. A. parade into the room and proceed to disrobe and then engage in simulated—I think it is simulated, although I try not to get too close—sexual relations. I sit there for the duration trying to imagine what medical emergency can possibly arise from this scene. I do carry condoms in my med cart, but . . .

As soon as the scene is over, Ms. A. makes a beeline for me, her eyes blazing with indignant rage. I go into a protective stance.

"I'm going to throw up." She heaves dramatically. "Give me something for my stomach."

"Was it something you ate?" I ask innocently, handing her a package of Tums.

She glowers at me and impatiently rolls her eyes. "I hate the man." She gags. "He literally makes me sick to my stomach." Taking the Tums, Ms. A. storms away into the loving, pampering arms of the makeup and wardrobe people.

As sweltering and muggy as the day was, the night is cold and windy. I spend my downtime at the craft service truck, downing cups of coffee, trying to stay awake and coherent, let alone warm.

At midnight, the craft service man leaves me sitting alone in the middle of the playground. The production crew have all gone off to watch the daily rushes; most of the crew is gone. I wait patiently for the transpo guys to finish cleaning the honey wagons, praying I will not fall asleep on the hour drive back to my rented room. I peek at the call sheet and see that I must be back here at 5:30 A.M. That means that I will get approximately three hours' sleep. Simultaneously, I realize that this twenty-hour day will be my schedule six days a week for the next four months. I wonder how sleep deprivation will manifest itself in Los Angeles.

Exhausted, I roll my TV cart to my car, feeling like I've been ridden hard and put away wet. On the way back to Sunset and Vine, I weigh the pros and cons—I mean, was eating, buying gas, and paying rent *really* so important? But at the same time, wasn't it exciting? Hobnobbing with, and being mauled by, the famous and neurotic on the front line? Hearing behind-the-scenes gossip firsthand? Having my name listed last in the credits?

And didn't I have autonomy? No sour faced nurse-manager hanging around, trying to make me feel worthless—just a bunch of alarmists who wouldn't know a real medical emergency unless the script said it was.

And the money was incredible. Regular time for the first eight hours. Time and a half for the next four, and then "golden time" for anything over twelve.

And it wasn't like I was having to do any real nursing—these were mostly healthy people . . . well, physically at least.

A limo passes and I see a set of bare feet hanging outside the window. Just as I am parallel with the window, the feet disappear and the window goes all the way down. D.H.—my favorite actor—sees the look on my face and blows me a kiss, then waves.

I wave back, sure that I'm awake and not hallucinating. Suddenly I feel less tired and a little happy. I decide that maybe being a Hollywood set nurse isn't going to be so bad. After all, there are worse things than sleep deprivation and having your name be last.

Shannon T.

"Birth and death. Traditionally, nurses have attended both occasions. I'm a tomb-to-womb kind of person, I guess, because I've worked on both ends of the spectrum."

—Shannon T., a thirty-five-year-old single mother from Rhode Island. After starting out in oncology, she has been a high-risk labor and delivery nurse since 1990.

Nurses are the most wonderful people in the world—they work so hard to take care of other people for long hours and little pay.

Nurses are the most horrible people in the world—some of them, I just want to slap. They tear each other down and refuse to stand up for themselves.

My mother was a nurse. She had seven kids and drove 160 miles every day to go to work. I was ten when my parents divorced, so I would have to come home and give total care to my three younger brothers, ages eight, six, and three.

I started out in oncology, but the work was so hard, and so draining, I couldn't stay with it. It was too much of a pull on my heart. Plus I always had a problem with the question of do I let them have hope or make them face reality now?

So, after spending a lot of time at the doorway of the tomb, I kind of did a one-eighty and decided to work with the womb. Mostly, labor and delivery is a joy, but sometimes it does have its horror stories.

I can smell that it's going to be one of those days. Trouble has an odor like flint and brimstone. It's in the air.

It's not even an hour into the shift and already trouble has brewed. A crack mom walked in off the street with the baby's head already out. She lay down on a gurney, popped out the rest of the body—a gorgeous baby boy. He's upstairs in pediatric ICU about to go through withdrawal.

While I'm trying to get information on this woman (who is stoned to the gills), I leave for two seconds, and when I come back to the room, she's put her clothes on and split, unofficially leaving her baby to the state.

Half an hour later, one of our infertility clinic women comes in— the one who has been trying to have a baby for over ten years—and tells me that she hasn't felt her baby moving all night.

And of course it has died in utero, and now she has to go through the hell of having a stillborn delivered. She has been placed in a section away from the other mothers in labor so that she cannot hear their cries or that first magical wail of the newborns.

I just have to shake my head and say, "Hey! This isn't fair! Who is in charge up there? Are you asleep at the friggin' wheel, or what?"

But want to know what *really* fries my ass? In this L&D there really are two systems of care: one for non-English speaking nonwhites, and another for the white and privileged. Like rooms 7 and 8? We have two women right next to each other and they got two completely different kinds of care yesterday when they both delivered. One is a Hispanic and the other is a wealthy white woman.

The Hispanic in room 7 came over the border to have her baby. Her course had been high-risk and complicated so that by the time the doctor showed up, the script ran something like this:

Nurse to the OB doc: "She's got a temp of 102.7. Can I call the pediatrician now?"

OB doc: "No."

Nurse, an hour later: "Okay, well, now she's passed meconium. Shall I call the pediatrician now?"

OB doc: "No."

Nurse, an hour later: "Well, now the fetal-monitor strip is looking crummy. Now can I call the pediatrician?"

OB: "Stop asking me that. I don't want a pediatrician here now or in the future!"

So, I of course called the pediatrician anyway. I mean, this lady could have been sectioned, she had so many options, but this man didn't care. Do you think he treated the white woman that way?

Of course, the baby ended up on a ventilator and then died within a few hours. It was a totally unnecessary death.

Two days ago I was sitting at the desk and I heard two of my colleagues moan and say, "Oh no, the patient's here."

The sound of it broke my heart. I turned around and saw this young pregnant woman with big brown eyes. She didn't know anyone, and I could tell she was really hoping there would be just one someone here she could connect with.

She was having a baby, and when she's old and drooly and doesn't remember who the President is, she will remember the day she had her baby. It is my belief that every woman deserves to have the best birthing experience she can get.

So, even though it wasn't my turn for an admission, I got up and smiled at her. She was grateful for the smile and took my hand to thank me.

I put her in the room next to Nellie. Nellie has been a patient in our infertility clinic for years, and now, after implantation of the ga-metes, she is finally pregnant with twins. This is the first pregnancy she has been able to carry for longer than twenty weeks.

Nellie has been a habitual aborter. She came in at twenty-eight weeks pouring out blood—one of the placentas had abrupted and one of the babies is dead. I'm not clear on why the docs want to keep the demised twin inside her, but they are. She had already named them— one is Natalie and one is Nan. Natalie is the twin who has died.

Although she was not my patient, I have taken care of her in the past, so she was very verbal with me about her concerns. She wondered a lot how Nan must feel, having spent so much time with her sister.

I recently lost my sister-in-law and best friend to a horrible death, so I felt comfortable talking about death with her. I tried to give her the answers I felt were closest to the truth.

On my break today, I looked out the window of the cafeteria at the panoramic view of the city and thought: *I have hundreds of children out there walking around.* It is a wonderful feeling.

I am not comfortable with this new obstetrician. He is young and too full of himself to be unassisted at this breech birth. The mother is full-term and healthy, and I have done many of them myself, so I'm not too worried. I think midwives have the best luck with breech births, and old-timey doctors who've done a lot of them. You must know what you're doing and this guy clearly does not have a lot of experience.

I tell him we need to do the delivery in the OR with a setup ready in case we needed to do a cesarean section, and he's agreeable to that. I know I'm fussing a lot, but it's because I know what I'm doing.

He snaps at me: "Why don't you just do it yourself!" and I snap back that I really would like to do just that.

The feet are delivered and I tell him, "Now you know that you have to get up there right away and grab the baby's mouth and kind of angle the head down so the cervix doesn't close around the baby's neck? You know that, right?"

He's really angry that I said that, and I can see how nervous he is.

I'm getting very worried. He's dawdling too much, and I realize for certain that he doesn't have a clue about what he is doing. The outward bravado and arrogance are cover-ups for his inexperience.

I force him out of the way and reach up to find the baby's mouth, and it is too late. The cervix is closed tight around the baby's neck, strangling him.

This is a full-term baby who was healthy and viable—this is pure negligence.

The tragedy and panic of the situation throws a hundred negative memories shooting through my brain. I recall the Sunday afternoon when the doctor on call was someone who truly hated to be called into the hospital on the weekends.

The patient was high-risk, preeclamptic, on magnesium sulfate with Pitocin. The fetal-monitor strips kept getting worse and worse, and the nurse taking care of this woman kept calling the doctor, who kept refusing to come in.

Finally, I took over and went to the charge nurse and said, "Look, we need to call the doctor *now*!" but she said, "But you know how much Dr. X hates to be called in on his weekends . . ."

So three hours later, the baby's heart rate went down to 30 and just stayed there. I rushed the bed to the OR like a flash and screamed to the other nurse to call the doctor and tell him to meet me in the OR.

The child was born without any brain stem activity at all.

I think about this kind of negligence and I get sick. Who has the right to take a family and string them out across a huge chasm of pain and despair and disability like that?

———

Sally is a big girl. She has been in labor for ten hours. She is eighteen and has told me that she is the girlfriend of a gang leader downtown. She rolls off his name as though I'm supposed to know who he is. I tell her I'm not up on my gang lore. She doesn't laugh.

The leader and father of this unborn child is dangerous and very obnoxious. For the past hour he has been "tagging" the walls in the labor room with a Magic Marker. I've asked him to stop, and he has begun screaming obscenities at me, threatening me with his knife.

I tell him very nicely that maybe he should take a walk and calm down outside. I tell him that his girlfriend needs him to be there *for* her, *not* upsetting her.

He tells me I am the cause of all his problems, and says he will find one of his members to have me "taken care of" when I get off duty tonight.

I call the supervisor and the doctor on the case, and I am told the father has rights and to allow him to do whatever he wants. The supervisor informs me I am in the wrong and not to "rock the boat."

The supervisor simply feels the need to go along with the doctor. The doctor—one of those macho docs—is retaliating because I wrote him up once.

We had this non-English-speaking patient go out of control on us while she was delivering. It was her first baby, and she was writhing around on the bed, screaming at the top of her lungs. All she really needed to do was take one deep breath and push, but she was so freaked out she just wouldn't do it. Instead of bearing down and keeping her bottom flat on the bed like the doc was insisting she do, she was arching her back up and holding her breath.

So Dr. Macho hauled off and slapped her a good one. Made her head roll until she saw stars. It left a welt the shape of his hand.

No one, of course, would confront this guy and write him up for assaulting a patient, so I finally did—which is why he's insisting this abusive jerk of a father be allowed to stay in the labor room now. I'm sure he's hoping I get killed—which seems like a distinct possibility.

When I go back in the room, the gang leader grabs at me and holds my throat while putting the point of his knife up one of my nostrils.

With a word from the girlfriend, I'm free. I immediately ask Johnna to switch patients with me. She gets Gangworld Baby and I get Nellie. It doesn't feel like a fair trade until Johnna informs me that Nellie is "bleeding a little more than before."

The daughter, suddenly frightened by having to make the decision on her own, called her brother who lived out of state.

Ambivalent, the brother would not make a decision after precious, wasted minutes of repeated explanations and the knowledge of his mother's recently expressed wishes.

The daughter broke down and began to sob. The doctor explained he needed a decision made—now.

The daughter became even more upset and looked to me—and then to him—for help. She pleaded with her eyes.

Then, she reached out to the doctor.

There was such a moment of silence—she holding out her arms, he wrestling with the buried emotions living inside him.

Finally, he took her into his embrace and comforted her, holding her, rocking her, gently speaking into her hair.

She decided to let her mother go in peace . . . to agree to what her mother had wished.

It was the first time I had ever seen him add that final touch of humanity to his work that is so necessary and so seldom given.

Sometimes irony can be the spice of nursing.

The private high school's choir was made up of thirty-five high school teens. I knew that, because I'd asked all of them to participate as "victims" in the hospital's staged annual disaster drill for the paramedics and emergency staff. That was on December 10.

The scenario I'd dreamed up was that a school bus carrying thirty-five choir students is hit by a truck, and the nearest ambulance is a long way away.

During the drill the students watched and listened carefully as the basics of triaging—locating and identifying all victims and prioritizing minor to major injuries—and assessing the ABCs [airway, breathing, circulation] were reviewed and then practiced—on them.

Each student had a card placed on them which listed their injuries. Some had obstructed airways from debris, some had minor cuts and fractures, others were to play dead.

All in all, it was a successful and informative drill. No one could have guessed at the time just how informative and successful it really was.

On December 7—one year later, minus three days—these same thirty-five students were coming back from a choral performance they'd given at another school. Their bus was on a two-lane road when a semi truck pulled right in front of them. The closest medical services were over twenty-two miles away.

The kids with minor injuries remembered and followed the drill exactly. Immediately they set out to locate every person involved, and prioritized them.

One student was unconscious under the bus, his face in a mud puddle. They pulled him out and cleared his airway, saving him from suffocation. Another had obvious abdominal injuries and was in shock. They elevated his legs and kept him warm while someone talked to him and held his hand to calm him. Airways were checked, pulses were taken. They did what they could for the four critically injured to protect their spines and make sure they kept breathing.

In the end, there was only one fatality. I like to think there weren't more because of that simple drill.

I'm not exactly superstitious or anything, but the next drill we have, I'll make sure the scenario I use will be something like a herd of African elephants falling from the sky.

Marcie O.

Standing four foot nine, Marcie O. is a forty-year-old mother of triplets. She has been a nurse for twenty years. Fifteen of those years have been spent as a geriatric nurse practitioner. She has recently earned her doctorate from the University of Maryland.

When she was sixteen and working in a nursing home, the director of nurses told her that the way she interacted with the elderly patients was very special. That wasn't news. Marcie had decided long before that she wanted a nursing career which involved geriatrics. She remembers thinking, at five, that there was always laughter with older people because they were so wise and kind.

A few weeks ago, I had a brittle diabetic patient who went into hypoglycemic shock and was quickly going out on me. Well, she was a dialysis patient as well, and didn't have any venous access, but because of my years in oncology, I found the tiniest little vein and managed to get in the smallest butterfly needle.

I gave her some IV-push dextrose and literally watched her come back to life. And I thought, well, you know, there's something to be said for emergency nursing and having the constant excitement of saving lives. But for me, letting a person live their life in the way they want to live it is more exciting than saving a life that doesn't want to be lived.

That is the key part of geriatric nursing. For the most part the patients are often ready and willing and anxious to die. What they want from me is to help them live the time they have left, comfortably and happily—getting out of it what *they* want to get out of it, not what *we* think they should get out of it.

As nurses we go beyond caring for the physical; we care for the whole person. There is great reciprocity in geriatric nursing. Yes, we give of ourselves physically and emotionally, but what I learn from these older adults is determination: how to grit your teeth and bear it—how to keep on and move on.

I remember a family in which the grandmother was being abused by one of the grandchildren. Every time I'd go there, she'd meet me at the door to show me her new bruises and give me the latest story of how she'd been pushed down the stairs.

What got my attention was that I had to inform the family that this was not acceptable behavior. They honestly didn't think there was a problem. Fortunately, just getting it out in the open was enough to stop the boy, but what the family did rather than modify the behavior, was to move him into a trailer on the property.

I remember one special lady who had bad rheumatoid arthritis. She was kind of crotchety, but her cognitive status was clear as a bell. She always kept her room very dark, and always wore dark sunglasses, since any kind of light bothered her eyes. So she would sit in her bed all day and basically direct life from that bed.

One day I went in to give her her meds, and she was lying there in a pool of sweat looking very dusky, complaining of a pain in her chest. This was before there were living wills, or any of the medical-hero mentality stuff. So, I sat on her bed and we talked and held hands. She told me that she wasn't scared at all; she was finished with life and ready to let go.

While she talked, I wiped her face, and rubbed her hands and arms. And when she got too weak to talk, I talked to her about the ocean and the forests and all free creatures who inhabit our world.

That night was one of the most incredible lessons for me. Thinking on how she died is such a contrast to the people nowadays who come into the emergency department or the hospital and spend their last hours being violated and treated badly.

I spent some years at the National Institutes of Health doing what was considered "real" nursing work in the medical and surgical oncology units. See, when you work geriatrics, you always have this anxiety that you should be doing "real" nursing work in the acute units. Part of the protocol on the oncology unit was that the patients had to be sixty-five or younger. However, I did get to have all the patients who were over sixty.

It was a real learning experience, getting to know the cancer patients and hearing them talk about what it meant for them to have cancer.

Since our unit was often the last-ditch try with experimental drugs, chemo, and surgery, it wasn't unusual to have two codes a night. For the most part, the patients were aggressively coded, so the nurses would, as we said then, "walk slowly to the phone."

You see, we knew that even if the code was successful, it only meant more chemo and more pain and more disappointment; there wasn't much quality of life for these people. Sure, there were those patients that you really fought for, but for the most part it was just hanging on.

I remember Tanya, a little sixteen-year-old who had ovarian cancer and, as a result, total obstruction of her bowel. She had this huge belly and skinny little arms and legs.

When we got her, her nasogastric tube was draining liquid feces. But oh boy, did Tanya love fried chicken. I remember going out and buying her buckets of fried chicken and letting her eat it [Marcie laughs] and then watching it all come right back out the nasogastric tube.

Day after day, her mother would sit by that bed while the two of them fought for life so desperately. We had to convince the mother to allow us to give the girl pain medication to keep her comfortable. You see, for the mother, that was like giving up hope and facing the reality of death.

The day Tanya finally died, the mother went out of her mind with grief; she was truly inconsolable. But the nurses rejoiced.

We had watched that young, beautiful girl spend her teenage years in that bed—no going to the prom with her boyfriend, no going to the mall with her best girlfriend, no necking in the back seat, no learning how to drive. She'd had nothing except physical and emotional trauma. All we could see was that Tanya was finally free of that pain. Finally free to move on.

There were other incidents wherein death was imminent that were not so joyful. Like the young mother who'd not recovered after the birth of her baby. She ended up in our unit with metastatic bowel cancer.

We knew she wasn't going to live, so we worked day and night with her, trying to get her to acknowledge what had happened, and then to accept it and make arrangements for her baby and her husband. You see, there was so little time, and she just never came to terms with this devastating thing that had happened to her.

God, how she fought [Marcie's voice breaks.] She never did accept. She died very soon, never having . . . [She is crying, and the tape is stopped.]

Another special little lady who came to us was . . . [She begins to cry again, but continues to talk.] Tiny bit of a thing. Young. Dark hair. Pretty healthy despite the fact that she had metastatic colon cancer and terrible pain. She was a widow who lived with this wonderful man who helped her do everything. On the days the pain would be so bad she couldn't move off the couch, he would clean the house and cook and tend to all of her needs.

During one of her many admissions, she shared with me the delicate matter of how they managed to have sex despite her colostomy, and asked me to help her purchase some fancy, sexy panties. That was one of the times when we both laughed so hard that we were told we had to be quiet or we'd be separated—like in grade school.

As the disease progressed, I watched her slip away a little at a time. And she would grab on to me and ask me the questions she couldn't ask the doctors. "How much time do I really have? What's it going to be like?" And even though she loved her physicians, they never told her what to expect.

There was so much that she needed to resolve. She talked a lot about her son who had died of sudden death syndrome at the age of ten. I never forgot her because even though she had this terrible disease, and she'd not had a great life, she was happy in her way; she had a loving relationship and she kept a stiff upper lip. Again, it was a testimony to the human will and strength.

This other patient I had during those NIH years was, I suppose, a testimony to the strength of the family. She was much loved and respected by her family, who seemed to always surround her—they were always present.

The woman herself was so loving and so kind it was easy to understand how everyone loved her, and how the connection, the lines of love, just seemed to spread out and include everyone.

Well, she had pancreatic cancer, but she wasn't considered to be near death at all. She'd had a surgery that was comparatively minor, but was supposed to have major, positive results, but suddenly she wasn't doing very well.

I don't know what went wrong—either she was too dry, or went into shock. I can't remember the details, but she lost her pressure. So the doctors decided they had to put a central-venous-pressure line in, and there was one try, and then another, and then another.

Then the doctors kicked the family out of the room.

It was clear to me then that this lady was going to die, and she'd been shut away from the most important part of her life. It made me crazy. I wanted to scream, "Hey, wait a minute! You can't take her family away from her. At least let someone stay to hold her hand and give her that lifeline!" But I was a nurse, and that sort of speaking out wasn't allowed from nurses. Back then, it was the "Be seen and not heard" principle.

The doctors eventually punctured her lung putting in the CVP line and she died. I was devastated and angry. While I was getting her ready for the morgue, I brought her family in. They dealt with her in such a lovely, dignified way. They placed a rose in her hands and each said their goodbye in turn. Then they all surrounded her so she lay within the circle of them.

When I felt I had sufficient acute-care-nursing skills, I went back for my master's and became a geriatric nurse practitioner in a three-hundred-resident facility. Besides taking care of them, doing routine nursing care—I let them know I cared.

Competency and caring—the two big C's—are what make the difference. I would try to imagine what it must have been like for most of them to come to these small apartments after moving out of their own beautiful homes, often after the loss of a spouse.

I spent a lot of time helping these very dignified people make this major adjustment—and then in the end, helping them obtain a death with dignity. One of the things that make a nurse practitioner better than a physician is that we really take the time to listen. We get the whole story, from complete, lifelong health history to current emotional goings-on.

While I worked there I discovered a wonderful way to provide care for the elderly, and that was to open my life and share it with them. There was one man who was just this vibrant happy soul. He and his wife—who was suffering from dementia—had had no children, so that when I would go visit, I'd bring the triplets along.

They'd call him Grandpa and snuggle on his lap. I can still recall one image of my little girls holding on to his legs, and that man just glowed with joy. It meant so much to him. It was so much more than just healthcare.

I have recently worked in a supportive care unit in the geriatric ward of a small orthopedic hospital. The objective of the unit is to get the patients functional and then get them home after they'd had an acute care stay.

One of the things I'd ask these people to do was to write their stories down about what life is like for them there.

I have one I want to read you. It's Emily's. She's a ninety-four-year-old who until recently ran her own farm quite efficiently. Listen to this:

Rehabilitation is like a nightmare. The therapy wears me out because at my age, I have no reserve strength. But I want to get better and I want to get home, so I do it. Old age does terrible things to a person.

I don't like it, but rehabilitation is something that I have to do. When you start a thing, you have a goal in mind. Like Sunday dinner: You have your breads ready, your five chickens to kill, and your cake to make. You don't sit around twiddling your thumbs, you do it. It's just the way it is.

Sometimes what they ask me to do here is ridiculous. Do they really think that a woman my age doesn't know how to bathe and dress? Sometimes the staff yells at me. I don't like that, so I say, "Just ask me nicely and I'll try," and I do.

Sometimes I feel that no one is listening to me. Sometimes the staff talks about me. Sometimes I feel like I'm not even present in the room. Sometimes I wish people would realize that I know what is best for me.

I know they love me and are worried about me, and they care about what will happen to me, but when my children decided to put me in a nursing home, I didn't want to go. They thought it was best for me, so I do what they tell me.

I no longer see the light at the end of the tunnel. I no longer think I'll ever get to go home.

Janet was a woman in her eighties who presented me with a dream she'd written down:

A nurse came into my room and sat down on the bed. She asked me what I wanted to get out of rehab, and what I need to be able to do when I get home. I tell her that I just want to sit in my chair and look at my pictures on the wall and at my sewing machine. I want to be free of pain. I want to transfer easily to the commode and to bed with just a little help from my husband.

Every morning I want to have my bowl of oatmeal with butter and salt. I then sit up for an hour or so and then lay down to read until I get up to eat the lunch my husband has prepared. Then I'll lay down to rest again and maybe, if I feel like it, get up for dinner.

I do not want to take any pills, because they make me sick. What I want is to be able to pick and choose what I want to eat and when, what pills I want to take.

Before she leaves, the nurse asks me about my sewing. I tell her about my piecework and how I can make a dress from just about anything. I also tell her that I draw portraits and tell her I will draw her if she lets me go home.

Eventually, I got Janet home. A couple of months later I went out to see her, only to find that she stopped taking her medication as soon as she got home, and had died shortly after.

What got to me was the apartment that she wanted so desperately to return to. It was this very sparse place. Very small—basically one room with a kitchen table and a few chairs and a bed and . . . her sewing machine.

I was hit so strongly when I saw the pictures Janet had drawn—pictures of people she'd loved, and places she'd been.

And I thought, this was all *Janet* wanted. It was her life, and she had chosen not to go on because of the constant pain in her hip, and she was ready to go. All she wanted to do was to die in a place and at a time of her own choosing.

Who are we to deny our elderly that?

David N.

Illinois-born David N. received a degree in mathematics in 1974. Taking off the cap and gown, he found himself graduated to a world that was not hiring mathematicians.

While I was job-hunting, I ran across this ad for a two-dollar-an-hour job as an orderly in a residential-care facility for cerebral palsy patients. So I thought okay, that's better than no job at all.

I worked there for six months, when, after having a lot of strange dreams about contorted people writhing around in various bed and bathroom situations, I realized I actually enjoyed going to work and feeling like I had some positive impact on other people.

I signed up for some business and accounting courses, but it just didn't seem to be very worthwhile ultimately, so I signed up for a two-year associate-degree nursing program instead. That was in 1979. I continued to work with the CP patients, went to nursing school, and took anatomy and physiology all at the same time. I know that it took more than a little patience on the part of my wife.

It didn't seem to be an issue for me about entering a female-dominated profession. It's been my custom throughout life to be different from everybody else anyway, so it wasn't at all odd.

One day when I was taking a class, I sat next to a Brit who asked what I was doing, and when I told him I was studying nursing, he said, "Ah, the noble profession!"

That always stuck with me, and I still believe it is true. It sets us apart—this ability to care for each other, to set aside time and resources to care.

Am I burned out? Well, gee—is there enough tape for this? Yes and no. I still work nights, but I keep coming back because I get the idea that the patients need the kind of care, intelligence, and skill I can give them. Despite all the obstacles the administrations throw up at nurses, I think it's worth it just to get next to the patients and keep my energy right there where they are.

If I do burn out, it will be because of the way institutions have treated me after I've made my best attempts to take care of patients.

I used to pack my mandolin and my tin whistle when I worked nights in the ER, where I was head nurse. I'd play to the patients while we waited for the doctors to come in.

Well, the night had been slow, and the LVN was off on a break and the doc on call had gone upstairs to ICU to help out with a patient up there. I was sitting in the back alone, playing my mandolin, when a young man—my age then, about thirty-one—came into the ER.

I will always remember the clerk saying, "David? We have a fellow who has chest pain here." I looked up and saw a man a few inches taller than me, pale as a sheet and wet as if he'd just crawled out of a pool. His right hand was over his chest and he said he was having some intense pain in his chest.

The feeling I had at that moment was very similar to the second just before a car accident when your foot moves from the accelerator to the brake, and the car goes into a spin.

You can bet I moved, although those first few seconds felt like hours. I called for an EKG, got him on the monitor, and was ready to put an IV in.

In the back of my mind, I was thinking about the policies that I had created for that ER about how the nurse shall act in the place of the physician in an emergency situation when the physician isn't available. And I was thinking this is okay—these are my policies. So I'm putting in the IV and I see the rhythm turn into ventricular fibrillation.

I hit him in the chest, and while I was charging up the defibrillator and putting the pads on his chest, I screamed out for the clerk to call the doctor stat.

Now, in my mind this is taking *forever* although it's really only a few seconds. So I shocked him with the full 360 joules. Then it took another forever in my mind to watch the flatline turn into a slow sinus rhythm, at which time I started to breathe again.

I finished the IV and bolused him with lidocaine.

That was when the doctor came in. It was also when my hands started to shake.

Well, of course, the stat page called the attention of everybody, including the nursing supervisor. Everybody showed up and I was being praised by everyone—including the ER doc and the cardiologist, who credited me for saving the man's life. It was generally a joyous time for everybody, especially me and the patient.

The next day it was more than a shock when the director of nurses came down to the ER to rake me over the coals. She said, "Now about this man that you defibrillated yesterday. I'm going to write you up. You should remember to use defib pads, because he's got burns on his chest."

That was it. No "Thank you," no "Good job." The man had some minor burns on his chest that he was too happy to be alive to even notice.

I restrained myself from beating her head into the wall and told her that in fact I did use pads.

And she said, "Well, you never know when they're going to get sued, so be more careful next time."

At that point all I could think of was what am I doing here working for people who have no recognition for what it's like to pull a patient from death's door, and then have the gall to belittle the nurse who did?

It wasn't long after that incident that I took the pediatric-events life support class, in which you are trained to get over your idiosyncratic aversion to breaking people's bones during CPR by practicing on dead chickens.

As it turned out, the day after the class, we got a baby in who looked more like a chubby eight-month-old than the fully developed sixteen-month-old that he was supposed to be.

This kid had multiple medical problems—respiratory failure, hyaline membrane disease, and other related problems. The pediatrician told us he had already outlived his life expectancy by many months.

Well, this baby had come in in full arrest and the parents were loudly and stridently calling out for the baby to come back.

"Come on Johnny, come on, you can do it. Come back, Johnny. You can do it. Come on back, Johnny. We love you, Johnny."

And it went on and on like that for the whole twenty or thirty minutes of the resuscitation. It was just torture.

I was doing an intraosseous cannulation of the baby's tibia in front of the parents who were cheering this baby on, and all these conflicting emotions were going on inside me.

I was wondering alternately whether or not what I was doing was any good, and feeling so very sad that the parents had been led to believe that their baby had a chance at survival when it was clear he didn't. Too, I was angry at them for thinking we could actually bring their child back from death. Then I was thinking that my experience with their child might help me develop some skills that might save someone who was viable someday. I was also thinking how wonderful it was that these people loved this boy enough to be cheering so hard for him to live.

He didn't live of course, but I couldn't shake the sound of those parents' cheering. It rattled around my head for months, every time a baby in trouble would come in.

I had my funnier moments in that ER too. I remember the day I took my wife to see *Born on the Fourth of July*. We happened to sit behind a guy who throughout the whole movie kept up a running commentary on the various artistic failures of Hollywood and the movie and how the film wasn't as good as it was supposed to be.

Well, that night the same guy walks into my ER and tells me that he's bleeding from his dick. And he is, in fact, doing just that in a big bad way. As it turns out, he was homeless—a Vietnam vet who had some liver failure and abdominal problems from alcohol abuse.

So I start talking to the guy about the movie and hear some more of his rather caustic critical commentary, when he adds that he actually lives in the crawl space under the theater.

Then he decides to share with me some of his nightmares.

The way he told me about them created this sense of tender intimacy, because you know that this guy isn't going to talk that way out on the streets.

He said he kept dreaming that his wife and kids were trying to chop his head off.

All I could think of was that this poor guy had a wife and kids, and gee, he must have loved them and now he misses them and he's living under this cold theater.

I mean, I'm really getting all sentimental and choked up over it.

"Yeah," he says with a sigh. "It's a chilling nightmare. It just kills me every time I have it."

"Well, sure," I said. "It must be, with them trying to chop your head off and all."

He shakes his head. "Not even that," he says. "The real nightmare is the idea of them ever showing up and trying to mess up my life just when I got it so good . . ."

Peggy W.

Ever wonder what really goes on in the operating room while you're under anesthesia?

Forty-three-year-old Peggy W. has been an operating room nurse since 1974. She has worked in North Carolina, Florida, California, Massachusetts, and Costa Rica.

Her mother and twin sister are also nurses, although she says she wouldn't wish the profession on her daughter. As she puts it: "While I was in nursing school trying to figure out what a Foley catheter was and where to put it, all my peers were in college having a good time. While my family and friends were all having social lives, I was working weekends, holidays, and nights in a hospital. I feel like I've missed part of life being a nurse, and I don't want my daughter to miss any part of life."

The catch-22 of working in an OR was that you had to have a year of OR experience before you could work there. I went into long-term care right out of nursing school but I hated it. The reason I hated it was phlegm. I hate phlegm, so that kind of ruled out long-term care.

Let me give you a quick rundown on personalities first.

Urologists are easygoing in the OR, plus they almost always have a bawdy sense of humor. Some of the jokes they tell? I blush just to think of it . . . but then again, look at the area of the body they deal with, right?

Cardiac surgeons are total prima donnas.

Orthopedic surgeons aren't usually considered to be very bright.

Neurosurgeons are usually eccentric, prima donnas, and very temperamental. We had one that was the meanest human being I've ever known. We've gone through at least five neurosurgery head nurses because of him in five years.

ENT [ear, nose, and throat] guys are okay, but they sometimes have a weird sense of humor. I'm really not too fond of ENT surgery—it kind of goes back to the phlegm thing—so I try to avoid it.

Vascular surgeons can be picky.

General surgeons are usually pretty nice.

And yes, we have surgeons who throw things and stamp their feet and jump up and down. I once had a surgeon throw a heavy piece of metal equipment at my head and miss by a few inches. Had it connected, I'd be talking to you from my palatial home in Bali right now.

But, I suppose, to be fair you have to look at what surgeons do. It's nerve-racking . . . absolutely nerve-racking—and very godlike.

I remember one surgeon who was older than the hills and had been doing surgery at this little hospital for years. He pretty much did as he pleased. I remember one of the things he used to do that would drive us crazy was—I swear on a Bible—orchiectomies [castrations—for prostate and testicular cancer] under local anesthesia. It was horrible.

Yes, ORs have music playing most all the time. The surgeon usually gets to choose the kind of music he likes. If there isn't a sound system actually in the OR, they'll bring in their own boom boxes and CD players.

I can remember in one Boston OR I worked at, we had a bad trauma case one night and we'd been working for maybe ten hours. It was about 4:00 A.M. and we were out of music, so we ended up playing yodeling music. I've got to tell you that when you have to resort to yodeling music, it's really bad.

I remember my first bowel resection when I was a student, and the surgeons had run the bowel [pulled out all the bowel to inspect it for perforations]. When they were done, they just smushed all the loops back in. In my naïveté, I asked, "Aren't you supposed to put them back exactly as you found them?"

The surgeon thought that was pretty funny and said, "Oh no, they settle themselves back to the way they were—they have a sort of memory."

All kinds of things have been dropped in the OR—I can't tell you how many hundreds of times I've heard: "Whatever you do, don't drop it!" A pause, and then: "Oops!"

I hate ophthalmic surgery . . . I can't do it. I remember this one surgeon who would come over to harvest the eyes from donor patients; he'd hold up the eyeball and say, "Hey, anybody want to look at this?" I couldn't even hold the metal bowl because I didn't want to feel the eyeball hit the metal—it kind of goes back to the phlegm thing again.

Sondra S.

"Management kept increasing the nurses' workloads, until it became impossible to give quality, compassionate care to the patients."

This was the reason Sondra S., a fifty-one-year-old mother of six, gave for quitting her job as a full-time oncology nurse in one of Detroit's largest healthcare facilities after ten years of service.

"I knew a long time ago that there was more to nursing sick people than just shoving a bunch of chemicals into their bodies. I'd secretly been practicing holistic healing on my hospital patients for ten years and had seen it work too many times to doubt it. After I'd finish the required nursing duties, I'd do a little acupressure or some visualization and healing-touch exercises with my patients, and the changes that took place were amazing.

"Of course, the docs never knew what I was doing (I would have been fired on the spot!), but they were impressed with how well their patients did under my care." She laughs. *"Sometimes they'd even make specific requests that I be assigned to their patients.*

"What it boils down to is that compassion is one of the most effective healing tools a nurse can use—it is the essence of a nurse."

Sondra left traditional nursing eight years ago in order to train as a holistic nurse. She is now the owner of a successful alternative medicine clinic in Detroit, Michigan.

One swing shift in the middle of summer about fifteen years ago, I was floated out of oncology to one of the medical floors, and believe me, to be a floor nurse in Detroit in the middle of summer is a miserable job. The regular staff immediately dumped ten patients on me, all of whom had intravenous lines and lots of medications. Of course, seven IVs out of the ten had infiltrated into the surrounding tissue, so I had to restart every one of those. Out of the seven, five were infected badly enough so that I had to notify the doctors in order to get permission to treat these folks. The other nurses didn't have time to help because they were all busy with their own loads, taking care of details that the previous shifts hadn't had time to get to.

So, by the time I got everyone settled and vital signs taken, it was 10:00 P.M. and I hadn't charted one word on anybody. On top of that, I didn't know the floor or where anything was kept, so I was running in circles. There wasn't any air-conditioning, and I'll bet that floor had to be about 103 degrees, no lie.

As soon as I sat down to chart, they told me I had a direct admit from emergency down in room 12. I objected, but they knew I had been floated in, plus they were so overworked they really didn't care much. So I went down to the room where the patient was and I just turned right around and walked out, because the smell was so bad I started to gag and my eyes watered.

Out in the hallway I gave myself a little talk and I said, *Now look, that's another one of God's creatures in there who needs some help. You can do this, because you're a nurse.*

So I went back in, and there on the bed where they dumped her was this seventeen-year-old black woman, IV drug user, HIV-positive, who the previous week had been in the emergency room.

Now, you know how druggies get those sores on their legs like big holes and they get really gross and infected? Well, this gal didn't have any insurance of course, so the ER had just wrapped them up and thrown her back out on the street.

Okay, so those bandages had been on for a week and it's been sweltering hot, and she's been living on the street, so you just know those legs are going to be full of maggots.

Nobody would help me bring her to the shower and all the wheelchairs were broken, so I picked her up myself and carried her into that shower.

While I was washing her down, pulling off the maggots, the gal starts bawling because the maggots scare her and she tells me she feels like the worms from the grave are already trying to get her and she doesn't want to die. I looked at those legs and the needle scars all over her hands and arms and I see this young black gal, sick and scared and so skinny it was pathetic. Nothing but bones—couldn't have weighed more than a hundred pounds—and all I could think of was that my oldest girl was just her age, and what if this was her?

So I start telling her that the maggots are her friends—of course they really were, because they ate away all that exudate in those sores.

Pretty soon, I got her talking and I was washing her hair and everything, telling her that she wouldn't be where she was if she had her choices back. I told her things like she had pretty hair, and nice eyes—trying to make her feel she was somebody, because you could see her eyes were filled up with pain and brutality. She'd been beaten down so bad she believed she was no more than an animal.

When we finally got the maggots out and those legs all wrapped up nice, I combed her hair and gave her a sample of perfume I got that afternoon at the gift shop. It was too late for her to get supper, and the supervisor wouldn't get a sandwich for the gal because she was a street person without insurance. The supervisor kept saying, "We don't give no free rides in this hospital, baby."

So, what the hell—I gave her my dinner. I've got lots of food at home and this gal was literally starving to death.

The whole time she ate, we just talked the way women do sometimes—down to earth. It was clear that she had been hurt real bad, but under all that hurt was an intelligent, sweet gal—and funny too! I told her she had a lot of valuable qualities that she could use to pull herself out of the street, and I gave her simple, concrete ways she could go about doing that. I didn't preach at her, I just told her matter-of-fact.

I was getting ready to go back to the desk when she took my hand and kissed it, so I kissed hers too. That seemed to shock the gal, but then she said, "You tell the Lord I got the message now and I won't forget."

Well, I walked out of that room at 1:00 A.M. feeling like I had been renewed. I felt very fortunate to have taken care of her. Now I don't know what happened to her, because I never saw her again, but I think I made some kind of positive difference in her life. It was through that gal that I realized for the first time that a nurse could touch people's souls with her compassion.

Two hours later, I floated out of that hospital still on cloud nine, really happy to be a healer. And that's the heart of who nurses are, you know—we're the ones with the power to heal.

Jane M.

"You know, there are many opportunities to be had in nursing. Not only is it flexible in terms of types of nursing to be done, but it is a profession which can be practiced anyplace in the world where there are people in need.

"Because of this, I've had some pretty far-reaching and wild experiences during my eleven years as a nurse—experiences I couldn't have had unless I was a nurse."

—Jane M., Washington, D.C.

Don't know why I wanted to become a nurse, exactly. I mean, I liked medicine, but it wasn't any burning need or anything. My dad was a Foreign Service agent, so growing up, I lived all over the world—the Soviet Union, Kenya, Saudi Arabia, all sorts of places like that.

I was in the Air Force Academy taking Soviet studies, but after a while I realized I wasn't cut out for that, so for want of a better thing to do, I went into nursing.

After I got my basics in med-surg, my husband and I decided I should use my skills and my international experiences to benefit others. In 1989, I received international reciprocity as an R.N., and my husband and I and our one-year-old son left for Papua New Guinea.

For the first few months, we settled in the lowlands, where I volunteered at a clinic. Mainly I just observed and learned the pidgin Malaysian and about the cultural differences. It is also there that I witnessed for the first time the most atrocious lack of sterility you could imagine. Things like using the same needle on patient after patient, soaking it in alcohol in between and then tweaking it with their fingers to make sure it was sharp enough for the next person. That was really the least of it. What I found hardest to deal with were things like the way they deal with people in comas. They don't understand the concept of prolonged unconsciousness, so they are convinced the person is actually dead. Many times people are buried alive like this.

Another belief is that maternal blood is extreme evil—never to be touched. If a woman dies in childbirth, the body is left for days. This concept sort of goes along with the fact that women are kept separate from men except for sexual relations, and frequently are bartered for with pigs and other livestock.

The belief that I came head-to-head with was the "evil twin" idea. If a woman has a set of twins, the first baby born is considered the good child. The second twin is thought of as the evil child and routinely killed.

One day a village woman ran up to me in the street with an infant in her arms. She'd recently had twins and had decided to defy her husband and try to keep both children alive. This was a very poor village, and most everyone was malnourished, so for a woman to successfully breast-feed two children at the same time was very difficult. Her sister had finally agreed to suckle the twin, and keep it out of the path of her brother-in-law's machete.

Through the interpreter she told me that her baby was sick and she wanted me to try and help him. I looked at this very tiny three-month-old and was sure this child was going to expire right there in my arms. His respiratory rate was fifty per minute, the pulse was about 180, and his temp was 104.

I told her to take the baby to the clinic, where there were four internationally trained registered nurses who were very skilled and had all the medications the baby would need.

The interpreter told me that the "sisters," as they are called, were on strike and had locked the clinic. Worse yet, the four sisters had taken the only transportation the village had—an old jeep—in order to go to the government and demand more money. The nearest hospital was a five-day walk.

Outraged, my husband gathered a group of village men together and began walking, knocking on every door and asking if anyone had a key to get into the clinic—he was determined not to let this baby die.

All I could think was that I was responsible for keeping this child alive, and I couldn't fathom what I would do if it came down to doing CPR on the child . . . I mean, it's not like you dial 911 and someone comes and intubates the child and starts an IV. So, I took the baby to our hut, where I kept a stock of medications for my family, and gave several I thought might help.

By that time, my husband came back with the keys, so I ran back to the clinic to see if perhaps there was something else I could give. But all the medicines they had had such toxic side effects there wasn't any way I could give them to an infant.

Of course, as my luck would have it, the four nurses came back while I was in the clinic. When they found this white woman wildly searching through their cabinets, they were shocked. I explained what had happened and begged them to give me some IVs and other equipment for this obviously dying infant. In answer, they simply said that they were on strike and they would not help in any way.

I went back to the mother and gave her a travel alarm I'd brought along so that she would know when to give her baby the medications. It was then that I learned that the Papua New Guineans have no concept of clocks and time. They have no need for time since everything they do is by the position of the sun in the sky.

Trying to teach the woman the concept of the clock in sign language took a major effort, but finally she understood that when the short black line was on this symbol, and the long black line was on *this* symbol, she was to give this medication.

We managed to keep the baby alive for two weeks. Finally, the mother gave in to the wishes of the father, completely distanced herself, and let the child die.

I'm a twin myself, so it was hard watching this baby die, but I quickly learned that in this society, death means very little—it is taken casually because it is so prevalent. To keep myself sane, I had to look at only the positives that came out of each death.

The villagers knew that I was married and had a child—this gave me some value. Without a husband or children, a woman is worth less than a pig. After this incident with the baby, they saw that I cared about their children enough to put in an effort.

My son had just turned two, and I was six and a half months pregnant with my second child. The hut we were living in was actually quite luxurious for the jungle. The walls were made from tightly woven mat, and there was a collecting tank for the rainwater that ran off the roof—which we used as our drinking water. We had a battery off which we could run five nine-volt lamps on special occasions. There was also a telephone that was run by a microwave repeater station. This one phone served a population of over two hundred people, including a government station.

Just before Thanksgiving, I had been working in the clinic, which was near an airstrip, and had just come home dead tired. I hadn't been asleep for more than a few minutes when someone knocked at the door.

My husband asked who it was and what they wanted. A man called back that someone was hurt down at the airstrip and that I needed to come down right away to the "sick house" and help.

My husband got up and went to the door, and a few minutes later there was a loud crash and my husband began to scream. I grabbed my son in one hand and the machete in the other. When I got to the door, I looked out and saw my husband being held by a group of men in war paint with bows and arrows and shotguns.

They demanded that I get him a coat and heavy shoes. Now, we were in the tropics, so all I thought was they were going to take him in a plane somewhere or perhaps imprison him in one of the caves.

Ten minutes after they left the house, I heard two gunshots.

So there I am alone in the hut. No electricity. No plumbing. No car. I tried to use the phone, but they had destroyed the satellite dish all the phones in the area were attached to. I didn't put the machete down for two days, crawling on the floor to get from room to room.

None of the villagers would help me, because they'd been threatened with their lives. The following day, I managed to get word out about what had happened, and several days after that, my son and I were airlifted out by an American pilot—at great risk to himself.

I found out that my husband, another American, two Australians, and a German were being held hostage by a rebel group from a neighboring country. The group was trying to make a statement to the United Nations about wanting status as an independent country. What they did not realize was that America absolutely does *not* negotiate for hostage release.

The Iraqi hotel hostage situation had occurred at exactly the same time, so they also didn't get any press or big media coverage. After thirteen days, the two Americans were released, and my husband and I continued our work until my thirtieth birthday, when I collapsed.

At first we thought I had dengue fever, because I had such bad joint pain, but I never broke out in the rash which accompanies it. I drew samples of my blood and gave them to a missionary who was going to a city that had a hospital. A few days later word came back that I had tested out both cerebral and vivax malaria simultaneously. I ended up being flown back to the States, where I delivered my second child and was treated for seven months with IV antibiotics for the malaria.

I always thought that after working in the jungle, nothing would beat it in terms of being tough or dangerous. I want to give first-person testimony that working in the jungle of Washington, D.C., with no backup support was, in fact, actually worse.

We have some areas and homes we go into that require us to have a police escort. We have to go into these crack houses sometimes, and the cops will just sit out in the living room while we do what we have to do with the patients and their families. A lot of our patients are down-and-outers and have weapons in their houses. If they're acting irrational at all, I make sure there are cops with me to watch my back while I'm starting an IV or inserting a catheter.

One of my first patients was Norma. She'd been a major alcoholic, and amazingly, had made it into her fifties; most of these women are dead by the time they hit their mid-forties.

Norma was thin as a rail and didn't have a liver left to speak of. Her brain was pretty well addled too. Her kids had walked out on her long ago, so she didn't have a whole lot of support, but for some reason, I developed a wonderful relationship with her.

She lived in a crack house which had been condemned. It didn't have electricity, but a mistake had been made and they still had water and there was gas to the stove. In the winter, Norma and all these down-and-outers would turn up the stove and everybody would huddle around it together. There'd be twenty people in there sometimes, trying to keep warm.

Norma had ulcers all over her legs and arms which would not heal. For months I went in there three times a week and soaked off the old dressings and put on the new ones. I could not, for the life of me, understand why they wouldn't heal. Then I got a brainstorm and went through her garbage one day. That was when I discovered she'd been drinking rubbing alcohol—the three-quarts-for-a-dollar variety.

In our contracts, the nurses have an R&R clause, which states in black and white that the nurses have the right to refuse to go into a home infested with reptiles and rodents. That should help give you an idea of the battlefield I work in. I have to say, though, that I have met some truly wonderful people in this war zone. One of those was my favorite patient, Mae.

The first time I was assigned to take care of Mae was in the middle of summer in a heat wave. I remember climbing up the stairs of this run-down slum building and the smell just about knocking me off my feet.

Mae was an older woman with bad congestive heart failure. She was crippled and almost blind, and the skin on her arms and legs would weep fluid. I mean, it would ooze off of her to the floor, so that my shoes stuck. I had to pour boric acid around her chair just to keep the roaches away while I examined her and cleaned out her sores.

Of course the roaches loved to feed on that stuff, plus the doctors loaded her up with diuretics, and she couldn't get to the commode, so she'd have to urinate in the chair she sat in. Well, she'd be swarming with those things and then she'd get infected and have to go to the hospital for IV antibiotics—those were the good times.

I think worse than the roaches was a nephew who fed off her. Mae had no food and no money. There was an income from her husband's pension—it came to about two hundred dollars a month. A hundred and eighty went to the landlord, and the other twenty went for food, except every month, the nephew would come into the apartment, take the twenty dollars and any food the neighbors and church sisters had brought in, and then leave her there to die.

I remember one time walking in and finding the gas stove was in flames. The nephew had made his monthly visit and cooked some food, then left the burners on. The grease had built up over the years, and had caught fire, and he left it like that. It was hard to say whether he was just careless or trying to kill the old woman.

I remember asking her to tell me what she wanted, and she said she didn't want to be a bother to anyone and that she was trying to die as quietly and as fast as she could. And oh God, she was so appreciative of the care I gave her. She would bless me up one side and down the other. I gave her clothes and always tried to clean her and the apartment up as best I could.

Once, when she really got bad, her blood pressure went up to 220 over 150 and I thought she was going to die. I called 911 and the paramedics who showed up really didn't want to come into the apartment. They refused to touch her, so I had to do most of the work of getting her on the carrier and out of the apartment. Once we got her in the ambulance, I remember two of them looking at me like I was crazy, and saying they could not believe I'd been going in there to treat her.

I suppose I could have taken the time to explain to them about how this was a fellow human being who needed their help, and it shouldn't matter how she smelled, or what bugs were eating off her, human and otherwise. I guess I could have told them what a beautiful soul this woman had, and how her smile was the light of my day. Or I imagine I could have told them that she really didn't want to bother them with her dying.

I could have, but the shame of it was that I don't think I would have gotten through, the same way I don't think I would have gotten through to those striking nurses in Papua New Guinea.

Hell, I don't know—sometimes I have a hard time believing what coldness humans are capable of.

Arthur B.

Arthur B. has dual professions. At night, the thirty-eight-year-old R.N. works in the ER of one of the largest trauma centers in the United States. During the day, he works as a risk management attorney for a large insurance company. He has been a nurse for two years and an attorney for eighteen. He makes four times the amount of money as an attorney, but as a nurse, he takes "ten times the grief."

So why does he continue to do nursing?

"I do it because there is some part of me that still wants to save the world. I'm a nurse because it feels like the right thing to do."

I guess that working in the emergency room should make me immune to the sorrow of seeing someone's loved one die, but somehow, I've never been able to escape the empathy factor. I don't have much of a social life, since my passion for "making the world a better place" consumes much of my time. Stolen moments with my rapidly aging children, who live with my ex-wife, take any free time I might have.

I work weekends and holidays at one of the busiest and largest trauma centers in the nation. As I drove the highway to the hospital last night, in addition to the usual feelings of *Sure wish I was out picnicking with someone I could love instead of working tonight*, there was a sobering overtone of *Gosh, maybe I fear love because I fear the loss of it once I have it*. It's sort of like winning the lottery and having your financial manager screw you out of all your assets—maybe it would be better not having won in the first place?

Anyway, my evening began as usual.

One. Show holographic ID to the guard. I mean, who would *want* to impersonate someone who works in this hellhole?

Two. Get used to ozone-conditioned air that is intended to mask smells of human blood and the McDonald's located down the hall.

Three. Put on my game face—the alter ego I must engage to hold down a job that is alien to my very being. Alien because in "real life," I get queasy when someone has a nosebleed near me. It is almost unimaginable to my parents that I could actually work on a gunshot wound, but then, parents are often the last to understand their children.

My first intake of the night was Bonnie, an early-fortyish woman to whom I felt an almost immediate attraction. Bonnie was five-six, slim, clear olive complexion, and had the most wonderful shoulder-length brunette hair. I noticed she wasn't wearing a wedding ring and I thought, *Hmm, is this fate knocking at my ER door?*

Bonnie showed no indication of needing medical attention, and it has been so long since I've been with a woman that my mind naturally raced toward other things . . . It was spring, after all.

"I was shopping with my daughter and I suddenly felt very dizzy," she said, smiling. It was a beautiful smile.

"Daughter?" I responded. "Does that mean your husband might be worried about where you are?" I thought this a rather clever way of finding out if she was available.

"Oh, he's not worried yet," she assured me, with another wonderful smile. "He's not expecting us back until nine-thirty."

Undaunted, I pressed on. One never knew nowadays what "husband" really meant. "Have you been married long?" I asked innocently enough.

Bonnie nodded. "Uh-huh. Seventeen years' and five daughters' worth. He's a great guy. Very creative and a good provider."

"Hey, that's great!" I said, feeling happy for her good fortune and a little disappointed for my own. I turned back to the task of filling out the intake questionnaire, not wanting to hear any more about the Husband Wonderful. This was a job, after all.

"How did you get to the ER tonight?"

"My oldest drove me from the mall. I was feeling too . . ."

I glanced up in time to see that Bonnie was beginning to perspire, even though the exam room was a brisk 67 degrees.

"May I lie down?" she asked, lying down on the gurney. "I'm sick to my stomach and I'm getting dizzy again."

Her complexion had changed from an elegant olive tan to a grayish green hue. I hooked her up to a pulse oximeter and took a blood pressure. The blood pressure had risen dramatically from the one I'd obtained when she first sat down. Something wasn't right. The clinical diagnosis hypertensive crisis came to mind.

"Have you started taking any new drugs or been doing any new activities lately?"

Bonnie nodded. "I just started taking Phen-Fen for weight loss? My husband is a real stickler about me staying in shape." She lowered her eyes, embarrassed. "After seventeen years of marriage, you begin to worry about your husband having a wandering eye. Gotta keep those buns tight and high, you know."

I nodded, amazed that someone so attractive and slender would be worried about a weight problem. I began thinking of the Husband Wonderful as Mr. Bluebeard. "Are you on any other medications?"

She nodded. "Nardil. For about three years."

In the back of my mind a bell went off . . . something about Nardil, which was an antidepressant, and weight loss medications never being given together. "Did the weight loss clinic know you were taking the Nardil?"

She shook her head. "They never asked."

I could see she was getting restless, and I turned up the oxygen again, then paged a resident for a stat evaluation.

"Could you go tell my girls that this is going to take a little while longer?" Bonnie asked. "They're going to be wondering what's taking so long."

As I walked into the waiting room, I saw three younger versions of Bonnie. Seventeen-year-old Tina was the photo image of her mother. I told her that her mother needed to be evaluated and we were waiting for the resident to show up.

"My dad is going to be so pissed off!" the teenager huffed. "He's working late tonight and he's going to want his dinner when he gets home."

Her response made me incredibly sad, but somewhere mixed with the gloom was anger. I massaged the knots in the back of my neck, telling myself to ignore it—and why should I care, anyway? "Your mom doesn't feel very well," I explained. "But I don't think it should be too much longer."

Somehow I instinctively knew as the words left my mouth that I was lying.

Tina stood up and looked off in the direction of McDonald's, twisting her fingers around each other. I noticed her nails were as long as knives and painted black. "Well, I guess I better get the brats some Cokes so they settle down for a while," she said, in that accusing, snotty tone that belongs exclusively to adolescents. It was as though her mother being ill had caused her and her father a life-threatening inconvenience.

When I returned to room 9, Bonnie was sweating profusely, gasping for air, and looking vaguely like a goldfish who had jumped out of her bowl. I shook her and called her name. Her response was slow and she was beginning to show signs of confusion.

I hit the call button and ran outside to the nurses' station, yelling for the resident as I went.

"Where the hell is the resident?" I asked the clerk, my face registering panic.

The clerk—possibly the most jaded of us all—had seen it all before. Nothing could fluster her anymore—not blood in any amount, or amputated limbs, or human hearts hanging out of bodies by their coronary arteries. In a voice I found unnervingly casual she said: "Oh, her boyfriend just come in from out of town 'bout twenty minutes ago. You prob'ly find 'em screwin' their brains out in the doctors' sleep room."

"We need a doc in room nine stat!" I started to run full steam toward room 9. "I don't care who you get, just get them now!"

My sixth sense told me what I would find before I pulled back the curtain to the room. One look at Bonnie's fully dilated pupils and the ashen gray color of her skin, and I knew that the simple, flat line dividing the monitor screen was for real.

My heart went to my throat as I hit the code alarm and began CPR. The motto of the hospital is "We're the Best." I kept that in mind as the respondents to the code call were a few first- and second-year med students lazily pushing the crash cart ahead of them, and a risk manager who wanted to know, "What's happenin', bubba?" as he strolled—not ran—into the room.

I asked God to help me, scoped Bonnie's airway, and intubated her. I pushed in the milligram of epinephrine and then the milligram of atropine. The CPR continued, as did the underlying rhythm of asystole. Flatline. Dead heart.

"Don't do this, Bonnie," I pleaded, taking over the chest compressions again. Under my hands, her skin felt soft and cool. "The Husband

Wonderful needs you to make dinner, and your snotty kids need you to pick out their prom dresses. Come on, damn it!"

One of the other nurses brought in a transcutaneous pacing setup and applied the electrodes. The machine was broken. Another was sent for, except we all knew it would be too late by the time another was found.

I gave another round of epi and atropine; then we stopped long enough to see what was going on under the CPR.

Flatline.

"Give me some hope, Bonnie." With the next chest compression, I felt one of her ribs crack. I had an instant flashback to being taught by my grandmother how to snap the necks of chickens, and felt sick to my stomach.

"I want to rescue you when the Husband Wonderful dumps you for a young bimbo with high, tight buns," I continued, not blind to the strange looks directed at me from the resident and a couple of the med students. "Don't do this," I begged. "Please don't do this."

A cardiologist arrived, ordered more lab work, and gave a few more drugs. He considered cracking her chest, then changed his mind. A working model of the transcutaneous pacer was applied.

None of it mattered. Bonnie remained a flatline—with the exception of the pacing spikes.

The resident called the code off at 10:22 P.M. and then added, "Oh well, shit happens."

The logistics technician, which is the new euphemism for an orderly, came and covered her body and left.

Alone with the body, I kicked away some of the postcode litter from around the gurney, pushed the various life support machines into the corner, took a deep breath, and uncovered Bonnie's face.

I stared at her for a long time, asking her to forgive me, knowing I would not be able to forgive myself. The one thing you learn right away is that there are no second chances in this business. The way I see it, you call it right the first time around, or you relinquish your right to play God.

Outside the flimsy curtains of exam room 9, I wondered—with a new surge of horror—what I was going to say to the three daughters in the waiting room.

I found the resident at the chart desk, getting ready to leave the unit again. "In the waiting room are this woman's three teenage daughters," I informed her. "Could you go out there and tell them? Could you explain what happened so that—"

The resident waved a hand in my face and started to move off, probably back to the boyfriend waiting in the doctors' sleep room. "Call the chaplain," she said in an indifferent tone. "It's not our job to inform the relatives."

When I thought I was ready, I walked out into the waiting room. Tina was on me before I could open my mouth.

"What's taking you so long, anyway?" she snapped impatiently. "You charge by the hour or something?"

The whole thing crashed down on my head . . . or maybe I should say my heart, because I started to cry and couldn't stop. I still don't know who I was crying for—the kids, Bonnie, the Husband Wonderful, or me.

I know I shouldn't, but I think about Bonnie a lot these days, almost in the same way I might think of a girlfriend who dumped me unexpectedly. I'm not an automaton. I can't always leave my patients at the hospital. I hurt because her death was such a waste. Mostly, I am tortured because I can't go back and save her.

JoAnna A.

When I put out the word for nurses to come forth and tell their stories, I made it a point to tell them that I wanted to touch on all branches of nursing.

Here's one you might not have heard before—a critical care R.N. who specializes in the care of sick and injured marine mammals.

I started out in Indiana and then moved to Florida in '85. Right out of nursing school, I cut my teeth on a step-down cardiac unit, which was in essence a "dump" floor [a unit that gets a wide variety of patients]. I learned all the insert-a-KAO-feed-tube-in-the-dark skills there, then transferred to acute cardiac care for four years, where I subbed for the IV team and floated to the ER. After that, I went to a cardiology office for a few years and then to home health, where I've been for four years.

I always thought that when I was old and gray, I would teach nursing, but now with nursing changing so much, who knows what kind of nursing school there would be—if any. I also don't know if I could honestly encourage people to go into nursing. I'd rather teach volunteers to care for marine mammals.

While I was working at the cardiology office I got a divorce. When I came out of my depressive phase, I decided I couldn't continue to sit at home and stare at the walls, so I volunteered at a local marine laboratory.

At the time, the lab had a dolphin named Matt who had been caught in a crab trap line until some fishermen found him and cut him free. Of course he was so debilitated that he sank to the bottom, so the fisherman pulled him up and brought him in.

Matt was my first dolphin—which is kind of like saying he was my first love. I'd work for home health in the mornings with my human patients, and then I'd go to the marine lab and work with Matt. He had to have around-the-clock care at the time, so I'd get into the water, help with the exam, give him tube feedings of water or Pedialyte or whatever medications the vet ordered, and then shower and go back and take care of humans.

On a few occasions, I was asked to stay for the postexam chat between the vet and the stranding program coordinator, who was also our marine mammal biologist. I remember that I'd sit there and stare at these vials of Matt's blood sitting out on the table. A couple of meetings went by before I got the nerve to speak up: "Hey, listen," I said. "About these vials of blood—what's going to happen to those, and when are they going to get to the lab? I mean, blood can't just sit all this time. The cells begin to degrade, and you lose valuable information. It isn't clinically correct."

So, I was elected to take the blood right away to the medical lab . . . which necessitated my "finding" a couple of small coolers and ice packs to transport the vials in. That was when I realized the marine lab was lacking a lot of real basic equipment. The first thing I did was to get a centrifuge machine donated by a local medical lab.

It was so nice for a change to have my knowledge and expertise instantly appreciated. There wasn't any of the usual hospital bureaucratic red tape involved, and it was very rewarding for me and the program because I had ties to the medical community that they didn't have before.

Matt did very well and was released in thirty-seven days to his original place of stranding.

Once the marine lab had the success of Matt's treatment and release under their belt, they were considering getting into long-term rehab care, which meant building a new facility. They were a nonprofit private organization, so in the next year I organized volunteers, started a newsletter, asked the scientists to give talks and lectures about the various mammals, raised funds which allowed the mammal program to buy equipment necessary to the keeping of any future live animals we might have.

And then, we got Freeway.

6/7/93 Monday: Wow. What a day! At 9:30 A.M. I got a page from the lab that there was a live animal stranded. When I asked its location, I was told the highway patrol had found him in a salt marsh that ran alongside Highway 75.

I had to check to make sure my socks were still on. First of all, the highway patrol isn't exactly who we usually hear about strandings from (!!), and second of all, how the hell could a dolphin get up there? He would have had to travel up the Manatee River for more than ten miles, go under the Manatee Bridge, and weave his way through the salt marshes. At low tide, there's barely a foot of water in some of those areas. Why the animal stranded so far up the river, we'll never know, although he could have just drifted with the tide.

Far-fetched though it sounded, I headed out the interstate and sure enough, there he was in a foot and a half of water, thirty feet below in a salt marsh. I estimated him at nine feet and about 350 pounds. I could also see he was desperately ill. He had rapid, shallow respirations and a lot of open wounds.

There were four people in the water already with him—including the fish and game officer for the area, who was still in his uniform. Thank God he'd had the good sense to drape the animal with the wet sheets. Dolphins dehydrate and sunburn as rapidly as human infants left on a hot beach. That beautiful skin is so fragile.

I knew we were going to have a major problem getting to him, so I suggested we call the fire department, who might be able to throw some kind of ladder over the edge so we could climb down to the marsh. I mean, they're good at cats in trees, right?

Eventually, the stranding program coordinator went up in a news helicopter to determine water-access possibilities, and in the end, it was decided to walk the animal to a trailer-park boat ramp that was about 750 yards from where he was stranded.

An off-duty fireman who had a jon boat [a utility boat] was called and met us at the boat ramp. With the fireman, we started at the boat ramp and backtracked through the maze of marshes to the bottlenose.

About six of us put a canvas sling under him and half carried, half dragged him the entire 750 yards to the ramp where all the equipment was.

What a job! First of all, I was the only female, so I had to work to keep up. That was nerve-racking, because one false step and I would have sunk up to my waist in the muck and not been able to get out. I didn't want to have to drop my part of the sling. I lost one of my shoes.

Halfway back to the ramp, the fish and game officer decides to tell us all about the terrible snakes that live in the marshes. I kind of wish he'd at least waited until we were a little closer to the ramp.

We were still a good ways out when I saw that crowds of people and several television crews had gathered on the ramp. Big news around here.

It was noon when we finally got to the ramp. The lab's marine biologist drew blood for the medical lab, and a vet did a five-minute assessment. We monitored his respirations carefully, because the weight of his chest could easily crush his lungs and make him go into respiratory distress and then shock and then possibly die. Their lungs are different from ours—not lobes but two huge balloons which have four times the capacity of ours.

I ran to a medical lab while the dolphin was transported to the marine lab by truck. As soon as the medical lab found out we had a live, stranded dolphin, they were thrilled to run the bloods—gratis!

Around 12:45 the animal (the volunteers have been calling him "Freeway") was placed in the same shark holding tank where Matt had been. An hour later blowhole and wound cultures were done. After that, we put a towel over his top and bottom teeth and then ran a stomach tube into the first of his three stomach chambers. The contents were tested and measured and he was rehydrated with a half-gallon of water.

The vet explained about the functions of the different chambers. The first chamber mashes the whole fish into chunks, the second grinds it down finer, the third sends it to the guts. They have no cough or gag reflex, so they don't throw up.

Around 4:00 P.M., Freeway had been identified as "Crumpled Edge" in a photo ID catalog. His dorsal fin, which is the dolphin equivalent to a human fingerprint (no two alike), gave us some information as to where he had been seen before.

The swim test was performed at 4:30 P.M., which he promptly failed by dropping like a stone and rolling all the way to the right without the ability to come up to the surface for air. He made no swimming motions. The vet is pretty sure he has pneumonia so he was given injections of penicillin G and Tagamet. The volunteers will have to hold him up twenty-four hours a day.

We cathed him for a urine specimen and counted his teeth so as to tell which species he is (bottlenose). I did a complete nose-to-tail assessment. Listening to his lungs was amazing. It wasn't the usual 0.8 to 2 breaths a minute—Freeway was breathing at a rate of 7 a minute! I really had to make sure of what I was hearing, so I took a long time with this.

The vets came to look at him again, and I shared the findings of my assessment, the most important of which was that I heard no lung sounds on the right. A collapsed lung! I told the vet that I thought Freeway had a pneumothorax—probably from blunt trauma from a shark. I also heard an S-3 gallop when listening to his heart. Tomorrow a.m., we're going to do an ultrasound of that right lung.

Freeway is in critical condition and no one here gives him much hope of surviving. He has very significant wounds—I think they're from a recent shark fight. The worst of the wounds is on his tail stalk—the area between the actual tail and the body itself. The wound is open all the way to the lateral spine. The vet found a piece of bone that had actually been broken off.

6/9/93: We did an ultrasound this morning and found a lot of fluid. The vet was just going to leave it, so I explained that in people with the same problem, we do a thoracentesis to aspirate the fluid. I told him how it was done, and he said we couldn't do that on a dolphin.

I asked him why not, and told him I could get all the equipment we needed from the hospital. I suggested we get a pulmonary specialist.

Picked up vacutainer bottles and tubing from the hospital. A marine mammal specialist called other vets and a human pulmonologist and got advice and method of procedure over the phone. There weren't really any physicians to assist, just an ultrasound company with some sophisticated equipment. Together, we performed the first thoracentesis ever done on a cetacean. We got three liters of fluid!

Freeway keeps his eyes closed. I think it's because dolphins' eyes are sensitive to the sun if exposed for long periods of time. He is still very attentive to his surroundings, though. He uses his other senses including echolocation to check things out.

6/10/93: We drained another three liters. I asked the vet if we could please start wound care. He said he didn't think it was important right now.

That bothers me, because it is SO important. I mean, when we do necropsies, how many times do we find out they died from septicemia from wounds?

We are doing major, fastidious charting. Freeway's respirations and behavior are recorded every half hour. I've been pushing the volunteers to describe what they see and hear instead of noting summations of their judgments. Don't label—describe! How many times did I hear that in nursing school?

When I assess an animal, I take in the whole picture—medications, diet, including the behavior and what environmental factors might be involved in the behavior.

6/11/93: Three more liters came off his lungs today. Got permission to begin wound care (FINALLY!). To properly care for the tail stalk wound, I had the volunteers rotate him onto his side, keeping his blow-hole above water. I found I could put my middle finger in to halfway between my proximal and middle joint, and it's about six inches wide. He's got gouge wounds and tooth rake wounds. I debrided them all, and scrubbed them down with Betadine.

When I ran my hands over his belly tonight, I found a tooth embedded in one of the wounds. We walked it across the street to the shark department, and asked them to identify it.

It belonged to a bull shark of about eight feet in length. Man, that must have been one hell of a fight. I wonder what came first, though. Was Freeway already sick and weakened, which might have caused the shark to attack, or did the attack come first and then he got sick?

Out in the wild, sick animals are easy prey.

6/15/93: Two more liters today for a total of eight. Freeway's breathing is much better and his heart rate has slowed down. He's getting feisty. He is NOT happy about being held by the volunteers all the time. He's temperamental, and he has a strong personality that is great in his own way. Whereas Matt was easygoing and friendly, this animal can be snotty—just like people. His disposition is wild. He truly makes me respect that he is a wild animal. If he doesn't want you in his pen, he can make that painfully clear. It's challenging. Today he bucked the volunteers off several times and then went after them with open mouth. Some of the volunteers are refusing to go into the tank with him.

I didn't give it a second thought—all I can see is that he is finally swimming on his own!

I noticed tonight how alert he is. Even though he doesn't open his eyes, he seems very curious about noises and sounds which come from the deck. We took a video of him, and it's obvious he's paying attention to who is walking down the deck.

6/93: I got to do an intramuscular injection on him. The challenge is to hit muscle—not blubber.

Also learned how to draw Freeway's blood. Seems that dolphins have cartilage tracks. The veins and arteries sit inside that track and you aim the needle at a 45-degree angle. Sometimes it's hard to know whether you have arterial or venous blood.

7/93 Wednesday: Freeway definitely swimming better, although he still takes lots of rest stops on the steps of the tank.

He's eating between ten and twenty-five pounds of fish a day—except he absolutely hates mullet. Doesn't matter how we serve it—filleted or headless or head-on—he will not eat it unless it weighs less than a pound. He will eat silver mullet, however.

The total amount of fluid we drained off his lungs came to fourteen liters!

7/93 Saturday: Today we brought Freeway to his new home—a thirty-by-thirty-foot pen made from construction netting that runs along one side of the lab. He, of course, swam immediately to the farthest, deepest corner and stayed there.

We're going to have to wait until low tide when we want to do exams on him.

The vet came to examine him today. We had about twelve people holding him. Someone was down at the tail drawing blood, and the vet was up at his head. The biologist got thrown off—about ten feet through the water. Three times in a row!

You never let an animal buck you off and get away with it. The best way to deal with it is usually to bear-hug the animal and hang on. With Freeway that was a nice thought, but it didn't work.

8/93 Thursday: Went down to the dock to do Freeway's morning assessment and give him his meds. When I looked in the water, I literally gasped—I thought sea grass must have grown overnight. The water had turned a mucky green. But as I got closer, I realized it wasn't sea grass at all, but masses and masses of minnows. The minnows had learned that they could get through the construction netting.

As Freeway swam around his pen, you'd see this sort of parting of the Red Sea. All the minnows would part and then form back together behind the animal. On close observation, I was amazed at the sudden healing rate of Freeway's wounds. When I really watched, I could see that he was slapping his tail a lot. I realized he was trying to shake off the minnows, who were actually serving as mechanical debriders by feeding off of the dead tissue, keeping those wounds clean.

He is still on a lot of meds, and although he's better, his blood work wasn't really improving. We looked at the meds. Tagamet to prevent stress ulcers—just like hospitalized human patients. Antibiotics, Mylanta for gas, plus a host of others.

I am so thrilled with the wound healing! God, they all look great—they're that beefy red color. He will always have an indentation on that tail stalk, and he will always have a scar, but it looks wonderful to me.

8/93 Tuesday: Freeway has colic. The night shift volunteers found him fidgety—doing pinwheels by spinning on his side. We took videos of his uncontrollable swimming around the tank—obvious pain. As the gas in his abdominal cavity grew, he began riding very high with his dorsal fin totally out of the water. At one point, he tucked into a crescent shape so that he couldn't get his blowhole out of the water. They jumped in and he actually let them lift him up without a fight so he could breathe. I guess that tells us how much pain he was in—normally, he wouldn't let them touch him.

They stomach-tubed him to relieve some of the gas.

This morning, we made the decision to take him off all medications. We'll see what happens.

8/93 Friday: Two weeks and nothing has changed. Freeway's white blood count, which usually remains around 10, started to climb a few days ago. We took him off all the other antibiotics and started him on good old-fashioned tetracycline.

8/93 Friday: Freeway drastically improved in every way. He's almost back to normal. His wounds are granulated about ninety-eight percent.

I am in awe of his fantastic acrobatic ability. Several times at sunrise, after Freeway "woke up" from the night, he'd begin zooming around the pen and then suddenly leap out of the water. Sometimes I notice that he does an intentional tail sweep of the dock—when there are volunteers sitting there. He'd create a huge wave that would soak everybody, then he'd circle back around eyeing the dock and laughing. What a character!

We should have a release date soon. I'll make sure every last one of the two hundred volunteers gets called so they can be there to observe.

———

9/22/93: What a fantastic day! I am so excited.

It's been 107 days. We released him just north of the Manatee River at Emerson Point.

The first thing he did was sort of meander around the boat, then he headed toward the mouth of the river. A huge roar went up from the crowd that lined the beach. The fish and game officer was there—he again waltzed right into the water with his uniform on—and the fireman who had come out the day he was found, and the medical lab workers . . . anyone who participated in any way, shape, or form.

Just as he got to the mouth of the river, he jumped and his whole body came out of the water—a complete breach—and he rotated and did a dorsal fin slap instead of a tail slap.

The evening paper said he was jumping for joy to be released, but the marine biologist said he was just trying to get that damned radio tag off his fin and that's the only way he knew how to do it.

We put zinc oxide on his dorsal fin (Freeway wore pink!)—to protect it and also so we could see him better while we tracked him.

We outfitted him with a transmitter, so I also got to go on the tracking boat. The only time we could hear him was when he surfaced for a breath, so we could also monitor his respirations. Just in case he started getting into any kind of trouble, we had obtained prior permission to recapture him. IF we could.

It took him about five hours to get to the Sunshine Skyway. We lost him a few times. He jumped frequently. He was in great shape.

So long, Freeway. See ya around.

Christine K.

A nurse since 1985, Christine K., forty-three, has worked in Colorado for most of those years. Formerly a teacher and counselor for the deaf and for the parents of handicapped patients, she is presently working full-time as a telephone triage nurse, and completing her third master's degree for clinical nurse specialist in pediatric education.

He had been a famous star of the screen. Even though he had aged rather badly, I recognized him through the wrinkles the multiple cosmetic surgeries had not nipped or tucked out of existence.

In the movies he was one of those handsome, robust though soft-spoken, romantic characters who always played the hero and savior to his equally robust (emphasis on bust) female leads. He was an actor everyone loved. The movie magazines swore in black and white that in real life, he was as kind and good-hearted as all his Hollywood characters.

Although he lived in one consistently foul mood, I don't know for certain what had put him into such an extremely loathsome mood this particular morning, but I guessed it was due to the fact he'd failed so miserably at dyeing. The disastrous attempt to cover what was left of his sparse, dull gray strands had left him an orangehead instead of a blackhead.

Or perhaps it was the fact that after being pampered and mooned over by an adoring nursing staff at a certain private and plush hospital, he had run out of insurance funds and was forced to live with his adoring daughter in her six-bedroom country estate.

When I walked into his room, he was staring at himself in a large mirror which had been propped up on a table over his bed. He frowned, but did not take his eyes away from his image.

I greeted him cheerily, exactly as I had for the last three weeks since his discharge from the hospital of the stars.

Glaring, he put his voice box against his throat. "What do you want?" he growled, as best he could in a mechanical monotone. "I didn't ring for you. You're allowed to enter this room at my command only."

I stared at him, wanting in the worst way to tell him he didn't need to take it out on me, and not to worry—his hair would grow out. Of course I didn't, but I wanted to.

"I just got here, Mr. X," I said, never once dropping my happy voice. "I thought I'd let you know I was here and offer a bath and a shave. It'll make you feel human again."

"Go to hell," he said, which I had learned was his way of saying okay.

I had already decided when I woke up that I would not let his abuse get to me on this day. Smiling, I backed away from the bed toward the drawers which held the clean linens for his bath and shave. You see, it was his number one rule that no one should ever turn their back on him. It made for interesting contortions sometimes.

After I had the water to the temperature he liked (he'd throw the basin of water at me or to the floor if it wasn't exactly the right temperature) and was ready to begin his shave, he demanded the mirror be removed and one of his movies be played so he could watch himself.

I did as he asked, glad for his choice of movies; the female lead had always been one of my favorite actresses. The movie hadn't even gotten to the opening scene, when he suddenly picked up the basin of soapy water and heaved it in my direction with the explanation that I'd blocked his view of the screen.

I hadn't seen it coming. The soap stung my eyes as I searched under the bed for the basin, but I still refused to let the incident ruin my resolve to remain if not cheerful then at least civil. I concentrated instead on how nice it was going to feel to change into the dry uniform I kept stashed in my car for just such an occasion as this.

A third of the way into the movie, I got back to the job of shaving and bathing Mr. X. He was doing his usual running commentary on his and everyone else's performance.

"I pulled this goddamned movie through. . . . The director was a worthless little man—stupid, really. I ended up directing the film myself. . . . Just listen to that! What a fabulous delivery I made there. . . . Her? Bah, she couldn't act her way out of a paper bag. She was so boozed up I had to save her in every scene. . . . Oh, just look at that shot of me, will you—best damned leading man there ever was since Valentino. . . . Him? He was a lousy actor. Had sexual problems with women, you know. Couldn't act for shit either. . . . Oh, I just can't believe how good I was there. Just listen to that voice . . . mesmerizing."

He wasn't, however, that mesmerized by his own performance not to kick me in the ribs while I was washing his feet. He didn't even look down when he told me I wasn't going fast enough.

I had slid off the back of a good mood and was holding on to its tail.

I did his oral care for him, because he had an aversion to touching his dentures (they reminded him of his own pearly whites, which had already crossed over and were waiting for the rest of his body to get there), then changed the dressing on his IV site, and hung new tubing and a fresh bag of fluid. I was about to take his blood pressure when he asked for his hairbrush.

The stand-up comedienne in my mind made an unkind joke about how the neon-orange color would come in handy in finding the three strands he had left to brush. I must have been momentarily distracted by the effort to bite my tongue, because I turned my back on him and walked toward the dresser.

I knew right away something was off—the straight-on view of that side of the room was new to me. I was in the middle of whipping around when he hurled the large TV remote control box at my head with all his might.

It hit its intended mark.

"How *dare* you turn your back on me!" he said, gripping his voice box with trembling hands. His face was a sea of fury and contempt. "You're an ingrate!"

Dazed, I swallowed, coughed, and spit into my hand.

The good mood fell into a deep, dark mud puddle of funk. The object had hit my head with such force as to cause me to slam my jaws together and break off two of my teeth. Staring at the pieces, I slowly turned around to face the leading man.

"I am leaving now," I said calmly, looking at him straight on—although I do believe one eye was narrowed somewhat by the swelling going on on that side of my face. "I'll find someone to cover me. I don't deserve this treatment from anyone."

He pointed a finger at me and snorted as best he could with his mechanical box. "You're just a nurse. A good-for-nothing, lazy woman who can't do anything."

I walked out of the room . . . face first, and began making calls.

My employer said two things. The first was that she had yet to set up with Labor and Industries because, as she put it, there hadn't been time to handle that "little hassle." The second thing she said was, "Don't be such a crybaby. You have to stay for the remaining four hours of your shift."

I explained to her that this wasn't possible because I was in terrific pain and needed to get to my dentist stat.

She hung up on me.

I called my assistant head nurse, who said he would come promptly to replace me. At that moment, Mr. X's daughter came into the room and demanded (it's in the genes, you know) to know why I had "abandoned" (a penchant for drama can also be passed through the genes) her father, who had been hurling obscenities at me since I left his room.

In response, I opened my hand to show her what had happened.

"Oh, but those *can't* be my father's teeth, my dear," she sniffed down at me. "Daddy wears dentures."

I assured her they were mine.

She grabbed the phone out of my hand and called my employer.

To this day my only regret is that I did not get a recording of that rather amazing three-way conversation. In the end, it was agreed by the daughter and my employer that I was at fault entirely—I must have done *something* horrible to have enraged the sweet old man to the extent he had to do such a thing to defend himself against me. The daughter billed him as the gentlest, most loving creature on earth . . . a true Bambi amongst men.

I gathered my wet uniform and walked straight to my dentist.

Fifteen hundred dollars of dental work later—out of my own pocket, of course—I can grind my teeth again.

Oh. Just for the record? The fellow who replaced me that day had both of his collarbones broken by Mr. X two weeks later. I never got the full story. I don't want to know.

Mary V.

As was my habit whenever I received recorded tapes from nurses, before sitting down to transcribe them I'd first listen to them straight through while taking my morning run.

While listening to Mary V.'s tape, a half-mile or so into it, I found myself slowing down in order to swallow down the lump and wipe away a tear or two, or then, a mile later, stopping to catch my breath from laughing so hard. It went on like this—an emotional roller-coaster ride—for the full seven miles.

Passing commuters must have thought I had just been released from the mothership (I was in Ojai, California, at the time), or that I was having a breakdown of one sort or another.

While you read this narrative, I have to ask you to imagine it in the way it was told—with a very thick Canadian accent, rich with aboot's and ooooot's.

I turn forty next month. I've been a nurse for over twenty years. Why did I chose nursing? Some days I wonder. At the time it was because Mum was a nurse, and I suppose, because I'd been a candy striper, which I enjoyed. I've worked as a rural nurse for most of my twenty years. I started out in a small, fifty-bed rural hospital. I've worked in med-surg, small-peds unit, obstetrics, outpatient care, emergency, and as an administrative supervisor. Since 1990, I've worked in home care and as a consultant in occupational health nursing. I also run a small independent practice that provides for home care, teaching, and assessments.

Nursing isn't a lot of fun anymore. It's more high-tech. A lot less caring. A lot busier. Many of the things of value have disappeared. I'm not burned out now, but I did about ten years ago. A change in practice areas helped.

My family accepts the strange things that happen to your life as a nurse. And too, my husband is a fisherman, which also makes for unpredictable hours and living in interesting times.

When my daughter was five years old she'd carry around a toy doctor's bag and say she was a doctor. Once I said, "Aren't you going to be a nurse like your mum?"

She looked at me horrified and said, "Oh no—nurses have to stay up all night!"

So I told her that doctors have to stay awake all night too, to which she replied: "Yeah, but they get paid more money for doing it." So even at that age, she'd figured it out. Unfortunately, I never did.

I go to school part-time now to study computers. It helps keep me sane.

1974

I worked my first full shift as a student in 1974. I was put in charge of a general ward. The only thing I wasn't allowed to do was to pass medications, which was unfortunate because at the time, it was the one thing I knew how to do. I had no idea how to manage a floor or be in charge, and I had only two nurse's aides working with me that night.

Of course, it was one of those crazy, crazy nights where everything happens all at once. Well, I was so busy that at one point I recall going into a room where there were these parents visiting their three-month-old daughter, who was hydrocephalic.

I remember wrapping her up and giving her and the bottle to the mother and saying, "Here. You'd better feed her, because I'm just too busy right now."

It came to light later that the parents had never touched this baby since the minute she was born. I had no idea what I'd done, but after that, they came in every night and held her. Eventually they brought her home.

In the middle of report there was a confusion down the hall, so we all went running down to see what the problem was only to find that one of the patients had been found dead in his bed.

Keeping in mind that I'd never seen a dead body in all my life— when we went to turn him over, he made that sound that happens sometimes in the dead when you move them, where the air rushes out of the body and the person makes that *ggguurrggghaaaah* noise?

It took about ten years off my life. I was beside myself. I was sure he'd come back from the dead and was going to rise up and spit.

Well, after having myself a good screech in the bathroom, I went back to the unit, which was getting more and more frantic. Also, it was hot as Hades—you know, one of those nights where the hair sticks to your neck. So I'm told to admit this little old lady. This woman was filthy . . . completely illiterate. She was one I'd seen downtown wandering around mumbling to herself. I go down with the admission sheet, and she makes an X at the bottom, and I'm trying not to breathe in the stench, and my eyes are watering because the smell is so bad I can't breathe.

That was the night that the supervisor, who was a rather nasty piece of work, made me give all the suppositories on the unit.

1978

Back then, there was no emergency department or outpatient clinic, so that meant that the supervisor handled all the incoming patients at night or on the evening shift. It also meant that patients coming into the hospital came directly to the wards.

There were five doctors for the area, mostly family practice physicians and one surgeon. In order to call in the doctor, even if he was on call, you had to be pretty darned sure of your facts, because the doctors were like gods back then, and the nurses were just dirt under their shoes.

So this one night I was in charge of medical. I was by myself when I got this seventeen-year-old boy who was intoxicated and had gone through the windshield of his car and had a questionable head injury.

For the first few hours, the boy's blood pressure was normal—120 over 80. He was conscious and, considering his age and circumstances, quite well-mannered.

As the night progressed, I noticed that the boy seemed to be more and more restless and he'd started up hollering. So, at one point, I took his blood pressure and found it was 40 over 0. Did I panic! I turned up his IV in a hurry and looked him over. He was pale, sweaty, shocky.

I was really scared now, since I was completely on my own. So, I call the doctor.

The doctor is in the middle of having a house party and isn't at all impressed with this new nurse who doesn't seem like she's too with it because she's so insecure she's stumbling over herself. So he bellows at me with this thick, Irish brogue: "And are you *sure* he's that sick, nursie?"

I tell him I'm sure and that he needs to come in.

As soon as I hang up, I walk down the hall to take the boy's blood pressure again and make sure he's not dead, when my life flashes before my eyes—his blood pressure is 120 over 80, and he looks pink and warm and dry, and he's saying please and thank you ma'am!

All I can figure out is that the boy must have been lying on his IV tubing earlier and pinched it off, and he hadn't been getting any fluids to support his pressure.

Outside I hear the doc's little red Austin convertible screech into the parking lot, and I look out the window. Sure enough, the old boy is in his cups—ran his sports car right up on the nursing supervisor's flower bed. He's tried to jump over the door, caught his foot, and he's facedown in the daisies.

All I can think is that this guy is going to stomp down the hall, see this boy looking tip-top, and kill me on the spot.

I would never, ever do this today—and I can't believe I did it then, but it will show you how scared I was of the doctors back then. I stopped the boy's IV, and by the time this doctor stomped into the unit seeing devils, the boy's blood pressure was back down to nothing.

1980

I was still working nights on the medical ward. This one night it was very quiet. I had only twenty-four patients, most of whom were older folks. Other than turning them at two, four, and six o'clock, there wasn't much to do. Not only that, but there was another R.N. with me, which was pretty unusual.

Now, this was an old, old hospital. It had been a tuberculosis sanitorium at one time and then had been a navy hospital for a long time. It was sort of falling apart and had that funny musty smell, like an old barracks.

This other R.N. didn't like working there at night because she was spooked by the building and this silly rumor that there was a night monster who stalked the nurses in the wee small hours.

Well, she asked if I'd go with her on her rounds, and I told her I would, even though I was thinking she was pretty silly. So, we're walking down through the wards, and I have to admit that the building was a little scary with all the creaks and the eerie shadows that those hanging lamps created.

Just before we got to the second men's ward, there was a noise coming from the EKG room.

Click, click, click—shuffle, shuffle, shuffle.

No one was allowed in the EKG room after 5:00 P.M., and so all the lights were off. We sort of held on to each other at that point, not quite sure of whether to scream or run. Then there was this slam and a long, ghostly groan. We just about climbed onto each other's heads. Finally, one of us found the strength to flick on the lights.

There stood Mr. T., an eighty-five-year-old alcoholic, teetering back and forth on his cane. Seems he'd gotten confused about where the bathroom was located and, as he described it, "taken a wrong turn at Albuquerque." Thinking the EKG room was the bathroom, he'd opened, and peed in, every single file drawer. What a mess.

We spent the rest of the night taking the files out and drying them all off and putting them all back. I think it would have been better if it *had* been the night monster.

1982

I had moved to another hospital up in the north country right on the edge of some pretty vast wilderness. One thing you have to know is that life up there is not easy.

Well, they got dogs up there in the north country that are mostly wolf. I think they use them for hunting. These animals are okay when they're under control, but when they get out, it's something else, let me tell you.

Apparently, from the way I heard it, someone had been out walking this pack of wolf-dogs and they'd gotten loose and escaped. So they were pretty wild and hungry when they came across this five-year-old boy playing in his backyard.

They had mauled him and were carrying him off, when the father saw them and shot his shotgun over their heads. Well, the dogs dropped the boy and the ambulance was called to go out and get him.

I was working in the pediatric ward that day. A lot of things I'll never forget about it, like the fact that the boy had graduated from kindergarten the day before, and that he was so small.

We were frantically working on this kid, doing CPR, trying like hell to do everything there was to do. It was the most horrible situation. Everyone was crying, and frantically working. Hands were flying, and all you could hear was the click of instruments, the hiss of the person bagging him, and people whispering hurriedly, "Get me this!" or, "Get me that!"

Finally the anesthesia student looked at the child's pupils and saw that they were huge and dilated, so he reached around the back of the boy to do something with his neck, and found . . . nothing. The child's whole posterior neck was gone from where these dogs had chewed him.

Of course it was clear that he was completely dead and there was no point in going on any further. I can remember looking up from this child's beautiful, delicate little face, and in the corner was the anesthesiologist sitting slumped over and crying his eyes out . . . sobbing and saying what a senseless, senseless death it was.

At the time I didn't have any children, and it was a good thing, because I really don't know how I would have been able to cope with it otherwise. Now that I'm a parent, I can't imagine.

It's unbelievable to me that it's been over fifteen years and I can close my eyes right now and describe vividly his little dark head and those perfect little features.

It's really something. I can still see his little face as clear as day.

1984

It was only a year later that we saw another tragedy patient that has stuck in my mind all these years. I was working in emergency on the day they brought in a seven-year-old boy. His parents both worked, and he'd decided to stay home from school. Well, he'd been playing with matches and had started the family couch on fire.

Someone finally called an alarm, and the firefighters went to rescue this child. Now there wasn't much fire, but the house had filled with this really toxic, black smoke. The child had tried to escape from it and had run upstairs and hid underneath the bed with his dog. Both he and the dog were found curled up together.

The firefighter who found them kept going back into the house time and time again, looking for this boy who he knew and who went to school with his son. His mask was steaming up and it was very difficult to see, so finally, he did something he never should have done; he picked his mask off.

He did find the child soon after, and he was brought to us. We worked and worked on this boy for a long time. The smell of that toxic soot was horrible, and the soot was all over our hands and our uniforms; it was everywhere, so that just from that little bit, we were all having a hard time breathing.

But the picture that stayed with me was this cute seven-year-old lying there like he was asleep, except for this black soot around his mouth.

Finally we gave up because there was nothing that would bring him back. I went to the outpatient department, where the fireman who had rescued this boy was.

The light from the overhead surgical lamp was shining down on him. They'd taken off his gear, and he was covered with that black soot. He wasn't breathing so good, but he was sobbing his heart out and could not stop. He kept saying, "If I'd just gone in sooner," and, "If I'd just found him quicker . . ."

This was in the days before post-trauma stress management, and I shudder to think of what happened to that man.

1986

I was working in emergency the night my next-door neighbor's one-and-a-half-year-old daughter was brought in with epiglottitis and sent down to the floor.

One of the nurses working there kept saying to us, and finally to the doctor, "This kid is going to code. I know it in my bones. She's getting worse and I've seen this too many times. We need to have her monitored."

The doctor in charge of her care was British and also the CEO of the hospital and he wasn't about ready to listen to some whippersnapper of a nurse telling him *anything*. He just said, "No. You're completely hysterical. There's absolutely nothing wrong with this child. I want her to go to the ward."

Despite the doctor's ruling that there was nothing wrong with the girl, the nurse was insistent. She told the rest of the nurses on the ward that she was sure if she left her, the girl would die, because the nurses were busy and didn't have time to take a watch over this one child.

So the nurse pulled a chair up and sat next to this kid's crib for the whole night—on her own time!

Well, sure enough, the baby went downhill until—bang!—she had a respiratory arrest! The nurse grabbed her, started CPR, and got an IV into her. Had that nurse not been there, this baby would have died.

Speaking of not listening to the physicians, I remember one night I was caring for this older gentleman who was having cardiac problems, and the doctor who was in charge of his case was one of those doctors who, again, thought little of the nurse's opinion.

Well, I noticed that the patient was having an increase in premature ventricular contractions, and was beginning to experience shortness of breath and some drop in his blood pressure.

When I told the doctor, he insisted the man was fine and that I was imagining all these things.

I insisted the man wasn't fine, and after we went around and around like that, the doctor says, "Okay, have it your own way! Put him on such and such dose of lidocaine."

The dose he gave was way too much—enough to drop a moose. I told him the dose was too much, but he wouldn't hear of it, and so I started this huge IV dose of lidocaine.

It certainly did stop the PVCs, I will say, but then the patient, who was a sweet, polite man, says to me: "Oh nurse, when you get a minute . . . Don't jump up and trouble yourself over it . . . but when you can find the time . . . do you think you could pick these dead frogs off the wall? They're getting kind of thick."

The doctor reduced the dose of lidocaine.

One night I was alone on the floor when one of my obese patients, who was upwards of four hundred pounds, asked me to help her get to the bathroom, a distance of about six feet. She couldn't wait until I summoned up some help, so we started off—she with her walker, and me following close behind to steady her.

Halfway to the bathroom, she declared that she could not go any further and promptly slid to the floor with me under her. It was very much like being the victim of an avalanche.

She lay quietly on the floor, uninjured since I had padded her descent.

The patient in the next bed watched the whole show.

After a pause she finally asked, "Do you need some help?"

I attempted to answer, but my voice was muffled, not to mention that the wind had been knocked out of me.

She rang the bell for assistance. A few seconds later, I could hear the switchboard operator ask if there was a problem.

The roommate finally said, "The nurse disappeared and only her legs are sticking out underneath."

This information prompted the operator to summon someone to help. After I had been extricated, the cardinal rule of always obtaining help before moving a large patient was brought home to me in its full wisdom.

1987

One night a sailor came into port and he'd gone up to the local bar and had a couple of drinks. It was February, and there'd been a bad ice storm, and on the way back from the bar, he'd slipped on the wharf and fallen into the water, which was frigid. Luckily, someone saw him and held his face out of the water, but still it took about fifteen minutes to get him out.

By the time he came to us, he was very hypothermic, and unconscious, and we were having a hell of a time getting him warmed and couldn't figure out why.

Now, this man appeared to us to be a bit chubby, and I said to the other nurse working with me that it was going to take a lot of warm blankets to thaw him out because of his weight. I turned him on his side and went down the hall to fetch some more blankets.

When I returned, I walked into the room and there was a gallon or two of water all over the floor. We couldn't figure out if a pipe had burst, or if a bucket had been spilled, but then we looked under the blankets. The chubby sailor was now thin. He had swallowed all that water, which was why we couldn't warm him up.

Well, as the night progressed, we were taking his temperature with a rectal thermometer, because his core body temperature was still very low, and at around two o'clock in the morning, we propped him on his side again and left the thermometer in place while we went off and did other things.

When we came back, we lifted the blankets, and he had produced a pile of feces that was—we measured it—seven inches high. And right on top of that peak was the thermometer—just like a flag at the north pole. The guy must have completely cleaned his bowel out with the salt water.

Thank God this man couldn't remember anything when he woke up the next day, because the two of us were absolutely no good to anyone as we lay on the floor screeching with laughter.

1988

This next story will tell you a little about nurses' attitudes and how they change over time.

One night there were three of us on the unit. One nurse had about five years' experience, I'd had about ten, and the other nurse had about twenty.

On the unit was a patient who was an alcoholic and well known to all the staff for being a really obnoxious old codger, and generally a nasty piece of work. Well, this gentleman was in for DTs, and for some reason, he decided about 3 A.M. that he's going to leave the hospital against medical advice.

So he comes out into the hall looking very wild-eyed. He's wearing a pair of bright blue BVDs, a ring of white Mylanta around his mouth, and a huge ghetto blaster under one arm. There's a touch of fire around his eyes, so we knew he was completely out of touch with reality. He says, "I'm getting out of here right now!"

The five-year nurse says, "Oh dear, oh dear. Hold on. You'll have to sign a release form and maybe we should sit down and think this over for a few minutes and then talk it through."

I said, "Oh. You're going now? Maybe you'd better sit down and sign this form first."

The twenty-year nurse said, "Forget the form. I'll call you a taxi right away!"

1989

One of the most distressing points of nursing are the ethical dilemmas we become involved in. Codes are noted for that. I remember one spring afternoon, an elderly man came into us from a nursing home.

Nursing homes have a policy of automatic no-codes, so if he'd been *there*, they would not have coded him, but when they admitted him to the hospital, no one addressed this issue because he wasn't expected to code.

He was settled in his bed, and we'd chatted a little before I'd left to get his armband. Well, of course, when I came back, he was dead. I remember looking at this peaceful old man in death and thinking what a terrible thing it was to call a code on him. I'd only spoken to him for about twenty minutes, but I had a sense that this man had made his peace and was perfectly willing to go anytime.

On reflex, I'd already done the appropriate thing—pushed the alarm, climbed up on the bed and started doing CPR. As soon as I pushed down, I could hear all the ribs crunch and break. It was the most sickening sound. Not that I hadn't heard it before, but for some reason, doing it on this old man felt really, really wrong.

The switchboard operator came on the intercom and asked how I needed help.

At that point I'd climbed down off the bed and was sitting down, looking out the window at this wonderful spring day. I didn't answer the operator.

She asked if I wished to call a code and did I have an emergency in that room?

I didn't answer her.

She asked what the heck was going on, and I mumbled that I didn't know and that I had to think about it.

She called a code.

I could hear the team coming down the hall with the crash cart and I still didn't move. Of course, they ran in and grabbed him and began the assault with the bagging and sticking tubes in him everywhere.

I still didn't move. I sat there continuing to look out the window. I wanted to scream.

The doctor arrived and asked what happened. So I told him.

He called off the code, and everyone just stopped what they were doing and left him there.

I covered him up and I sat at the end of that bed and cried and cried. You know, that could have been my grandfather, or my father. To think what we do sometimes, it just seems like the sickest thing.

That was the closest I have ever come to just walking away from nursing and not returning. To this day, I still beat myself up for not letting that poor man be.

Eighty-nine was also the year I had quite a few experiences in the neonatal unit. I remember two very clearly.

One was a child who had been born a beautiful, healthy looking baby, but unknown to us at the time, had contracted listeriosis—an unusual bacterial infection—in utero.

Dad was this big brawny fisherman who was just tickled silly about his newborn daughter. He's so excited he sleeps next to the crib, waking up every once in a while to stare at his baby in complete wonder. The next morning, he goes out on the boat to bring in a haul of fish, because he still has to earn a living, and this is a decent, hardworking man.

Well, that day, the baby becomes sick and the neonatal team is called to come down and pick up this child—who is now septic—and take her back to the intensive care unit.

The next day here comes Dad loaded down with about ten packages, all wrapped in pink paper, and he doesn't know that the mother has just been given word that the baby is dead.

He's so upset, we don't dare let him drive home, so we give him a cot and set it up next to his wife's bed. He lies there crying all night long holding on to her hand.

So there they were. This couple who had been trying to have a baby for about ten years. The dad was a down-to-earth man who had worked hard to provide a nice house and a decent life for his wife and this child they'd tried so hard to have.

And when the doctor came down and went in to explain what had happened, this father took a deep breath and drew himself up to his full height. He put his hand out and shook the doctor's hand and said, "I want to thank you, Doctor, because I know you did the very best you could to save my baby."

Let me tell you, if you hadn't been affected by the situation until then, you couldn't help but take notice. To think of the terrible thing that had happened and that this man still had enough class to realize what effort had been made. I've seen a lot of people with a lot more money and education who wouldn't have had that much class.

It's really amazing the strength of human spirit you see as a nurse.

———

The other story is about a Vietnamese couple who'd come to live in our area. Neither of them spoke English very well, but they did manage to tell us that they had a daughter who was about a year and a half old. They had brought the child over on the boat with them, taking extreme care to keep her close to them at all times, because apparently there was so little space many babies had been smothered by the crush of the crowd.

So the mom becomes pregnant again and doesn't tell anyone because she's afraid the group who is sponsoring the family will make her get rid of the child. She is a tiny woman, but somehow she managed to keep the pregnancy a secret.

Well, one night she's out shopping, and she gets this ache in her back, and comes into emergency fully dilated. A few minutes later, without any labor pains, we deliver her of the most gorgeous baby boy you have ever seen. I mean, this is one big, healthy baby with a shock of black hair and great color.

Well, the parents are just tickled pink because in that culture the accent is on the male child and this is one incredible baby boy.

So the nurses are all making a big fuss because this baby is so beautiful, and the mother has actual breast milk—the only mother I've ever seen in my whole career who had breast milk inside of twenty-four hours. So she feeds him right away, and then she puts the baby down in the crib next to her bed.

Well, back in those days, when a delivering mother already had a child at home, we used to take the babies back to the nursery so the mom could get a good, full night of sleep. And that's what we did; we took the baby back to the nursery. We never had to bring the baby back, because he'd fed well, and basically he slept right through the night. The mother—who had her back to the door—appeared to be asleep as well, so nobody bothered her.

The next day the baby wakes up at 6:00 A.M. on the dot, and we wash him and dress him all up.

So I go to the mom's room to tell her we're bringing down her baby, and I find her hysterically crying. Her face is puffy, and I can see that she's been biting her fingers to keep herself quiet, and it hits me that she's been crying all night long.

Well, I'm confused, so I go up and bring down the newborn, and the minute she sees him, she lets out this screech, grabs him, and starts kissing him everywhere—his fingers, his toes—and really making quite a fuss. She doesn't speak English as well as the father, so when he comes in, he tells us that because the nurses made such a fuss over the baby, she thought we'd taken him away and sold him.

I don't think I'd ever felt lower in my life. Of course she forgave us, but I still think about the fact that as a nurse, I caused that woman so much anguish.

Brenda S.

When she was growing up, this forty-year-old ICU and ER nurse had a friend whose mother worked as an R.N.

"Yes, I was impressed by the sense of independence this woman seemed to have, but I was more fascinated by the white hose, hat, and uniform. It seemed like there was such authority in that uniform.

"How sad it was to realize there was no command to the profession at all, and what there was is being stripped away from us. People go to the hospital for nursing care. I wonder what they're going to do when all the nurses have been cut and there's nobody left to take care of them?"

It was two days before Christmas and the mad rush was on. Outside, the stores and streets were packed with last-minute holiday shoppers. Parking lots and restaurants were full. Highways were jammed. There wasn't a parking space to be had within blocks of any front door.

The hospital was busy with holiday drunks and those of fragile health who had already overextended themselves on their booze, salt, and stress intakes.

I was lucky. I'd finished my shopping early. Very early. By July 31, I had most of it done and wrapped. This year I'd been good and not given in to my temptation to give people their presents before the end of August.

It didn't bother me to work the holidays, especially Christmas. I've been afraid of Christmas since my first year out of nursing school, and my first Christmas Eve on the job. I lived in a small, rural town where the only "ambulance" was a meat wagon. No EMTs. No paramedics. I was just getting ready to get off shift at midnight when we heard there was a head-on collision on the main road. The wagon just went out there, scooped them all up, and brought them in. We didn't have a trauma team or a surgeon. We called as many surgeons as we could, but it was Christmas Eve and nobody was available.

Everybody in the crash died. Grandma, grandpa, mom, dad, two small kids, and the driver of the other car. The whole family wiped out in one second. That was when I knew for certain how important those paramedics and their "golden hour" really are. . . .

I was working in ICU on this night, and was glad of it. It was, to my way of thinking, a whole lot better than working someplace like pediatrics or oncology or psych during Christmas—or any time, for that matter.

I've never been confident dealing with children. There were other nurses who could handle them better, just like there were nurses who could handle the constant death march of oncology and the insanity of psych—no pun intended there. I did try once to work in a psych unit. I lasted for about a week. Then a psychotic walked in off the street in full-blown peritonitis. He'd opened himself up with a pocketknife and eaten eighteen inches of his own intestine. I walked off the unit and never looked back.

Charlotte, one of our day nurses, called around 8:30. Three of us picked up extensions to chat and hear the Christmas madness horror stories and feel glad we weren't out there. She didn't disappoint us. She said that the mall was so crowded she and her husband had to park almost a half-mile away.

"I got this bad feeling," she said. "Like something really terrible was going to happen."

"Probably the crowds," I said. "Claustrophobia."

"No. It was more than that. I told my husband we had to leave immediately. He wasn't happy about that, but he'll get over it."

One of the other nurses was asking her about the sales when our supervisor, Anita, walked into the unit. Her face was as white as one of our sheets. The last time I'd seen her that pale was the night sixteen nurses called in sick.

"Put your disaster plan into effect," Anita said. "A plane crashed into the mall. There are lots of injuries and fatalities."

No one moved or said anything. It was as if we were all frozen into place. For me, it was an exact replay of that Christmas Eve so many years before.

I can't say I'd never thought about why our county's only mall had been built so close to an approach runway of the airport. Considering how busy the airport was, and the amount of dense fog we got, I had a hard time believing it hadn't happened before.

Joan, one of the other ICU nurses, stood in slow motion, her hand covering her mouth. "Oh my God," she whispered through her fingers. "Ron took the kids there tonight to see Santa Claus."

She ran to the phone and dialed her number. We waited with her, our stomachs in our throats. The phone rang three times, which to us was like an hour. On the fourth ring someone answered and she broke down and sobbed.

I took the phone out of her hand and explained to a confused Ron what had happened. He was, like the rest of us, in shock at the news.

"I left thirty minutes ago—the place was packed." His voice broke. "Oh my God, all those kids . . ."

We flew into action, turfing out as many patients as we could to the floors. As soon as most of the beds were free, we left Joan—the only mom of our group—behind and ran to the ER.

All the way down, I kept thinking, *Please no kids. Please no kids.* The first thing I saw—and heard—as I entered the emergency department was a little boy of about two. He was sitting on a gurney and screaming at the top of his lungs for his mother.

He had some first degree burns on his arms and legs, with a scatter of second degree, but he was okay. A volunteer was trying to comfort him, but he wasn't having any of that. He wanted Mommy, and no one else would do. I didn't want to think of where Mommy was.

The main smells that filled the ER were burned flesh and airplane fuel. Everywhere I looked was burned flesh in shades of second and third degree. Melted clothes, melted hair. The screams were deafening.

At least a hundred doctors and nurses were crowded into the treatment rooms and the halls. It was, I thought, identical to a war zone. I started IVs and gave narcotics like it was water. The ER docs were on the phones, in constant contact with burn centers in the surrounding counties.

"Do they know what happened yet?" I asked the ER nurse, helping cut charred strips of clothing from a screaming teenager so I could start an IV—provided I could find a vein through the burns.

"Private plane misjudged the runway through the fog," she said without looking at me. "Plowed directly into Macy's."

Macy's was in the center of the mall. Santa was stationed in front of Macy's. I bit the inside of my lip and concentrated on getting an IV into the boy as fast as I could. I wanted to quiet those screams before they split my sanity.

One patient after the other was transported to burn units in the three counties surrounding ours. The chaos had settled enough so I could allow myself to take one, deep breath. When I let it out, the supervisor came in to tell me I had been assigned a patient who I was to take back to ICU with me.

"I think she's in her twenties," Anita said in a monotone. "She was intubated at the scene. She was near the plane. Got completely soaked in fuel. She has third degree burns over ninety-five percent of her body."

My mouth dropped open in shock. "Why isn't she in a burn center? Why . . ."

Anita looked at me; I read the answer in her eyes. The woman was going to die. No one survived those kind of burns over that much of the body.

"Make her comfortable until she goes," Anita said. "Nothing heroic."

"But who is she?" I asked, not believing that was all there was to tell. "Where are her family? What's her name? Is she—"

"We don't know," Anita said. "She's conscious and alert, but she can't talk and she can't move. She's completely unrecognizable."

Horror-stricken, my face must have gone through some pretty amazing changes, because Anita gave me a hug and told me it would be okay.

What, I thought, could possibly be okay about what had happened here tonight?

To this day I don't know how she remained conscious and alert. I had never given any one human being so much morphine all at once. She was so small, and the morphine doses were so big, that I wondered more than once if maybe the morphine had been tampered with and I was actually giving water.

I walked gingerly around the bed, making sure not to jar her body or cause any added unnecessary pain. "Hi," I said softly. Her eyes were a pretty grayish blue. "My name is Brenda. I'm your nurse. I know you can't talk, so I'll talk for us both."

And I did. I told her what time it was and what had happened, and what I was giving her, and told her about all the equipment around her bed and what it was for. I *didn't* tell her I was her death watch.

I was running out of things to say when Gail, one of the senior ICU nurses, who had come in as soon as she heard about the disaster on the news, came over to the bed.

Gail has been in nursing a long time. The profession seems to have had a profound effect on her. It hasn't hardened her like it does many nurses, but it has served to make her a wise and most compassionate soul. She is a great nurse and a wonderful, loving person.

Gail zeroed right in on my patient. Then she pulled me into the nurses' lounge. "We have to find out what her name is," she said urgently. "We can't let her die alone."

"How? She can't—"

Gail was already at the girl's side. With the gentleness of handling a newborn, she touched the girl's right hand, then slid her hand under it. "If you can move any of the fingers on your right hand, press down. My hand is right underneath."

I held my breath. Slowly the middle digit pushed down.

"Good." Gail laughed. "Now, when I come to the letters of the alphabet that spell your name, press down. I'll go very slowly. A . . . B . . ."

Forty-five minutes later, Gail had patiently gathered the girl's full name. Cindy T.

I proceeded with what I had to do while Gail tracked down Cindy's family and fiancé. None of them knew she had been at the mall.

Her sister told me later that Cindy's wedding was the following Saturday. Cindy had told her sister the day before that she needed to go to the mall to pick up the ring she'd had engraved for her husband-to-be, but didn't think she'd be able to get around to it until later in the week.

Cindy, twenty-four years old, died within an hour of the arrival of those who loved her.

I didn't leave Cindy at the hospital door the way a good nurse is supposed to leave her patients behind. I carried her with me for a long time. I replayed the details of that night over in my head, trying to make sense of why God arranges some things to happen the way they do.

I've seen so many tragedies and I still can't figure it out. Maybe it is to test us—the survivors. I don't know, but I don't think it's healthy to dwell on that too long.

All I do know is that I'm a nurse. I tend to the suffering and the dying and I do it the best, most compassionate way I know how.

Echo Heron

For the record, I went to work as a critical care nurse in 1977 and quit in 1994 when I could no longer tolerate putting my license and the lives of my patients in jeopardy because corporate CEOs and insurance companies felt the need to increase their already grossly swollen profits.

With seventeen years' experience under my belt, I believed myself to be a valuable critical care nurse—compassionate, capable, and intuitive. In the best of times things were rushed, always stressful, but the nurses always managed to deliver good, nurturing care to the patients. Those were the days in which a nurse had time for a word of reassurance or a simple touch that said: "I care. Don't be afraid and don't worry. I am here for you."

When managed care and mass downsizing began, the focus rapidly shifted from the well-being of the patient to the bottom line—the almighty dollar. Hundreds of thousands of R.N.s and LVNs were no longer allowed to practice nursing the way nursing was meant to be practiced. R.N.s, including critical care R.N.s, were fired and replaced with less expensive personnel who had as little as two hours to a few weeks of training. Nurses became replaceable grunts in the healthcare mills . . . helping the prospering few to exchange patient safety for dollars, keeping silent for fear of losing our jobs.

I feel bad that I allowed the politics of greed to force me out of nursing. I miss nursing. I miss the patients. I miss the feeling that I made a difference in someone's life. I miss the adrenaline rushes and the joys and the sorrows. I ask the nurses who have hung in there and live this nightmare every day, and the patients whom I might have helped, to forgive me for jumping ship. My only excuse is that I felt I could do more good for both the patient and the profession through giving a voice to the truth.

The following is an account of my last shift. It is not a unique story by any means—most nurses who are still working in the trenches live this, and much worse, every single day.

It's July and San Francisco is cold and foggy. I have lived here since the summer before the summer of love, and I can't remember a July when I didn't have to dig out my wool socks and turtleneck sweaters.

I have driven my beat-up '78 Pontiac station wagon around the block six or seven times, looking for a parking place. Because I am just a nurse, I am not allowed to park in the hospital's three-story parking building, the ground floor of which is reserved for the physicians' and administrators' cars. I can see that most of the slots are empty, so I attempt to bargain with the guard on duty at the gate. His name tag reads "Julio." To lighten the mood, I ask if his last name is Iglesias. My attempt at humor fails, although I think he appreciates the effort.

He tells me in broken English that doctors park free but nurses and visitors must pay sixteen dollars for eight hours. When I tell him I think this is unfair, he shrugs and says the lower working classes always pay the most—it is the way of the world.

I have five minutes before I have to report to the nursing office when I find a space three blocks from the hospital. It is one of the sections of San Francisco that isn't mentioned in the travel brochures. Six days ago, a thirty-seven-year-old Asian-American nurse was sexually assaulted and then shot to death in this block as she walked to the hospital at 11:00 P.M.

I stuff my purse and lunch sack under my wool jacket and hope that my "pregnant" belly will act as some sort of deterrent for stray bullets and would-be rapists. I try not to think about the terror I'm going to feel when I walk back to my car at midnight.

I run faster than I did in high school and I'm still five minutes late. In the nursing office I find my name and next to it the notation "ICU/CCU." I do not like working in this particular unit at this particular hospital, but too bad—twenty-five dollars an hour is twenty-five dollars an hour. It pays the rent and keeps my cat supplied with kibble.

Despite my work assignment, I smile. For every unit I work, one of my fellow nurses will, at some point during the shift, ask me why I continue to work as a nurse; they assume, because I have been published, that I must be wealthy.

I will sigh and point out to them that contrary to popular belief, writers don't make a whole lot of money unless their name happens to be King or Krantz or Grisham. Not only am I just a nurse, I am only small potatoes in the megaworld of publishing. I tell them that I am a very pragmatic person—I earn more money working as a nurse than I do as a writer.

I push open the double doors of ICU/CCU and find my patient assignment. I have five patients.

My heart sinks like a hot rock into my gut. I don't know why it hits me this way: I'm used to this type of assignment.

But I also know from experience that I will not get a bathroom or dinner break, which means I will not be able to get off my feet for the next nine or ten hours. Sitting is aggressively discouraged among all personnel. The unit is designed so that a chart stand—which looks very much like a podium—is placed at the end of each bed or outside each isolation cubicle. There is a chair for the clerk, and four more for residents and interns to use when having a patient conference. That's it. Nurses do not sit.

Momentarily I fantasize about faking illness and going home and finding a job as a telemarketer. I think this every time I come here.

The head nurse, a male R.N. with a doctor-wannabe chip, asks me why I'm late, and before I can answer, tells me to find Andrea and Kerri for my report.

I go to my first station, where Andrea, who has three of my five patients, waits to give me report. She starts with bed D, Alan Rodriquez. Twenty-four-year-old AIDS patient with MRSA (methicillin-resistant staphylococcus aureus) pneumonia—highly contagious and difficult to treat. Alan is intubated and is having severe heroin withdrawal. His lungs are failing, he is in total isolation, and he's coming off the walls. Alan also has a long history of psychosis.

Andrea relates details from the night before when he broke out of his restraints and climbed to the windowsill, where he pulled out his IVs and defecated. When the nurses entered his room, he jumped on one and forced a handful of his feces into her face. Before they could pull him off, he'd broken his captive's nose and torn off the top part of her uniform.

I don't know why the nurse feels it is necessary to warn me not to turn my back on him for a second.

I chance a peek at the monster and see a head of bleached hair with black roots, an ear that has at least fifteen earrings going through it, a pierced nipple, and a high tattoo-to-tooth ratio—about six to one is my guess.

Bed E—another total-isolation cubicle—is a nineteen-year-old girl who attempted suicide with an unknown agent which has destroyed her kidneys. During the course of her hospitalization it has been determined she has tuberculosis. She is demanding more and more pain medication, and has become ventilator-dependent.

The doctors think the pain is psychological, though they continue to increase her doses of morphine and Valium.

Andrea instructs me to keep her "snowed" so that I will have time for my other patients.

Bed G is an eighty-seven-year-old woman who is having an anterior MI. The yahoo residents have used her as a teaching tool and given her a powerful drug known as streptokinase, which not only dissolves the clot in the coronary arteries but thins the blood tremendously, so that the risk of internal bleeding is high. Because her hematocrit is low, and no source of bleeding can be found, she is to be given two units of packed cells. Almost as an aside, the nurse tells me the woman is a diabetic and has a couple of gangrenous toes on one foot.

Before I run to my next station, Andrea tells me she doesn't think my assignment is safe and that I need to complain to the head nurse. She says, "If one nurse lets them get away with it, then they think they can do it to all of us."

On the other side of the unit, Kerri is furious that I am late. She has to pick up her kids from day care which charges unaffordable rates by the quarter hour. I explain that I had to get report on beds D, E, and G.

Immediately she softens and then gets angry again. "You can't take these five patients together," she insists. "You can't have compromised patients with buggy ones."

I sigh. "Tell that to the head nurse."

"You tell the head nurse," she says bitterly, and begins report.

Bed P is a forty-five-year-old fresh postoperative craniotomy who has had a cardiac infarct during the neurosurgery. She is intubated and, luckily for me, not conscious. Not so lucky for me is that she is on more medications and blood tests than even God knows about. The residents and interns have made a sort of research project out of her and keep ordering new procedures and medications to assault her with. She is a whale of a woman at 281 pounds. She must be turned once an hour.

Off the main room is a small alcove. Bed R has been moved to this hidden, out-of-the-way cave. She's a forty-two-year-old pregnant woman in her first trimester who was admitted after a come-and-go breast biopsy which her doctor had previously assured her would be a benign cyst.

Her sister and ten-year-old son are in the waiting room thinking she will be ready to go anytime. They have been waiting since one.

No one has bothered to tell the patient why she is in ICU instead of the come-and-go recovery room. No one has mentioned that the cyst has turned out to be a malignant tumor.

I jump ahead and wonder if there are lymph nodes involved, and then wonder if the surgery will have to be extensive and if there has been metastasis. I also hope there is a husband involved who is loving and supportive.

The patient has asked several times if her sister is here yet, and shouldn't she be getting dressed, and what is wrong, and why is she here? Kerri says she has managed to evade the questions.

"But why *is* she in ICU instead of come-and-go recovery?"

Kerri shrugs. "I don't know, and I haven't had time to go through the chart to find out. I've asked both attending blade and two residents to tell her what they found and give her some kind of game plan, but they keep putting it off."

Of all the information that has been shoved at me in the last twenty minutes, I find this the most infuriating. I want to scream out of frustration—instead, my eyes well with tears of rage.

Kerri sees my tears and misinterprets them. "Oh for Christ's sake," she snarls, rolling her eyes. "Grow up!"

A resident stands in front of me asking if I've drawn the blood work on Mr. Rodriquez and why hasn't he received his 2:00 P.M. vancomycin? I explain that I've just come on duty. I skim through my patient information sheets while I'm speaking, and realize that three of them have thirty-minute vitals.

The head nurse approaches and asks why the blood hasn't been hung on bed G yet. I tell him that I have just finished getting report and repeat what Kerri has said about my assignment.

He reacts. He shoves his finger in my face, holding it very stiff, and says: "Too bad. If you want to work here, keep your mouth shut and do what's asked of you. If you can't cut it, don't come back."

Kerri happens to pass us at this moment. She steps into the fray and snarls again—at him. They walk off arguing about buggy patients with fresh postop patients. At the door, they both shake their heads and walk in opposite directions.

I run to hang the packed cells on bed G, and find that the unit hasn't been ordered yet from the blood farm. I fill out a detailed order form and ask the clerk to get the blood. He says he will when he's not so busy. I tell him it was supposed to be hung an hour ago, and he laughs at me and tells me the next time I want blood stat, I need to order it two to three hours in advance.

I dress in isolation garb and enter Mr. Rodriquez's cubicle. He is pulling at his wrist and ankle restraints. His respirator is alarming because he's biting down on the endotracheal tube. I go to the med cabinet and find his med box empty. I do as much of an assessment as I can and try to draw blood on him. His veins are blown from years of drug use. I try three times and finally motion to the third-year resident who is observing through the viewing window.

I tell her through the window she's going to have to draw the blood because I can't, and lab has noted on his chart that they refuse to draw his blood.

She acts as though I am a defective because I can't access a vein and agrees to draw if I sedate him. I degown and run to the med supply room and gather two of his six overdue meds. The rest, including his vancomycin, have not been delivered and are not in stock. No one knows who has the only narcotics cabinet key, so I must run from nurse to nurse.

News is that a day nurse has taken the key home. The supervisor with the master set of keys must be called. Forms and incident reports must be filled out. The resident doesn't want to hear excuses.

I decide not to wait for the supervisor, and go to my next priority, the TB patient, who is banging on her side rails for attention.

The IV cartridge which delivers a constant amount of narcotic is dry. I tell her she has to be patient, and explain about the missing keys. She shakes her head, perspiring like an addict in withdrawal. I notice she is ashen.

A nurse comes to the door and bangs on the window. Before I turn around, she hollers that bed G is having chest pain and wants to use the bedpan. She also tells me that bed R is asking again about when she's going to be discharged, and can't I please answer my own damned call lights?

I stick my head out the door and ask the nurse to please put bed G on the bedpan and slip a nitro under her tongue. The nurse says she only has time to put her on the bedpan.

I do a cursory set of vitals on the teenager. I can feel her staring at me, and I wonder what she thinks of this skinny white nurse who won't look her in the eyes. I wish I had the time to explain to her that I am mortified and ashamed of not being able to give her the care she deserves—the care that I went into nursing to give.

I degown and run to see if the narcotics key is home. It is not, but the clerk hands me the unit of blood for bed G. I run into that room and see a full bedpan on the bedside table where the other nurse has left it rather than walk two steps to empty it. The tech delivering the patients' dinner trays has placed bed G's tray next to the full bedpan.

Bed G says good evening and to call her Kitty. Kitty says her heart is aching. I turn up her oxygen, take her BP, and slip a nitroglycerine tab under her tongue. I commit a major safety mortal sin and double-check the blood myself. I do this because each nurse I ask to do the standard two-nurse blood check refuses for lack of two minutes to spare.

I hang the blood and set the blood pump at a slow rate; Kitty is eighty-seven after all.

The resident comes into the room and demands to know what's going on with Mr. Rodriquez.

I rush to see if the narcotic cabinet key has been delivered—it has. Because I am an outside agency nurse, I am required to fill out two forms before one of the regular staff can open the cabinet for me. I get various narcotics for Mr. Rodriquez, Kitty, and my nineteen-year-old TB/suicide.

I medicate Kitty for angina, Mr. Rodriquez for agitation, and my nineteen-year-old TB/suicide for hopelessness. I feel like a drug pusher. I break more laws, and instead of wasting leftover drugs, hide them in the patients' med boxes—this will save me the trouble of having to track down the key and fill out forms for a while.

All the regular meds are overdue by an hour. I run to the surgical resident and plead with him to at least tell bed R's relatives to go home. I ask for permission to inform her that she will be staying, and I am refused with the statement "Nurses don't have that authority."

I run to the crainy, whose cardiac monitor is showing an increase in premature ventricular contractions, take her vital signs, and try to turn her by myself. I can barely lift her leg. Her neuro checks are the same. Another resident approaches, chart in hand, and asks why beds D, E, and G haven't had their thirty-minute vitals for the last hour.

To cover my feelings of inadequacy and embarrassment, I laugh in his young, handsome face and inform him that if he wants some done, he's going to have to do them himself or do without.

I run to bed R for a quick set of vitals. She is anxious and crying. She wants to know why she's received a dinner tray when she was supposed to be discharged several hours ago. I tell her I'll have the doctor come and talk to her. She says she's been told the same thing by the other nurses, and begs me to tell her what is going on. I lie and say I don't know.

I run back to the med room and try to find my patients' medications. On the way, I see the resident still working over Mr. Rodriquez's arm. She waves me in and tells me to set up for a cut-down.

I call pharmacy and am told there's only one pharmacist for the whole hospital and he's backed up for hours. He tells me to beg, borrow, and steal from other patients' cabinets. I know he has given this same advice to every nurse who calls, which is why my patients don't have their drugs.

As I run to gather equipment for the cut-down, a really foul smell invades the unit. My crainy/MI lady has expelled a massive amount of diarrhea stool, which is literally dripping off the side of the bed onto the floor.

I cannot move her without help. One nurse—a tall woman with lots of curly hair—says she will help me in an hour.

Kitty is crying. I run over and see that someone has readjusted the flow rate on the blood line so that it is running in wide open. She complains of itching and feeling short of breath—classic signs of an adverse blood reaction. At once, I stop the blood and must fill out a form stating that there has been a blood reaction. Rather than wait for orders, I draw a clot on my own, do vital signs, give her the standard dose of Benadryl—which I take from my own personal stock in my purse. A resident comes in, hands on hips (which is how I know he's not a new intern; he's already taken Arrogance 101), and demands to know why the blood has been removed.

I ask if he's the one who opened the blood line.

"Yeah," he says challengingly. "I wanted her to have it before next year."

I have been encouraged to instruct residents on nursing procedure, so I explain about the reaction and start to explain about basic precautions when giving blood.

He walks away before I finish the second sentence.

I finish finding the cut-down equipment and run back to bed D. I gown up, and as I am about ready to enter the room, a resident and an attending want to know the results of bed P's last lab tests, and his last set of vitals. I tell them I don't know.

I get the "defective" look again.

During the cut-down, the window is knocked on a total of seven times: three nurses, the clerk, two residents, and one intern. They shout through the glass about things I must do stat, or ask why something hasn't been done.

The resident doing the cut-down tells me to attend to my other work. She says she'll finish up on Mr. Rodriquez and chart a set of vitals for me. I thank her profusely, promising my second-born child in payment.

I decide I must get things in hand and take each patient and attached residents, interns, and attendings one at a time. I begin with Kitty, who is resting without pain. I medicate (borrowed and stolen meds), do an assessment (rapid), chart (cursorily), empty and measure (urine, blood, IV fluid), hang more blood (illegally, without the two-nurse check), change the dressings on her gangrenous toes, check her serum glucose, give her insulin, and start to run for my next patient, when Kitty crooks her finger at me.

I go close, but she wants me closer. I move closer. She kisses my cheek and says, "Thank you, girlie, for being so nice."

I echo her words right back to her and she giggles like a girlie. At the sound and the kiss, I get a rush of energy.

Next the crainy/MI. I tell the tall nurse I need help now and not in an hour or ten minutes. She hears my tone and sees my expression and does not put me off again, although she does not speak to me during the bed change.

She does, however, insert a rectal tube and drainage bag to the patient without being asked. She also helps me turn the mammoth body. I change IV tubing, check the patient's blood sugar, hang new antibiotics, do an ICP reading, suction, medicate, and chart.

I run next to the TB/suicide and quickly flip to the summary page of her admission notes. My eyes get snagged by the lines:

Social Service reports patient has had increase in use of heroin/?crack/self-destructive behavior since she witnessed the murder of her three-year-old son who was shot through the head—execution style—by the father.

This is thirteenth suicide attempt.

I flip ahead to the most recent notes and am shocked to read that her prognosis is nil.

Patient's request to be removed from life support and be allowed to die is up for a third review by Ethics. Will recommend regardless of young age, patient should be allowed to die with dignity.

She stares at my eyes and I see a young girl who has been to places I can't even dream of. I lay a hand on her arm and gently ask if she has pain. She nods and I understand exactly where the pain is.

I assess her quickly and give her an extra dose of pain medication that I will not document. All the while, I talk to her about anything that comes into my head—the weather, her hair, the lighting, my other patients. I tell her I'll be back and ask her if she wants anything.

I untie her hands and give her a pen and pad. She writes big, slow, shaky letters, like a child.

"PLEASE LET ME DIE."

I push myself to look into her eyes. The despair is so raw it leaves no room for bullshit.

I say, "I wish I could give you peace, but I can't."

As I am degowning, the emergency alarms shriek through the air. I look frantically for the source of trouble, and out of the corner of my eye, I see a human form where it shouldn't be.

Mr. Rodriquez is standing on top of the med cabinet, his endotracheal tube hanging off the side of his face by a length of adhesive tape. His new cut-down is gushing blood, so that the room looks like several chickens have recently been beheaded there. His urinary catheter, still in his bladder, is hanging free of the drainage bag, dribbling urine.

He is taunting the crowd that has formed outside the cubicle window. Though he's been intubated, there is no hoarse whisper. He is yelling in a loud, clear voice. He isn't just calling us names, he's threatening to hurt us unless he is given his freedom. He tells us he needs to get some real drugs.

As an afterthought, he adds that the first person who enters the room is going to get a mouth full of his blood and shit.

The man—or this animal that is passing for one—is like something from the Far Side, and I don't mean Gary Larson.

The supervisor wants to know who is responsible for allowing this to happen.

"He's my patient," I say. I take a deep breath.

"It's my mistake," says the resident who did the cut-down. "I left his hand unrestrained."

People wander away. I don't know what to do. I also wonder who they expect to go inside the patient's room.

The resident reads my mind. "Don't worry," she says, watching the madman. "He'll have a respiratory arrest in a minute or so."

I look at Mr. Rodriquez, who has jumped down from the cabinet and is ripping open small vials of saline, and I think she has miscalculated. Mr. Rodriquez isn't going to arrest soon enough or anytime soon.

The supervisor tells me to medicate him stat and walks away. I ask the resident—whom I see now as more human than doctor—what she wants me to do.

She says she'll reason with him.

Another miscalculation.

I call security and tell them to come stat and bring a few male psych-unit people and a tranquilizer gun.

I run to the breast cancer lady, and while I do a set of vitals tell her she probably isn't going home.

Of course, she asks why.

I say it is because the surgeon found something in her breast tissue and wanted to run more tests before sending her home.

She asks what was found, and runs a hand over her belly—a protective maternal gesture.

I tell her I don't know and run to the desk and call the attending blade in the party room—the staff's name for the physicians' lounge. I tell him to get his ass upstairs and talk to her, or I'll . . . I don't know what, but I will.

While I'm on the phone, I notice that one of the tall nurse's patients has expired. I watch the wife and the son limp away from the bedside in tears.

Once I would have felt compassion. Now, I can only think about unloading one of my patients onto the nurse who now has only two cases.

Instead, she is immediately assigned two of three new admits.

The supervisor gives me the third.

The tall nurse protests on my behalf, and is reminded of the hospital's policy not to "load up" regular staff nurses with too many patients, so they can be free for emergencies.

I glance around the unit and see nothing but emergencies taking place in every corner. "What exactly do you mean by emergencies?" I ask. I am told I have an attitude problem.

The tall nurse says not to worry.

I'm not worried—I'm freaking out. I'm thinking of all the things that must be done for the patients I have now, and even if I carve those down to the basic necessities, I know I can't do it all because it is humanly impossible to do it all.

I am running now from bed to bed, suctioning, vitaling, checking monitors and pain levels.

Two policemen, and three psych unit guys are gowning and masking and gloving up outside Mr. Rodriquez's room, like some specialized SWAT team.

I see Mr. Rodriquez discover the med cabinet. I remember the half-filled syringe of Valium hidden inside. I pray to any available higher power that he shoots it up before the SWAT team gets in there.

As I watch, he does exactly that. I make note of where the empty syringe lands when he hurls it at the wall, and run to prepare bed L for my new patient.

I have only just turned down the bed when the double doors crash open and a gurney is raced in. The crowd of people surrounding the bed are all yelling at once. The patient has coded in the elevator.

I run for the crash cart, while the patient is wheeled into the first available space which can be hidden from the view of the other patients.

While I am charging up the defibrillators, I grab a paper off the floor which has fallen out of the chart. The name is Middleman, John. My new patient.

A 53-year-old tourist from Lansing, Michigan. Here with his wife on a six-day vacation package. First vacation in ten years.

And last.

John stepped into the crosswalk at Market and Hyde Streets and was hit by a speeding taxi. Every major bone, including his skull, has been broken or crushed. Spleen, liver, bladder, brain, heart—there is damage of varying degrees to each one. The guy is not much more than a bag of mashed potatoes.

I deliver 300 watts to his protesting cardiac muscle and we are back in business. The fourth-year surgical resident begins report by giving odds for the man's survival. They are not encouraging, and I find myself praying he will die because I know I don't have the time to care for him properly. If he lives, none of my other patients will get any attention.

Several of us hook the man to the advanced-life-support machines. I am starting another IV line when a sudden outburst of yells and screams freezes everyone in place.

The emergency alarms pierce the air as Mr. Rodriquez runs out the double doors, growling like an animal. He is naked. The urinary catheter is still hanging from the end of his penis, but now it's dribbling blood instead of urine. So much for the Valium.

The SWAT team runs out after him. As they pass me, I shout: "Let him go! Please!"

I go back to inserting the IV on Mr. Taxi-Mashed Potatoes, wondering if Mr. Rodriquez dies, will it be blamed on me?

Once John is stabilized, I run to check on the woman in Bed R. who I have come to think of as my forgotten patient. As I approach the alcove, I see she is quietly weeping as is the worn looking man embracing her.

I back away, thankful they have each other for comfort, yet simultaneously feeling frustrated that I have no time to spare for them.

Probably.

Kitty's blood has run in, and I draw postblood bloods. Four of my call lights are buzzing, when John goes into ventricular tachycardia.

The resident in charge is no longer cool and collected—he's anxious that he might lose this one, and he doesn't want to be responsible.

I recharge and go for 360 watts. Again. Then again.

Pop goes the weasel—John comes back.

More medications, more equipment is brought in.

I tell the supervisor I need someone to cover my call lights, and that I have to pee. She pretends not to hear.

I am growing more panicky about leaving my other patients unattended for so long. Kitty could be holding her bladder, or vomiting, or having angina or another blood reaction. Bed E might get a hand free and extubate herself and die. Bed P's ICP could be increasing, or perhaps she's extending her infarct. Bed R might try to leave against medical advice, although it is not a bad idea to my way of thinking. Mr. Rodriquez has already done everything he could do.

Except here he is again, strapped to a gurney like a deer to a car fender. The victors, still gowned and masked, are pushing him back to his room, laughing and making jokes at Mr. Rodriquez's expense.

The supervisor taps me—hard—on the shoulder and tells me to get in there with him.

I turn to follow her orders, when John has another cardiac arrest. The resident tells me to get a drug that I know is not on the cart but in a special cabinet.

I run.

In front of the cabinet stands an intern and an attending. I say, "Excuse me. I need to get in there stat," kneel down, and grab the handle. The attending pauses, looks at me as though I am some kind of insect floating in his soup, and resumes his conversation.

I ask again, stressing the word "stat." Again my request is ignored. I pull the cabinet door against the backs of the attending's legs, and with a firm, steady pressure, push him, inch by laborious inch, out of the way.

I return with the medicine, but the resident has changed his mind. He wants something else, which must be fetched from pharmacy five floors below.

The clock on the defibrillator says it is only 7:00 P.M.

I am feeling used up.

It is 2:00 A.M. I am a block away from the hospital when I start to cry. My two bruised ribs, courtesy of Mr. Rodriquez, hurt like hell with every sob, but I cry anyway.

For seventeen years, I have practiced the art of healing and compassion. I have saved lives, eased pain and suffering, given hope, comforted, brought joy and peace, and provided dignified deaths. And because of this, I have reaped the rewards of love, joy, spirituality, peace, respect, and fulfillment.

Now, as I have been for some time, I am filled with guilt, worry, anger, frustration, anxiety, and shame. I am no longer the instrument of healing, but the doer of harm. I am no longer able to give compassion, because there is no time for such nonessentials. I am no longer able to fight for my patients' right to good, safe care and well-being. I feel ashamed of myself because I allow the money powers to degrade my profession by forcing me to flirt with disaster and act inhuman.

I sit in my car and shiver with the cold, damp air until I stop crying. I have done this probably ten times in the last two years.

I start the car and turn on the wipers—as if to clear my inner vision.

"You can't do this anymore," I say, knowing that this time I mean it—for real.

"No more of this abuse for you, Ec. You don't need abuse to be happy, okay?"

I take a big breath and let it out in a sigh of release. My heart is pounding in my throat.

"Okay. No more."

I pull out of the parking space and suddenly remember where I am and that I have walked to the car alone without mishap.

"Ha!" I laugh quietly. "You forgot to be scared."

Steve R.

Steve R., forty-six, has worked in Florida, California, Okinawa, New York, and Tennessee. His work history is even more varied. He has been a flight nurse with a fixed-wing company, the nursing director of an emergency room, charge nurse of an eighteen-bed pediatric critical care unit, and a freelance agency nurse for ER and trauma ICU. He has a master's degree in human relations and is presently working on a second master's degree in order to attain a family nurse practitioner credential.

In our interview, I asked Steve what he thought about the profession of nursing in general. Without missing a beat, he gave me his answer:

"Nursing is as sensual an occupation as one can be in. You see the patient's injuries, wounds, illnesses, and imperfections. You see their emotions and triumphs.

"You can hear them when they moan or cry, hear their lungs and the way they breathe, listen to their bowels, listen to their hearts working . . . or not.

"You can smell them—the foul urine, the musty damp smell of blood, the perspiration, and the stench of death.

"You touch every inch of a body from the toes to the head, feeling for heat or cold, soft or hard, dry or wet, full or empty.

"The only thing we don't do—anymore—is taste the patient.

"Four of your five senses are intimately involved in absorbing another person's pain and suffering.

"I think that is pretty amazing, don't you?"

It wasn't until I transcribed his tape and read the words that the full extent of what he'd said sank in.

I was tired. As if there was any other way to feel after seven hours of running my buns off in a major trauma center. I'd been on since 7:00 A.M.

It was just a few minutes before 2:00 when the radio announced that an ambulance was coming in from one of the nursing homes with a patient who had a fever. I yawned. Considering what I had to deal with most of the time, a little old person with a fever was nothing.

I stripped a bloody sheet from a gurney—recently vacated by a minor stab wound who had been stitched up and sent back out on the street to incite someone into doing a better, deeper job next time—and put a fresh white one down. I don't know—maybe it was the smell of the fresh linen and the fact it was close to Christmas, but it reminded me of the starched white cloths they'd put on the chapel altar at Christmas.

When I thought about it, it really didn't seem too far from the truth—a gurney could be seen as a sort of altar. Lots of people had prayed around and on them, that was for sure.

I'd just sat down again when the EMTs came in with their feverish patient—a small mound under a sheet. With an involuntary groan, I got up and sauntered over to the gurney, thermometer in hand. I casually flipped back the sheet, and there, lying on her side in a fetal position, was a young, blue-eyed woman.

Something inside my chest dropped and I winced.

She had on a hospital gown and a soaked adult diaper, which smelled strongly of urine. There were the spastic muscle fasciculations consistent with a severe cerebral palsy.

I put up the side rails and listened to the EMTs' report. Lucy was thirty-five, completely lucid, had a raging urinary tract infection and an elevated temp of 102.2. On top of everything else, she suffered from severe rheumatoid arthritis in all joints. Verbalization was almost impossible for her.

I walked over to the gurney, and although it was awkward, put my face directly in front of hers. "Hi. I'm Steve, your nurse. I'm going to help you as much as I can."

In that halting voice of the CP patient, she said she understood.

There was something tugging at my heart, my brain, my spirit, but I didn't want to stop and listen to what it was saying. I simply began my assessment, listening to her lungs, taking a temp, getting a blood pressure.

Then I got to her pulses. Her hands. Fingers that were bent backward, swollen and red from the rheumatoid arthritis. I could remember being told by other patients who suffered from this crippling disease how painful each and every movement was.

I checked her pedal pulses. Again, misshapen toes, red and swollen.

I began removing the wet diaper, feeling how hot and dry her skin was. She would have to have an IV started and blood work drawn, which would mean holding her down and causing more pain. I assessed her veins, which were really bad, then pulled back and just took her in as she jerked around the gurney in constant, spastic motion.

Suddenly, out of the thousands of patients I'd ever had who paraded through my life, this woman crystallized in my heart. My mind was tortured with the unfairness of it: Here was a human being who could not control her movements, and yet every movement had to be agonizing, tremendous pain. Here was an intelligent woman trapped inside a body that could not communicate. Now, to add to her misery, we were going to have to start an IV and lab would have to draw blood and she was spastic and we'd have to hold her down causing even more pain.

I felt the lump in my chest rising to the point where I knew I was going to be overcome . . . a strange thing in and of itself because I'd been involved in trauma work for a lot of years. And now, for some reason, in rolls this one patient who decides to stay forever in my mind.

I asked Belle, the other R.N. on with me, to finish taking and recording vital signs on Lucy. I went to the back lounge and poured myself an apple juice.

How grossly unfair it was for this woman to be imprisoned, trapped. Yet, no matter how hard I wished or prayed, I wasn't going to be able to get her out—no one could get her out—now or ever.

It tortured me. I was a nurse, someone who alleviated pain, helped to heal, and returned a wounded person to their former level of wellness—not to a prison of pain and suffering.

And then I began to sob, the whole time thinking: *Good. Good for you, Steve. You haven't become callous yet. You have served in some of the most stressful environments in healthcare, and yet there is still the emotional heart which beats under the professional umbrella of your place as a nurse.*

Good boy. The heart is still open and functioning.

Finally, I went back out and got the IV-insertion tray ready. When I approached the gurney, I told Lucy that I was going to have to start an IV and that someone would have to hold her arm steady.

She blinked her eyes in understanding.

Dear God, please just let me get in on the first try. Please don't let me hurt this woman any more than she's already hurting.

Belle came over and, without having to be told, held Lucy's arm as steady as she could. I propped the hand holding the angiocath against her arm very steady, and by God, I slid the angiocath directly into the vein, taped it up, and began running in the fluid.

Afterwards, I asked the ER doc to give her some IV Demerol besides the Tylenol suppository—just so she could have some rest from her arthritis pain. It didn't surprise me at all that he refused.

I kept at him, hounding him until he relented. When I told her that I was going to give her some Demerol to relieve her pain, tears spilled down her face.

"Thank . . . you . . . so . . . much." It took her a full minute to say those four words, but it was the highlight of my day, my month, my year.

At 5:00 P.M., Joseph Williams replaced Lucy in room 2B. Joseph stated on his intake form that he was suffering from a flare-up of arthritis pain.

Hobbling into the treatment room, the things I noticed first about him were his madras plaid shirt, his Stetson cowboy hat, his cane, and the look of pain on his face. His wife, an attractive woman who appeared to be a good twenty or more years younger than he, handed me a paper bag filled with his medications.

"The pain," she said, helping him unbutton his shirt, "started this morning. We did everything—medications, hot wax dips, mild exercise, football videos—but he just couldn't stand it anymore, so we came here."

I nodded and asked more questions pertaining to his health history. Then I noticed his cane again. It was very strange-looking, to say the least. It was tan-colored, and kind of gnarled-looking. It had been coated with something clear.

Mr. Williams saw that my attention had wandered, and despite the pain, he smiled ever so slightly and gave me the cane to put aside.

As I walked over to the rack where the rest of his clothes were, I couldn't help but notice it was quite heavy—a lot heavier than most canes I'd ever seen.

I hung it on the pole next to the madras shirt.

"Okay," I said, after I'd taken his vital signs and signed off his chart. "I'll rack up your chart and come back after the doctor sees you. We'll get some medication into you that'll take care of this pain."

I left, taking one more look at that cane.

Outside, Belle was dealing with Mr. Paravoni, the eighty-four-year-old who'd come to us seriously dehydrated and with a lower than low blood sugar level. After pumping a couple of liters of glucose and water into him, he seemed to have revived to the point of friskiness.

Belle had just asked one of the male volunteers to help the gentleman off gurney R and take him for a walk down the hall.

Mr. Paravoni seemed like an interesting old guy. At five foot three inches tall, with a full head of white, curly hair and a big, cherubic face, he looked like a character in a play. He didn't speak English very well, but his facial expressions more than made up for that.

Within three minutes, the volunteer came back to tell Belle that Mr. Paravoni wouldn't budge, so Belle motioned over the other, older volunteer and told *him* to take Mr. Paravoni for a walk. I could tell her patience was wearing thin by the way she was writing in the chart—dotting all her *i*'s and *j*'s with hard slashes.

I went back into room 2B to take Mr. Williams's temperature, and there was the damned cane staring me in the face. When I finished with his temperature, I couldn't help myself—I went over and, under the guise of moving it to another part of the room, kind of picked it off the pole and ran a finger over the length of it. I even brought it up to my nose and sniffed it to see if I could detect some scent of a particular kind of wood.

"I'll bet you're wondering what the hell that thing is made of, aren't you, boy?"

I noticed that Mr. Williams was kind of chuckling even though he was obviously hurting.

"Well, yes sir, I guess I am. I don't think I've seen anything like it before."

Mr. Williams rolled the tip of his tongue around the inside of his cheek. "Well, why don't you think about it some more?"

His wife clucked her tongue and shook her head. It was my guess that I wasn't the first person who he'd put through this particular drill.

When I went back out to the desk, the second volunteer had just returned from Mr. Paravoni. He told Belle that Mr. P. again refused to try and walk.

Belle rolled her baby blues and crooked her finger at both the volunteers. "Okay you guys, now I want you to watch how this is done. Follow me."

As the trio headed toward Mr. Paravoni, I saw the doctor coming out of 2B. Handing me Mr. Williams's chart, he told me to give the patient seventy-five milligrams of Demerol.

"It's gotta be some kind of wood . . ." I said later, as I was injecting the drug into Mr. Williams's buttock. "Something heavy like ironwood or mahogany, right?"

Mr. Williams shook his head and laughed. "Nope. Think some more, son."

Back at the main desk, I overheard Belle as she finished her explanation to Mr. Paravoni about how he must walk on his own before we can let him go home.

I noticed that the whole time Belle is talking, Mr. Paravoni has this big silly grin on his face and he's nodding like a wild man.

Belle turned to the two volunteers and in her Miss Perfect Nurse voice said, "See? You must explain things to the patient. This is how you motivate the patient to walk."

Mr. Paravoni, aided by Belle, begins to put on his shoes. I notice how thin and bony he is and think of the cane again.

It actually isn't grainy like a wood, so it's got to be bone. I'd seen canes made from giraffe bones before.

I went back into Mr. Williams's room.

"Bone," I said, smiling, sure that I'd hit it on the old noggin. "Gotta be giraffe bone."

Mr. Williams shook his head, trying to keep the grin down to a minimum. "Nope."

I went back out to the desk in time to see Belle positioning herself with one hand under Mr. P's armpit and the other on his arm. The odd couple began to move toward the door.

I can see that Mr. Paravoni is beaming, and suddenly, three steps into the walk, he reaches over with his right hand and grabs Belle's breast, giving it a loving, gentle squeeze.

"You really shouldn't do that, Mr. Paravoni," Belle said, removing his hand with her one free hand.

Immediately, his other hand slips around her backside and grabs a buttock.

Belle, who couldn't very well let go of him, swatted as best she could at the hand on her butt. Except, as soon as Mr. P. removed one hand from one target, the other hand went for the other target.

So there they were—a five-foot-eight blond, attractive woman being groped quite successfully by a five-foot-three Italian Jimmy Durante kind of guy. They did this little dance about halfway to the door, when Belle handed him off to me and, red with embarrassment and anger, stomped off to the back lounge.

I got Mr. Paravoni back to his gurney, when I realize that the cane didn't have any sort of tuberosities, so it can't be a bone.

I went back into Mr. Williams's room and just outright took the damned cane down and started tapping it and smelling it. I felt like I was going to go nuts if I didn't figure it out.

Well, Mr. Williams was just enthralled at my interest and starts to laugh right out loud. Not only has the Demerol kicked in, but he was pleased that he'd hooked somebody with this cane.

Then it hit me. "It's a horn," I say, smiling. "A horn from some animal you hunted in Africa."

"Nope," he said. "I'm telling you, it's not anything you have ever seen."

"Okay," I said, hoping to God he wouldn't try to tell me some story about space aliens leaving behind a leg or a piece of spacecraft. "I give up. What the hell is it?"

Mrs. Williams waved a hand at him. "Oh for God's sake, Joe. Stop torturing the poor boy and tell him."

Mr. Williams adjusted himself on the gurney. If he'd been standing, he would have hitched up his pants.

"Son," he said, grinning, "you're holding on to a genuine bull penis."

"Huh?"

"See, I got a friend who works down in the slaughterhouse and he takes them bull penises and pokes a rod down the middle and lets it dry in the sun, and then he takes some polyurethane and . . ."

Betty G.

"There are so many love stories in what nurses do. It's inspiring to see people reaching out to other people. I don't expect to see it much anymore, but when it happens it's a gift," says New Hampshirite Betty G., a thirty-five-year-old ICU staff nurse, writer, publisher, and married mother of two.

"I've learned how ill prepared we are for death. In this country there is so much denial and such a lack of communication about death. People are terrified of it, and I find that amazing. In my practice, it is inspiring when I see a person transcend fear and denial and connect with someone who is suffering. I've learned a lot about human nature from the people who are dying and those who surround them."

The patient had come to the United States from Canada. He'd worked in an environment in which he was exposed to a material that caused the outer layer around his lungs to thicken. The disease had progressed to the point that he wasn't able to expand his lungs fully to breathe.

This man and his wife had had a very hard life just trying to survive, but what struck me most about them was that they had such a romantic relationship. They were truly soul mates.

While he was in ICU, the wife lived out of her car with their seven-year-old son. Because of the length of his hospitalization, any other housing would have been too much of a financial burden. She spent a whole summer living like this until I invited her to come and stay with me. I asked her because I liked her and respected her. This woman was a very private and proud woman, so she would only come to my house to shower and sleep, but oh, how she appreciated that. The management didn't approve of my taking her into my home, but I didn't really care—it was something I had to do as a caring human being.

She was difficult for some of the other staff members to deal with. Much of the time, people willingly assigned her husband over to me because they found her irritatingly hypervigilant and demanding.

Everything always had to be perfect for her husband. She was very particular about his mouth care, and suctioning, and how the nurses transferred him from the bed to the chair, and how his dressings were changed, and even what the right attitude of his caretakers should be. What the nurses failed to see was that this woman went in there with an agenda of making her husband's day livable for him—which was not easy to do, since the quality of his life as it was was horrible. He was vent-dependent, had chest tubes, and developed various infections and pneumonias. He underwent two decortication surgeries of his lungs, which were difficult at best.

The surgeon who did the surgeries described them as "trying to take the skin off a ripe peach without harming the fruit inside." It's impossible. There was never much hope for cure, and as long as he was on the vent, he wasn't a candidate for a lung transplant.

I kept up with this woman's demands because I understood that it wasn't her underlying nature to be demanding. It didn't come from any other place than her sincere desire to make his immediate life and surroundings livable. I admired that about her and felt that I had to try to live up to those expectations as well.

She was really something—like an island unto herself. She'd be there, working alongside me, helping to bathe him and take care of him. She would constantly talk to him about what was going on in the world. Her sole function [Betty laughs and says, "Perhaps that should be spelled s-o-u-l?"] was to be a support for him.

She had a true romantic love for this man. He'd have his endotracheal tube coming out of his mouth and he'd be bubbling with really disgusting-looking secretions that didn't smell very nice, and she'd kiss him on the lips.

But one of the most amazing things was she insisted on bringing in her son in order to promote her son's understanding of what was happening to his father. She made sure he saw that although his father was ill, he was still treated like a human being with dignity.

For the four months her husband was in ICU, she never allowed him to be dehumanized. She constantly made us see the person her husband was, and not just the sick person decompensating each day. It is very easy for staff to forget that person under the equipment.

It wasn't only her either. The husband was as much a husband and supportive helpmate as he could be to her. No matter how sick he was, he always expressed an interest in her life and what she did aside from him. He was concerned because of the amount of time she devoted to him.

The love between them was so strong. I think he felt just how deeply he was loved for the first time in his life, and I know she . . . [She starts to cry and stops the tape.]

This experience was remarkable, not so much for the story but for what this woman taught us. For me, she was an example of incredible strength in a traumatic life event. To put aside her own needs and be compassionate and giving.

He died in our unit, and even then she was wonderful. She did as much as she could to prepare her son and get him some psychological support to deal with his father's death. It is such a wonderful story of caring and romantic love and what it means to put someone above your own needs for an extended period of time.

Now, in polar opposite to this story is a story about isolation.

The patient was a distinguished-looking man about sixty-seven, well educated, and very prosperous. He'd had a severe cerebral bleed, and was on full life support, vent and all.

The game plan was to stabilize him and see if he could reabsorb some of that blood, and then assess whether or not he would become operable. The neurosurgeons were pessimistic at best. They felt he was a huge risk for a rebleed and painted a sort of doom-and-gloom picture.

So the family was called in. There was a loving, gracious wife and two daughters from different cities. All were well dressed, perfectly groomed, extremely well educated. Between the three of them, they tried to create an environment to facilitate a "good death for Dad."

They were very concerned about the physical environment; they kept the lights dim, made sure his favorite classical music was playing, and were constantly wanting to change the position of the bed. When we'd enter the room, they'd want us to speak in soft, hushed tones. So, we tried to help in the creation of this atmosphere they thought was necessary for "Dad's perfect exit."

What was striking to me was that they never spoke to him. The lack of conversation with the patient or between themselves was eerie—it was as if he was already dead and they were holding services for him at a funeral parlor—open coffin.

Gradually his mental status improved, although the prognosis for a rebleed remained the same. One day in this time frame, I went into the room to do my assessment and had asked the family to step out for a few minutes.

While I was taking his blood pressure, he opened his eyes and looked at me with such intensity and urgency that I knew he was trying to connect.

Then he mouthed the words, "Am I going to die?"

I could not back off from the question. So, I did what some people would do in the same situation, and I said, "Huh? What?" stalling for more time to think about this.

It was very emotional for me. I remember just looking at him and saying very softly, "Yes, I think so."

He maintained eye contact with me for a few seconds, and then he looked away and his whole face contorted into this silent sob. I felt all the psychological pain of this man who truly heard what I had said and understood the meaning of it. It was devastating.

I sobbed in my car all the way home that night, wondering whether or not I'd done the right thing.

When I think back on it now, I remember feeling so sad about the room control and environment that the family was maintaining.

Yes, it was beautiful, but at that moment in the scheme of things, it didn't really hold as much importance as everyone thought it did. The more important thing would have been for him to have the human contact instead of the lighting and the music. This man's isolation was so great that I can still feel it in my soul.

God save me from that kind of death.

Amelia M.

When asked her age, the nurse from Ohio laughs and states simply that she's old. At the age of four, she saw several nurses dressed in starched white uniforms, white caps, and white stockings, and wanted to be a nurse ever since. At six, she was declared a natural since she was the only kid on the block who could—or cared to—say "immunization." There was a brief time in high school, however, when Amelia changed her mind to wanting to be a teacher, a switchboard operator, a scientist, a librarian, a secretary, a housecleaner, even a nun. When she looks back now, she realizes that being a nurse has encompassed all those professions and many more.

After she graduated from nursing school, her first job was in a nursing home. Describing her second night there, she states: "So there I was finally . . . wearing an all-white uniform and being splashed with puke and urine. It didn't exactly fit the vision I'd had since childhood, but I didn't care—I was a nurse and that was all that mattered."

Since that time, Amelia has worked in med-surg, ICU-CCU, transitional psych, and alcohol rehab.

"Someday, when I'm through with nursing," she says, "I'd really like to work in a bakery."

I went back to school after I'd had my family. It was quite a change. All through college I didn't clean the bathtub except on quarter break. The dishes sat in the sink for weeks on end and by the end of the quarter, the hair on my legs was about an inch and a half long and the dining room table was covered in research books.

I loved it. My two teenage girls loved it—Mom was off their backs. My marriage did not love it, so that was the end of that. Over the years I'd noticed that most nurses have pretty poor marriages, so I was just one of the many. Face it—not a lot of husbands, or nonmedical people for that matter, can understand the psychology behind our jobs. We work shifts, weekends, and holidays and we're tired all the time.

When I started out, nursing was everything. For me nursing was clean green soap, a numbing quiet, and cool, green hallways. I made twenty-five cents an hour as a student, and after graduation I moved up to the whopping financial reward of two dollars and thirty-five cents an hour!

At that time, antibiotics and the Salk vaccine were miracle drugs that were saving lives, and intensive care and coronary care units were just being developed as places to treat the life-threatening diseases. Those were the days when we used the autoclave for sterilizing only certain instruments, and we were still dissolving morphine tablets which had to be calculated, liquefied, and then drawn up for injection.

And, oh my God, remember the Sippy Diet the docs used to put some of the patients on? Milk and cream every half hour around the clock—and of course, *every* patient you had was on that damned stupid diet! By the end of the shift you smelled and looked like a wet nurse.

We didn't have automatic IV pumps back then—we had to calculate the drip and constantly keep an eye on it. Death to the nurse who should ever let one of those IVs run dry, because we weren't allowed to start IVs—the doctor had to be called for that because it was considered so far beyond the nurse's mentality, let alone her capability.

Through all this we wore our perky white caps and were considered part of the mystery of the hospital. Nurses weren't respected then, but they never have been. I don't think the public has a clue as to what it takes to be a critical care nurse. Very few people have a clue what goes on behind the closed doors of a critical care unit.

And now, God forbid, we've got the "new" nurse—with her two-inch-long fingernails painted red, and hair that's been whipped with an eggbeater and varnished into place, not to mention her underwear showing through her uniform . . . assuming she's even wearing a uniform—or underwear. These days it might be a pair of jeans so tight you can see her labia, and a scrub top with a *really* deep V cut and no bra.

We didn't question—we obeyed. We stood when anyone entered the room, we said hello with a smile, we gave our seat to the doctor. The doctors were and still are considered the all-powerful gods on the scene. They did and do look down on the nurses as threats—someone who will steal their thunder. They continue to keep us two paces behind, treating us like imbeciles in front of the patients. That part never changes.

The satisfactions we get as nurses are small, but huge at the same time. Like starting an IV that the anesthesiologist couldn't get, or the fifty times a shift that the M.D.s come asking for your opinion on one thing or another, or could one of us please interpret this EKG for him?

Personally, I always keep in mind that a nurse is in a unique position with God. She is there holding the baby as it begins its new life, and we hold our patients as they die. In essence, we are spectators of the soul as it journeys to and from this life. How much closer to the highest power can you be? I am not a religious person, but thirty years in the nursing profession has made me feel that my life has been touched by God's presence.

Nursing is changing now. There are less nurses left in the hospital to give care, and the patients are sicker. Businessmen with no medical background are the ones making decisions on how medical care is delivered and to whom. Through all the changes, I see the morale declining. Now the attitude of "It's a job" is replacing a pride of profession in which sacrifice, nurturing, and healing are truly prized.

It makes me sad to admit that I'm disillusioned with nursing. Maybe I'm an old dog who can't learn new tricks. Maybe I'm just old. But from what I see, we have the capacity to give such quality care and yet we're taking away the most important thing that nursing has always offered, and that's the human touch and the emotional component that goes with one person caring for another.

As all nurses who have been in the profession for many years, my mind travels back to small incidents that we tuck away deep in our emotional baskets. Without our weird sense of humor and the ability to filter out the horrific, we could never survive.

Gee, there've been so many memorable things—I mean, I've had a miscarriage while lifting a patient, I've had my cap flushed down a toilet once. I even helped corral a bat in the middle of the night while the patients all screamed around me.

There is one incident that never left me—I guess because it reminds me that as a nurse I am a professional witness to the human condition. It took place when I was a new nurse. I'd gone to work on a midnight shift in a nursing home, and as anybody knows, when you work in a nursing home, you're pretty much on your own.

To begin with, I had the feeling something terrible was going to happen to me that night. The place itself was scary. It was a big place and we turned all the lights off or down at night. In those rooms the elderly barely moved and it was almost like walking through a morgue. You'd go by the ends of their beds, and you were never sure whether or not they were alive.

Not that I hadn't seen my share of people die. I've held their hands as they took their last breath. I saw one woman—while sitting naked on a shower chair—hemorrhage from ruptured esophageal varices from her mouth, while the nurse's aides screamed in horror.

I made rounds every hour to make sure all forty-two [she laughs— "Yes, I said forty-two!"] of my patients were breathing, or not hanging over the side rails looking for a drink of water, or lying in a puddle of something of their own making.

Even though the night was pretty quiet, the knot in my stomach wouldn't go away, no matter how I tried to kid myself out of it. Still, I was aware of the fact that I was working with nurse's aides who weren't going to go out of their way for two-fifty an hour to help me out if something did go wrong.

On my 3:00 A.M. rounds, I was going past a room, when out of the corner of my eye, I saw that the clothes closet was open a crack. That was unusual because I always made sure the closets were closed, because sometimes those folks would wake up and see a dress or a robe hanging in the closet and they'd think it was a ghost and just wig out.

Then I noticed something sort of moving inside the closet. It scared me, you know, because I'd had this premonition and all I could think was that an intruder had broken in and I was being stalked. But rather than run screaming down the hall, which was my first inclination, I decided to take on the situation face-to-face.

I walked to the closet and slid back the door a little.

There was Mildred, eighty-five years old—a longtime resident of the facility. Initially I felt relief that it wasn't a stalker, but then the next thing I noticed was the motion she was making, which was sort of like she was swaying back and forth.

You know how old people sometimes rock themselves if they're upset or afraid? Well, I started talking to her right away in a soothing voice, except I'm starting to put things together—like the fact that Mildred is a paraplegic and how did she get to the closet?

I managed to pull the door open all the way and there she was in her hospital gown, and tied around her head was a sort of turban hat.

It was the turban that held my attention. You could tell she'd made it herself. She'd fashioned it out of a pair of pink tricot panties, secured in place with a big, gaudy rhinestone brooch.

It was a very impressive getup, despite the puke and poop all over the place. Oh yeah—that and the fact that she was hanging from the clothes rod by her neck.

Poor woman had wrapped a draw sheet around her neck, knotted it, then tied the other end around the rod. I admired her for her strength of resolve, when I sat down and thought about it. Here this elderly woman, who was paralyzed, had gotten herself over the side rails, then maneuvered herself into a wheelchair; then she had to roll to the closet, tie the knots, secure them, and then push the wheelchair out from under herself.

That takes determination mixed with some desperation.

After a few minutes, what I was looking at jelled in my mind, and I started screaming for help. Two aides came running. One passed out on the spot; the one left standing and I untied the knots and got the old lady onto the floor. I started CPR and waited for the ambulance.

We didn't have paramedics then, but we did have some EMTs. These were a group of wild and woolly young fellows. Two of them arrived a few minutes later and hooked her up to the monitor, and started an IV.

All I could think of was: *How long are we going to do CPR on this poor old dead woman?* but I was new, and didn't know what I could or couldn't say to anybody.

The next thing I know, I'm in the rig doing chest compressions, and the EMT in the back is defibrillating this lady over and over and over again . . . and all you can smell is burned flesh.

Meanwhile, the cowboy up front is driving like hell with sirens and lights down the freeway at three o'clock in the morning, and there isn't another car within sixty miles. All of a sudden, he looks at the speedometer and scares himself, so he slams on the brakes and we go sliding off the freeway, over an embankment. All the cabinets in the back of the ambulance flew open and emptied onto our heads. There's boxes of medications and bandages and equipment scattered everywhere—but we didn't stop our CPR, by God, not for one solitary beat.

And through this all, my little white nurse's cap stayed perched neatly on my head.

Of course, she was pronounced within thirty seconds after we arrived in the emergency department. After I was grilled by the coroner, I couldn't get a ride back to the nursing home, because we didn't have taxi service at that time of the morning and neither of the two nurse's aides at the nursing home would come pick me up, because that meant leaving the other one all alone in that scary place.

I ended up talking the nursing supervisor at the receiving hospital into driving me back. I remember as we were leaving, the orderly wheeled Mildred out of the department.

The urge to peek under the sheet was too strong to resist. I knew I'd wonder about it forever if I didn't check to see if she was still wearing the panties with the brooch wrapped around her head.

She was. I just hope whoever was in charge of her arrangements had the good sense to let her wear that magnificent turban creation during her final rest.

Kate J.

Kate J., a nurse in her early forties, started in pediatrics twenty years ago. Since then, she has worked primarily in pediatric ICU, pediatric and adult open-heart unit, and pediatric and adult organ-transplant unit. She is presently in her final year of study for becoming a nurse anesthetist.

She is, without a doubt, the most stunningly beautiful woman I have ever seen in person. I asked why she had become a nurse when it was obvious she could have done anything with her looks and her multitudinous talents.

"In 1972 I sat down and evaluated myself in regard to what I wanted to do," she told me. "What I came up with was: I had an innate ability to take care of people. I wanted to be able to do something I could do well and do anywhere and not be tied down. Nursing was a positive means to an end— others would benefit from what I had to offer, and I would make a decent living and have my own schedule.

"I did quit nursing for about seven years and went to New York City. I got into the public relations scene, I sailed and traveled, got married and divorced, became an alcoholic and got sober.

"Then I realized nursing was where I needed to be, so I went back. It is where I make a difference."

Kate began her stories with this statement:

"As an intensive care nurse, there are two kinds of patients who tend to stick out in your mind—those who might have died if it hadn't been for your intervention and those who would not have died with dignity if it hadn't been for your intervention."

SEATTLE, 1979

They tell me that the twenty-four-year-old woman on the gurney was thrown off a loading dock two hours ago. She landed on her chest. She

328

is a waitress. She was going in the back door of the restaurant, and a man attacked her and threw her off. No one knows why for sure. He just did, says Rose.

Rose has multiple pulmonary contusions along with a lot of other problems. Like a fractured neck and two broken legs.

I tell her to wiggle her toes. She does. I pinch her legs all the way up to her waist—not a very long distance because she can't be much taller than five feet. She tells me to stop pinching and scowls at me.

I am joyously happy that I do not have to tell her she will never walk again and that she will be stuck in a wheelchair for the rest of her life. I really hate it when that happens.

I take off her size 2 dress and see a tattoo over her left breast. A red rose. I don't label her as a lowlife, as will the surgeon and the neurologist. In her sad blue eyes I recognize a fellow survivor, and I know, for unknown reasons, that this small and delicate person is going to be my "special patient," the way no other person ever has been before. I know that she and I will connect on a deep heart level, and I will come to know her heart better than I know my own.

What I don't know is that after twenty years of intensive care nursing, she will remain the one closest to my heart and foremost in my memory.

She asks about her son. Six years old. The light of her existence. Father unknown. The child is staying with the next-door neighbor until she gets home from work. I call the next-door neighbor and tell her what has happened. The next-door neighbor is not surprised and I wonder why.

I tell the next-door neighbor she may have to care for the boy for a while longer. I am relieved when she says not to worry, she will care for him as long as necessary.

As I ready Rose for the surgeon, she talks about her life. She talks about experiences I cannot fathom. Like delivering her son by herself in a Texas oil field in the middle of the night. Like working to feed herself from the age of eight, doing things that make my mind spin around like the blades of a Maytag.

She says that being small and blond, she has managed to get away with being tough without looking the part.

I tell her she is going to have to be tough now. I tell her she is critically ill. I try to explain about her lungs, avoiding words like "pneumothorax" and "hypoxia." I go with her to surgery, holding her hand the whole way.

At the surgery doors, she gives my hand a squeeze and asks if I will be around when she comes out.

Needlessly I look at my watch, and tell her yes.

It is Rose's one-month anniversary in ICU. We have a celebration. *I* have a blueberry muffin—*she* has her intravenous antibiotic.

Rose also has three chest tubes. She knows more about pneumothoraxes and chest tubes than most pulmonary specialists. I tell her she could probably insert a chest tube in a warthog if she had to. Rose laughs, and I revel in the sound of it.

She has had so many pneumos we've lost count. She is the only patient I've ever had who knows immediately when she's getting a pneumothorax. Every time I go off duty, I make it a point to tell the doctor and the nurse taking over her care: "If this patient tells you she has a pneumo, believe it. She's qualified to know, so get an X ray and get ready with the chest tube."

She is getting better, even though she does not believe it. Like most long-term patients, there are days she gets depressed and says she doesn't care what happens to her.

On those days, I tell her everything will be fine. I promise that she will have a life again soon, only better than before.

What she does not tell me is that there are days she wants to die.

Two and one half months after the day Rose told me to stop pinching, she is transferred to a rehab hospital. It is only a few miles out of my way. I go to see her almost every day.

In a sunny kitchen eight years later, I am laughing over a story Rose has told me about one of her physical therapy patients, when she touches my hand and says: "Have I ever told you that it was knowing you would take care of me, and listen to me, which gave me the will to live? The sight of you walking into my room kept me hanging on."

She hugs her seven-year-old daughter—who is named after me—and I am filled with an emotion I don't know how to put into words.

SAN FRANCISCO, 1989

Esther is in her mid-eighties. She wears size 3 shoes, is four feet nine inches tall, and weighs fifty-nine pounds. She has lived her entire life doing things her own way. Everything has been, is, and will be done her way or no way at all. She is tyrannical, selfish, and obstinate. Very seldom has she ever been compassionate or giving. I do not particularly like her, nor do I care much for the way she has chosen to live her life.

She is in the hospital because the doctors are trying to fatten her up so she can withstand surgery for the tumor they have found in her throat. She has been here for a long time. Esther continues to lose weight.

I walk into her room and the tiny, birdlike woman is curled into a ball. Her respirations are shallow and rapid, and her color is grayish white. Esther looks like she is going to code.

The nurse in charge tells me that her code status has never been discussed. She has refused all care and it is unclear to everyone what they would do if she does code.

Twelve hours later she codes. A respiratory arrest. She is intubated and on a respirator in ICU, but she continues to refuse all care, including lab work.

I spend the entire day with her, trying to communicate. I know from her eyes and what is behind them that she is completely lucid. God knows she won't give up one bit of control—even in death. At the end of my day, she writes me a note:

"I want to go home, damn it!!!"

I assure her that if she is able to breathe on her own with the tube in, I will take her home. It is Thursday.

Friday very early—Esther is breathing without the aid of the respirator. I tell the ICU nurses that she wants to go home. As usual, they are the patient's advocate one hundred percent and begin the red tape ball rolling in order to give her what she wants.

The stumbling block is Esther's physician. He tells me I cannot take her out of the hospital with an endotracheal tube in place. He says it is against the law.

I feel myself bristle at his arrogance and sense of command, and I say, "Is it in fact against the law, or is it just something that you don't want to do? If it is truly against the law, then you need to inform me of exactly what law it is and then tell me who I need to contact to get it changed, because I intend to take Esther home so she can die there instead of here."

"Just give us this weekend," he says. "Just two more days."

I laugh in his bewhiskered face. His expression betrays his ignorance.

"Why?" I ask. "You want the weekend for *what*? Face it, there is nothing more you can do for her here. She won't let you, and she's running the show."

Thus we dance around the ring, throwing verbal punches above and below the waist, for ten more rounds. The ongoing title bout: nurse versus doctor. With a few words of legalese I connect with the fear portion of his solar plexus and he's down for the count.

Four hours later, I am riding in the back of an ambulance with Esther. I am as careful about keeping her endotracheal tube suctioned as I am about keeping her comfortable with drugs. I pray that the hospice nurses will have already set up the morphine drip in her room.

She has lived in this house for over fifty years with her cousin, Jack. Jack is a stout, balding gay man, who in his earlier years had been a famous jazz pianist who played with the likes of Dorsey and Miller.

She is in her bed, in her room. In the next room there is a grand piano. Jack is practicing while she listens intently, waiting.

I wait for the anesthesiologist who will come at 1:00 P.M. and extubate her.

It is 1:30 and the anesthesiologist has just arrived. Esther is anxious to get the tube out. I tell her daughter that I do not know how long she will live after the tube is out. Maybe a few minutes, maybe a few hours, I say. I think about who she is and correct myself: Or, she might hang on for days.

The anesthesiologist lets the air out of the endotracheal tube cuff and slips the tube out of her throat.

The tube isn't even out of the doctor's hand before Esther says, "Oh thank God *that's* over with! Jack, play something for the doctor."

We laugh politely. Jack smiles and says, "What's your pleasure, doc?"

The anesthesiologist is a rather queer-looking fellow to begin with. Now he's confused and looking even more queer, because he doesn't know Jack, nor that there is a grand piano in the next room. He thinks we're all crazy.

I tell the doctor he must choose a piece of music for Jack to play on the piano.

Because he cannot let down and be human even for this, he says in a very clipped, cold tone: "I don't care. 'Chopsticks.' "

Jack leaves and all of a sudden this incredibly beautiful music fills the air. Mozart. Chopin. Gershwin.

"Chopsticks," indeed.

We all stare down at this tiny little woman waving long, red finger-nails in the air in time to the music. She is smiling widely, saying, "Oh thank you God, oh thank you God, oh thank you God, oh thank you God. . . ."

And why not? She is going to die soon, and she is so happy to be dy-ing here, in her own bed, in surroundings she loves, with Jack in the other room playing her favorite tunes.

And besides, she has gotten her own way.

At 2:00 A.M. she sits up suddenly and asks for water. Because her hands are shaking so badly I hold the cut-crystal glass for her, bringing it to her lips. Before it reaches her mouth, she has slapped my hands away and taken the glass. Water is spilling out everywhere. An edge of the peach taffeta quilt is soaked. Her nightgown is sticking to her chest.

I am lying next to her at 3:00 A.M. listening carefully for the rattling noise in her throat, watching for any sign of discomfort. I stare at her face, and I see the beginning of a furrow between her eyes. It is the pre-cursor of the fear that people have when they cannot breathe.

Every fiber of my consciousness is aware of what I am doing when I reach over and give her another 2.5 milligrams of Valium and another dose of morphine. I know her low blood pressure will dip even lower and her respirations will become more shallow and farther apart.

I lie with her, one hand on her arm, the other over my heart while my soul engages in a moral battle. I know I am cheating her out of time. I know I am also giving her a gift.

At 5:00 she is again restless and complaining of pain. I give her an-other round of morphine and Valium. When she lies down this time, she takes my hand.

She is holding my hand when she takes her last breath.

I must be honest. I am not sure even now that I did the right thing. The quality and quantity of her life was in my hands. I weighed quality against quantity, and I decided dignity was the best I could give her.

And yet knowing that, and knowing in my heart I made the right decision, it often crosses my mind that I cheated her out of some amount of time that may have been comfortable for her.

But that is always the bottom question, isn't it?

Her daughter often tells me that had it not been for my being there, this never would have happened, because she did not have the knowledge or the guts to stand up to the physicians and say no—she wants it *this* way, not your way.

I have to believe I did the right thing. But you know, even when it isn't your grandmother, it's never easy. . . .

Kellie H.

One of my more animated interviewees was Kellie H., forty-four, a lively, petite woman with sparkling green eyes. Though she has stayed at the same institution in upstate New York, the R.N. has moved over, under, around, and through all branches of nursing for twenty-four years, and still manages to keep a positive attitude.

Not only was her body in constant motion when she spoke, she is by far the fastest talker I've ever met.

Why did I become a nurse? You know, I don't have any idea. I could call my mother and ask her if she remembers.

I know my parents didn't want me to do it. I think if they'd wanted me to be a nurse, I would've gone into sales or been a bartender or something completely different. I don't know for sure, but sicko that I was, I probably wanted to help people.

I remember that when I was five years old, I had a respiratory arrest from scarlet fever. My brother found me and told my mother by asking her if it was normal for girls to turn blue when they slept. I remember going to the hospital and being packed in ice cubes for five days, but I don't remember the nurses. I'm sure the sight of them carrying in those tubs of ice cubes was so traumatic that I've repressed all my innermost feelings about them. My guess is that whatever it is I've repressed, it's damned ugly.

I loved nursing school because I was good at it. I got straight A's— compared to my high school grades, it was like comparing Albert Einstein to the brain-damaged.

I love the patients, but I'm not so sure about nursing anymore. I think nursing is a dying art—the insurance companies and the bureaucratic red tape killed it.

Nurses are soon to be gone, but I don't think they'll be forgotten for a long time.

For the sake of confidentiality, let's call the patient Florence. Flo was a fifty-five-year-old catatonic who'd been on the psych ward for two and a half months before she came to the med-surg floor. According to her chart, she'd become catatonic when her husband of thirty-five years dumped her for a twenty-five-year-old waitress with a set of fake tits. Of course it didn't say that in the chart—the part about the tits—but the psych tech was a neighbor, and he knew the whole story.

Anyway, over the course of a year before he left, the husband bamboozled Flo into signing over the house she'd put the down payment on thirty years before. Then he gave her some cock-and-bull tax story about why he had to put all their savings and assets into his name. I suppose you could say Florence was to blame for being so stupid, but she trusted the guy. I mean, if you can't trust the man you've been married to for thirty-five years, who can you trust?

So the husband comes home one day with this young blond babe and tells Flo she's got one hour to pack her clothes and get out of his house. He doesn't let her take anything except her clothes—not even the photo albums.

She has to call a taxi because the old man won't give her a ride anywhere, and she's standing there in the snow, and . . . Oh, wait. Back up. Did I mention that this is a week before Christmas?

Okay, so it's the week before Christmas and she's standing there in the snow without a dime to her name, and she goes to her daughter's apartment, and the daughter won't take her in because the daughter's boyfriend—who's the lowest form of sewer scum—doesn't want her cutting into the cozy deal he has, which is sitting home smoking and drinking beer while the daughter works to support him.

The daughter pays the cab fare, however, and then drives the mother to a fleabag flophouse in the worst part of town and drops her off.

So Florence is at this flophouse and the first thing that happens is someone breaks into her room and beats the crap out of her and steals her clothes.

The next day two guys break into her room, rape her, and break her leg.

Apparently that was the last straw, because she went catatonic. About two days later, someone else broke into her room to rob her and found her like that. They cut off her finger to get her wedding ring, then called nine-one-one to report a dead body.

Believe it or not, things went from bad to worse from there. I don't know how this happened, but the people working in the psych ward didn't bother with her at all once she was admitted. They let her lie around in her own waste and never cleaned her. It makes me furious to think how they could do that—the whole lot of them are jerks if you ask me.

Anyway, the skin on her back and buttocks got excoriated and broke down so bad that she had to have skin grafts. That was how we ended up with her on the med-surg floor.

I admitted her the first day she came back from surgery, so I kind of got assigned to her permanently. I don't know what it was about Florence that made people not care about her—it was like she was just one of those people that sometimes fall through the cracks . . . like a nonentity?

I made sure she was put on a special mattress to help with the circulation to her skin, and of course she was on reverse isolation since her resistance to infection was zilch. Once you went into her room, there was so much to do you could never, ever get out of there if you were the nurse. Once you entered that room, that was where you stayed.

She didn't talk, she didn't make any expressions, she didn't move. She was so far gone into the catatonic state that the psych people gave up on her ever coming out of it. Somehow I never believed that. I'd go home and read all this stuff about catalepsy and catatonic states, until I swear I could have done a master's thesis on the subject.

For three months I took care of Flo every day. One of the ways I found to pass my time while I was working with Florence was to talk.

As you can tell, I do like to talk. My husband says it drives him nuts the way I go on sometimes, but I just can't stop my mouth once it gets going. So I'd go into Flo's room and I'd talk nonstop. Constantly. Yakety-yak. I talked about what I'd done the day before, I'd talk about my husband and our problems, and about my son and his Little League games, and our dog, Miaow, and the cat, Toto, and about fishing and about all my friends and my life. I think I even went back to my earliest childhood memories and told her about my parents and their problems and then worked my way up to the present day. I probably did more self-psychotherapy during those three months of taking care of her than if I'd gone to a shrink for the rest of my life. I could really be honest with

Florence—you know, let down and be myself, because I knew she wasn't going to judge me.

During this whole time, Florence would lay there and drool, without any indication that she was on the same planet. The only thing I could ever be a hundred percent sure of was that she liked ice chips. . . . I think she did, anyway.

I'd come in at seven in the morning and none of the nurses would have touched this woman all night, and her lips would be all gunked up and glued shut she'd be so dry, so I'd put a chunk of ice between her lips and she'd suck it right down. She'd go through four or five bowls of ice chips that way in a shift.

So one day I'd been in there for about two hours, and as usual I was going on about some problem that had come up with the house . . . maybe when the water heater blew and we couldn't afford to get a new one?

No. No, wait. It was when Toto had her litter under our bed and we couldn't sleep for all the noise going on? Or maybe it was the time that the barn burned down? I can't remember. Anyway, there I am in the middle of a dressing change on her butt, and all of a sudden she turns and looks me right in the eyes and says: "I hate the sound of your god-damned voice. Would you please shut the hell up? I can't stand it anymore. You're making me insane."

Just like that. I was so psyched that I started yelling at the top of my lungs. "Oh my God, you spoke! Florence, my friend Florence! You spoke to me!" Then I ran out in the hall and yelled until everybody on the floor was running to see what had happened.

About two weeks later she went to a rehab nursing home and now she's doing fine. She's got a part-time job cleaning houses and gets some sort of government aid.

But can you imagine that? Poor Florence had to listen to my voice five days a week, eight hours a day, for three months, hating it the whole time?

Mostly people have told me that my talking drives them crazy, so the best part of that was that I get to say that once I literally talked a patient out of a catatonic state.

But . . . but wait. Don't turn off the tape machine. I've got another one for you. This is the weirdest thing that ever happened to me in my whole life, let alone my whole nursing career.

Here, let me turn the tape over—this one is gonna freak you out.

———

I'd been working up in cardiac rehab for about a year when I got this train wreck of a guy from the CCU. He'd had a triple bypass and was doing okay. He looked exactly like the guy on the Quaker Oats box, right? He was about a hundred years old, and at first, he was meaner than cats because he'd never been sick a day in his life before his infarction, but as he got more used to us, he was the sweetest guy in the world.

I don't know what it was about him, but I loved the man like my own father. His wife even looked like Mrs. Claus with the rosy cheeks and the pure white hair. She was just like him . . . they were like Mother Goose grandparents.

Anyway, I'd been taking care of George for about a week, and we'd gotten really close. It turns out that they lived on the same rural route that we did, so we made some plans about getting together after he was out, because he was working on his family tree and I knew a little about how to go about looking up genealogical information on the Internet.

So Friday is the day he's scheduled to go home, which was my day off. I promised that after I picked up my son from school at three, I'd drive out and check on him to make sure he'd gotten all settled in.

I spent most of Friday running around doing errands, and when I got home at one, I was suddenly so tired that I had to lie down.

If you know me, you know that isn't normal for me . . . I don't go down unless I'm sick or dead. So I lay down, thinking that I'd just lay there for a few minutes and then finish my chores before I left to fetch my boy from school.

Now, as God is my witness, I'm not making this up, nor am I a drinking woman, so you know this is the straight deal.

I start to doze, but I'm not asleep because I can hear Miaow barking and I'm trying to think of what could be upsetting him, when as fast as mercury, I'm looking into this beautiful bright light and I'm hearing this noise like—don't laugh—hundreds of angels' wings flapping.

I felt like I've never felt before or since in my life, which is peaceful and joyous and like I'm floating on air without a care in the world. Over the sound of the flapping wings, I can hear hundreds of voices whispering to me. The light softened and I saw all these angels—probably about two hundred or more—floating over me, telling me that I need to go to the hospital immediately because George is going to code.

Oooh boy. I'm starting to get goose bumps. I always do when I tell this story. It does me in every time.

So all of a sudden I jumped off the couch and ran—barefoot, mind you—to the car. No purse, no coat . . . nothing. Thank God I was dressed, or I would have gone buck naked.

I made it to the hospital in twenty minutes—it usually takes me forty. I left the car still running in the parking lot and ran to the back door. It was locked. In all of my years at that hospital, that door had never been locked. Not before, nor since that day. Okay, so I run to the front door and fly to the elevators. The elevators, all six of them, are not running—again, an unprecedented event.

So I found the stairway and ran up the stairs to rehab. In the stairwell I heard the announcement on the PA system that there was a code ninety-nine in cardiac rehab. Of course I knew who it was.

By the time I got into George's room, they were defibrillating him and Dr. Turner—our chief cardiologist—was shaking his head at the cardiac monitor strips rolling out. I took a step in his direction and tapped him on the shoulder, careful to avoid the big smear of toothpaste on the back of his navy-blue cardigan. Just as the doc turned around, I looked up over George's bed and saw the angels again—hundreds of them going up and coming down over the bed . . . up and down, up and down.

They were talking to each other in that windy kind of whisper and their wings were still flapping. Right out loud I asked them what the verdict was. And they told me and disappeared.

Dr. Turner was staring at me weird, but he answered the question I'd asked the angels. "Not good," he said, and then started telling the drug cart nurse to push a couple more drugs into George's IV line.

I told her not to bother with the drugs.

Everybody stopped and stared at me in my bare feet and my old work jeans like I had gone off to Buffalo and forgotten to pack my mind.

"They don't want him now" is exactly what I told Dr. Turner.

So Turner asks: "Who doesn't want him, Kellie?" He sounded like a shrink from crisis unit.

I told him that the angels had had a discussion right over George's bed and they'd just now decided not to take him after all—in short, he wasn't ready for the final vinyl [the body bag].

Nobody said anything, so I did. I told the nurse doing CPR to stop. When she did, George had a normal sinus rhythm, and he was breathing on his own. He woke up about thirty seconds later and asked what the hell was going on.

Dr. Turner—who is the coolest doc I've ever worked with in my whole career—believed me when I told him the whole story. He said stranger things have happened, and to keep paying attention to the angels.

I know I saw the angels, and I wasn't asleep. I know I sound a little nutty sometimes, but I'm a rational person. I have never told George or his wife, though, because I thought I would leave well enough alone. They've got enough to worry about without having to worry about angels holding court over their heads.

Now, let me tell you the time when I was working in the ICU and I had a head injury patient who thought he was Gandhi reincarnated . . .

About the Author

ECHO HERON is the author of the bestselling *Intensive Care: The Story of a Nurse*; *Condition Critical: The Story of a Nurse Continues*; the novel *Mercy*; and the medical mystery *Pulse*. A critical care nurse in the San Francisco Bay area for seventeen years, she is an advocate and spokesperson for nurses' and patients' rights.

Ms. Heron and her amazing cat, Mooshie, currently reside in California.